VOLUME THREE

Current concepts in radiology

VOLUME THREE

Current concepts in
RADIOLOGY

Edited by

E. James Potchen, M.D.

Chairman, Department of Radiology
Michigan State University
East Lansing, Michigan

with 487 illustrations

The C. V. Mosby Company

Saint Louis   1977

VOLUME THREE

Copyright © 1977 by The C. V. Mosby Company

Printed in the United States of America

Distributed in Great Britain by Henry Kimpton, London

The C. V. Mosby Company
11830 Westline Industrial Drive, St. Louis, Missouri 63141

Library of Congress Cataloging in Publication Data

Potchen, E   James.
   Current concepts in radiology.

   Includes bibliographies and index.
   1. Radiography.   I.   Title.   [DNLM: 1.   Radiography.
2.   Radiology.   WN100 C976]
RC78.P667   616.07′57   72-83971
ISBN   0-8016-3987-5

CB/CB/B   9   8   7   6   5   4   3   2   1

CONTRIBUTORS

S. James Adelstein, M.D., Ph.D.

Professor of Radiology, Harvard Medical School;
Director, Joint Program in Nuclear Medicine,
Charles A. Dana Cancer Center, Children's Hospital Medical Center,
and Peter Bent Brigham Hospital,
Boston, Massachusetts

Ralph J. Alfidi, M.D.

Director, Diagnostic Radiology,
Cleveland Clinic Hospital,
Cleveland, Ohio

John H. M. Austin, M.D.

Associate Professor, Department of Radiology,
Columbia-Presbyterian Medical Center,
New York, New York

Frederick J. Bonte, M.D.

Dean and Professor of Radiology, Southwestern Medical School,
University of Texas Health Science Center at Dallas,
Dallas, Texas

Colin B. Carrig, B.V.Sc., Ph.D.

Associate Professor, Michigan State University
College of Veterinary Medicine,
East Lansing, Michigan

Gregory M. Carsen, M.D.

Assistant Professor, Department of Radiology,
Columbia-Presbyterian Medical Center,
New York, New York

Tuhin K. Chaudhuri, M.D.

Chief of Nuclear Medicine, Audie Murphy Memorial V.A. Hospital;
Associate Professor of Radiology,
University of Texas Health Science Center at San Antonio,
San Antonio, Texas

James H. Christie, M.D.

Professor and Head, Department of Radiology,
The University of Iowa Hospitals and Clinics,
Iowa City, Iowa

R. Edward Coleman, M.D.

Assistant Professor of Radiology, Department of Radiology,
University of Utah Medical Center,
Salt Lake City, Utah

Kenneth R. Davis, M.D.

Assistant Professor, Harvard Medical School;
Department of Radiology, Massachusetts General Hospital,
Boston, Massachusetts

Hugh Davson, Sc.D.

Professor, Department of Physiology,
University College,
London, England

Samuel J. Dwyer, III, Ph.D.

Professor and Director, The Image Analysis Laboratory
Bioengineering and Advanced Automation Program,
College of Engineering, University of Missouri-Columbia,
Columbia, Missouri

Jack Edeiken, M.D.

Professor and Chairman, Department of Radiology,
Thomas Jefferson University Hospital,
Philadelphia, Pennsylvania

William V. Glenn, Jr., M.D.

Director of Computerized Tomography, Department of Radiology,
Memorial Hospital Medical Center,
Long Beach, California

David J. Goodenough, Ph.D.

Director, Radiation Physics,
The George Washington University Medical Center,
The University Hospital,
Washington, D.C.

John Haaga, M.D.

Radiologist, Cleveland Clinic,
Cleveland, Ohio

Ernest L. Hall, Ph.D.

Associate Professor, Department of Electrical Engineering, University of Tennessee,
Knoxville, Tennessee

John F. Harwig, Ph.D.

Assistant Professor in Radiopharmacy, University of Southern California,
Los Angeles, California

Gerald C. Huth, Ph.D.

Director, Medical Imaging Science Group,
University of Southern California School of Medicine,
Marina del Rey, California

A. Everette James, Jr., Sc.M., M.D.

Professor and Chairman, Department of Radiology and Radiological Sciences,
Vanderbilt University School of Medicine,
Nashville, Tennessee

Gerald S. Johnston, M.D.

Chief, Nuclear Medicine, Clinical Center,
National Institutes of Health,
Bethesda, Maryland

Alfred Eric Jones, M.D.

Assistant Chief, Nuclear Medicine, Clinical Center,
National Institutes of Health,
Bethesda, Maryland

Lennart Krook, D.V.M., Ph.D.

Professor of Pathology, New York State Veterinary College, Cornell University;
Professor of Pathology and Radiology, Cornell University Medical College,
Ithaca, New York

Gregory N. Larsen, Ph.D.

Assistant Professor of Bioengineering and Advanced Automation Program,
College of Engineering, University of Missouri-Columbia,
Columbia, Missouri

Barbara J. McNeil, M.D., Ph.D.

Assistant Professor of Radiology (Nuclear Medicine), Harvard Medical School;
Radiologist, Joint Program in Nuclear Medicine,
Charles A. Dana Cancer Center, Children's Hospital Medical Center, and
Peter Bent Brigham Hospital,
Boston, Massachusetts

John R. Milbrath, M.D.

Assistant Professor of Radiology, The Medical College of Wisconsin;
Director, Breast Cancer Detection Center,
Milwaukee County Medical Complex,
Milwaukee, Wisconsin

Björn E. W. Nordenström, M.D.

Professor of Radiology, Karolinska Institutet, University of Stockholm;
Chairman, Department of Radiology, Karolinska Hospital,
Stockholm, Sweden

Eladio A. Nunez, Ph.D.

Associate Professor of Anatomy,
Columbia University College of Physicians and Surgeons;
Adjunct Associate Professor of Radiology, Cornell University Medical College,
New York, New York

Robert W. Parkey, M.D.

Professor of Radiology and Chief, Nuclear Medicine,
Southwestern Medical School,
University of Texas Health Science Center at Dallas,
Dallas, Texas

M. Sandy Schwartz, M.B.A.

Project Manager, Department of Radiology,
Thomas Jefferson University,
Philadelphia, Pennsylvania

Katherine A. Shaffer, M.D.

Assistant Professor of Radiology, The Medical College of Wisconsin,
Milwaukee, Wisconsin

David H. Trapnell, M.D., F.R.C.P., F.R.C.R.

Consultant Radiologist, Westminster Hospital,
London, England

Michael J. Welch, Ph.D.

Professor of Radiation Chemistry,
Edward Mallinckrodt Institute of Radiology,
Washington University School of Medicine,
St. Louis, Missouri

Joseph P. Whalen, M.D.

Professor and Chairman, Department of Radiology,
Cornell University Medical College;
Radiologist-in-Chief, The New York Hospital,
New York, New York

James E. Youker, M.D.

Professor and Chairman, Department of Radiology,
The Medical College of Wisconsin,
Milwaukee, Wisconsin

TO

TEACHERS OF RADIOLOGY

PREFACE

As has been said so many times in the past, the field of radiology is at the turning point, leading to exciting, remarkable, and increasingly important contributions to health care. Much of the recent excitement in radiology revolves around the potential impact of computed tomography. Equally important is the increasing concern for greater operational efficiency and better evaluation of the contributions of this diagnostic tool to the health care system.

When asked to define what is current in radiology, one is left with an ambivalence relating to the improved developments of older technologies (e.g., chest x-ray studies, bone radiology) and enthusiasm for the new technologies exemplified in computed tomography and nuclear radiology. To attain a balance for these enthusiasms is difficult indeed. Therefore, in preparing for this third volume of Current Concepts, I am forced to make a personal assessment, hopefully eclectic, of the many developments in radiology in the past two years. This personal impression of the relative priorities and major developments and the importance of more widespread dissemination of specific concepts in radiology results in this book's being a mixture of a state of the art in computed tomography with nuclear radiology and a review of the more traditional radiologic procedures.

Since its inception, the Current Concepts series has been dedicated to providing a bridge between the current journal publications and the more formalized textbooks in the field. I acknowledge that this effort is made by others in differing formats, but the previous acceptance by the radiologic community of the Current Concepts publications has led us to continue in this effort with renewed enthusiasm as the field of radiology continues to expand in many dimensions at the same time. Much of what is current has of necessity not been included in this book, but hopefully the essays provide a somewhat balanced appreciation of the excitement engendered by reevaluation of past experiences in an amalgamation of the newer technologies.

I would like to take this opportunity to extend my sincere appreciation to the distinguished group of essayists who have contributed to this volume. I would also like to extend my personal appreciation to Diane Torrance and Linda Gard for their efforts in completing this book. It is hoped that it will provide

xiii

readers with additional insight into current concepts of the new technologies of computed tomography and developing technologies of nuclear radiology as well as the more traditional radiologic procedures.

E. James Potchen

CONTENTS

VOLUME THREE
Current concepts in radiology

1 Information systems in departmental operations

M. Sandy Schwartz and Jack Edeiken

The objective of an effort at Thomas Jefferson University Hospital was to determine the advisability of developing systems that would control activities associated with the operational environment of the radiology department. Specifically, the investigation was guided by two major premises: (1) definition of a system that would provide the best balance between maximum beneficial impact on operations and procedures and minimum development and operational cost, and (2) delineation of a modular system that realistically could be developed to achieve the stated goals and objectives. It would provide successive operational supports during the three-year span of the project as unit phases were implemented. As a result of the study, it was determined that by including several key support functions in a proposed automated system, the following significant improvements in operational capability could be achieved:

1. Increased efficiency in patient scheduling and processing
2. Monitored film library storage on retrieval techniques
3. Provision of 24-hour diagnostic report capability by interfacing the radiologist to the computer
4. Improved timeliness of records through automated file edits and updates
5. Increased efficiencies through control of staff procedures and work processes
6. Improved statistical reporting

To maintain control and anticipate future development, an automated data-processing system installed in the immediate future would be an accepted managerial instrumentality for the next decade. The design, development, and installation of the computer system created to support the needs of the radiology department could embody an innovative combination of sophisticated approaches and conceptual features that would serve as a model for future development in the field of x-ray automation.

The performance of the radiology department amid the demand for more complex examinations and sharply increased requisitions for radiologic services during a period of spiraling costs prompted a study to seek solutions that would bring effective management controls, improve the quality of service, and maintain cost constraints.

The growth in demand for health care services has intensified the volume of radiographic explorations to be conducted within a facility designed for the 1950s and yet satisfy the need for an installation allowing increasing numbers of patients to be examined or treated more reliably in less time and at reduced risks. A streamlining of the flow of work must be patterned within present space limitations; the stay of the patients in the radiology department must be short and not unpleasant; the examination must be easy for the physician and the technician and ensure maximum results.

To meet these requirements, there is the choice of systems development and counseling combined with electronic data processing, as a total department enterprise. The following demands and interactions of the department's requirements should be considered in a design philosophy for constructing a conceptual model:

1. Equipment to meet the needs of the systems that are readily available
2. A system conceived and designed as a total enterprise starting with the developmental stage
3. Installations and accessory facilities that are systematically planned and constructed

The areas of the department where systems controls may be applied to attain the most improved operational results are Patient Registration and Scheduling, Film Library, and Diagnostic Reporting. The department has attempted to identify the problems of these areas and discover solutions that could be accomplished by the application of sound management policies and systems techniques.

MANAGEMENT CONSIDERATIONS

It was believed that proposed improvements in departmental organization coupled with better systems and procedures would promote the development of an improved working environment. The application of cybernetics to the solution of managerial problems should stress the human aspect of improvement with automation. A total systems design should be constructed for comfortable operation by the entire team—the symbiosis of the staff and their apparatus must be perceived in conceptual model planning.

To achieve success in the introduction of new techniques, methods, and procedures, staff involvement must be attained to assure support. Involvement between the radiologist and the system that services his requirements is predicated on an understanding of the automated procedures. For example, to facilitate rapid reporting, the diagnostician must dictate the report on completion of a study by the following consultation session and be present for verification and signature when the typewritten report is completed. The scheduling and coordination-control functions exercise a central control on case actions to ensure their completion on a timely basis. The success of this function may vary directly with the judgment, experience, and intuitive understanding of the coordinator in the performance of the assigned role. The technicians performing the x-ray study and the film quality control become involved with the system by providing data inputs. The film library is a support system requiring continuous, accurate, and controlled inputs. The role of the librarians within an automated environment depends on their understanding, involvement, and motivation in interacting with the system. The human aspect—the interaction between the system and the people involved—is the strategic consideration. Indoctrination should endeavor to illustrate and explain to all staff members their roles in the total system. Communication channels between staff and management should permit a cross-fertilization of ideas and concerns. Management objectives and staff problems should be expounded and resolved jointly in the decision-making process.

Implementation of the control elements requires increased coordination and cooperation among a variety of diverse areas. This coordination can in itself be a source of problems insofar as it increases the work of the area managers or supersedes and/or contravenes organizational groupings. As a person's status, recognition, esteem, and sense of achievement are primarily dependent on his relationship to organizational and social environments, the implementation of control elements that require increased cooperation necessitates the use of methods other than those required for eliminating resistance to change.

The implementation of new resources and the resultant changes in work loads and manpower patterns should ultimately be beneficial for the staff. Positive personnel efforts will in turn benefit patient care and the department. Comprehending the relevance of one's role in the team effort should engender a sense of commitment, spur work attitudes, and heighten motivations. The goal to be reached is a well-organized, efficient department staffed by cooperative and willing personnel.

PROBLEM IDENTIFICATION AND SOLUTION
Quality of diagnostic reports

One objective in evaluating the quality of diagnostic reports is to return to the physician correct and accurate diagnostic reports for the studies ordered.

Accuracy of diagnostic reports

Problem. The previous film of a related study must be available at the time of the study diagnosis. The present system does not ensure accountability or provide total inventory control; films are misfiled, misplaced, and borrowed for private use and sometimes not returned. Thus the radiologist may not be provided with the complete, comparative data necessary to make a highly accurate x-ray report.

solution. Improve film library access and retrieval methods. Film loss can be reduced by the application of automated monitoring controls. The rapid delivery of previous studies will also provide all available data for the rendering of an accurate diagnostic report. Automated storage of previous films will ensure that films are delivered on request. The timely presentation of supportive data allows the referring physician to prescribe patient treatment without delay.

Processing of patient data

Problem. The present system for processing patient data is a clerical operation. The element of human error in transposing information, sorting, filing and refiling, updating, and recording is time-consuming and tedious and creates delays in patient processing. The effort required to keep the files updated results in substantial delays between case action and record update. Thus keeping the files current is a plaguing problem. A serious clerical activity waste is attributable to incomplete and/or lost information, duplicate records, and multiple medical record numbers for each patient. On a daily basis there are approximately 25,000 manual actions to process. With current methods, handling 250 patient records a day requires 138.2 man-hours.

SOLUTION. An automated system should provide a 40% reduction in clerical activity and manual processing as well as instantaneous data availability. It can minimize the possibility of human error in clerical and control functions and significantly reduce the number of daily manipulations. With automation the clerical process is reduced to the actual time required to key-in and verify basic data to the terminal. Processing 250 patient records a day would require approximately 83 man-hours, and overtime payments attributed to this activity would be minimized.

With computerization, data can be recalled, edited, or added at any stage of processing, and provision can be afforded to enter basic data cases not previously scheduled. In addition, patient identification and previous radiologic history verification may be facilitated by access to the central hospital information system.

Any approach to the design of a central hospital information system must consider the unit record. A single patient data base containing a patient identification number system would aid in the centralization of all records for each patient. For the physician, a single, complete record file would furnish supporting data for making medical decisions. There are several other advantages. The scheduling and patient-coordination function can be reduced. Automated clerical controls can eliminate the loss of patient data, omissions, and transcription errors in patient data handling. Reduction in clerical data transfers, paper processing, sorting, and filing can save many man-hours a day. By reporting the existence of previous related or future conflicting x-ray studies, automation can reduce unnecessary duplication of x-ray studies. Monthly administrative schedules and logs produced by a computer would be accurate and timely and provide savings in labor.

Incomplete examination

Problem. The equipment and/or the technician that performs the examination may produce a defective film. Present quality controls spot the errors, but manual analysis of the data is not always performed in time to identify the cause. Also patients not properly prepared in advance for special examinations must be rescheduled for examination or require additional x-ray studies. Time-consuming x-ray retakes account for an unnecessary increase in total x-ray volume.

SOLUTION. With a control station in each examination room linked to the computer, a statistical check can help determine the cause of the film's not attaining acceptable standards. Statistical data will provide feedback for control decisions by management, and a reduction in retakes results. A statistical check can also pinpoint possible failures or breakdowns in the central darkroom equipment and possible x-ray equipment malfunctions or maladjustments in each room. It may identify a need to modify a technique, procedure, or preparation or to provide additional technician-training seminars.

Emergency room procedures

Problem. A mechanism for retrieval of information (previous medical record number and film studies) on patients using radiologic services in the emergency room does not presently exist. Patient information from the emergency room is not immediately available to the radiology department for file update, charging, inquiries, and diagnostic reporting. The temporary patient number issued by the emergency room must be checked against the patient file by the radiology department for permanent number assignment.

SOLUTION. Installation of a terminal in the emergency room would provide for inquiry to the patient file for retrieval of patient medical record number and previous examinations, if any. On completion of an x-ray examination, patient information, type of study, and the date are entered into the system through the terminal for file update, patient charging, inquiries, notification to pull comparison films for interpretation, and dispatch of a messenger for film delivery to the diagnostician.

Speed in processing diagnostic reports

Another objective is to return to the physician the correct diagnostic report in the shortest possible time.

Diagnostic report delays

Problem. Delays associated with the present manual diagnostic reporting process impede the attending and/or referring physician. The average time between the initiation of an x-ray request and the distribution of the report is approximately 4 days. The usual time between report dictation and final distribution of the approved report copy is from 39 to 67 hours for the general hospital and clinic areas.

SOLUTION. An initial approach envisioned the installation of a sophisticated word-processing system to produce typewritten reports rapidly. Specific recommendations allowed for an increase of total paperwork production along with the elimination of approximately three secretarial positions. A word-processing system would allow for greater staff flexibility and increased secretarial productivity. It would permit open time for physicians and administrative personnel to perform additional support tasks. While producing higher-quality documents and an increase in productivity, it would also lower costs. Future work volume increases could be handled without an increase in staff. The success of this innovation depends on the cooperative response of the radiologists; the diagnostician must be available to dictate the report on completion of a study by the following consultation session and be available for verification and signature on completion of the typewritten report.

A word-processing system interfaced to a computer could store diagnostic reports (or portions of reports), with retrieval potential determined by the the communication network. The stored reports, which can supply data for statistical report analysis, teaching, and research, could be transmitted to any terminal linked into the system.

A further enhancement and a singular contribution toward the creation of an improved diagnostic reporting method is the incorporation of unique, innovative designs and techniques developed by Dr. Paul Wheeler of Johns Hopkins University. An electro-optical input unit to assist in the reporting and diagnosis-processing of radiologic studies has been developed and will be commercially available soon. The radiologist probes appropriate information points projected onto the surface of the unit. The parameters of the reference data available for input are contained in a synoptic lexicon of anatomic, pathologic, support, and related functional terms. The data are put into format and processed on completion of the probing phase.

Although the system has the capability of producing automatic reports, uncommon discoveries or extraordinary amplifying information may be inserted into standard terms by conventional typewriting. All input terms and phrases introduced during the report preparation are visually monitored on a cathode-ray-tube (CRT) screen.

A major design concept features an automated diagnostic reporting system that can produce a completed report in the time used to dictate a diagnosis. By interfacing the radiologist directly with the system, concise, clearly defined reports with improved appearance and readability are produced. Upon display on the CRT, they are reviewed, corrected, and verified by the radiologist with an electronically coded signature and entered into the system. The final copy is prepared by the system for immediate transmission to the patient care unit.

A major benefit of this approach is the ability to identify the information entered; the potential for subsequent retrieval of entire reports or specific diagnoses or studies can be made readily available. This feature is useful both for developing a computer-based medical record and for purposes of utilization review, medical audit, clinical investigation, and preparing teaching material.

Management concerns

A third objective is to maintain a high level of management planning and control.

Scheduling and coordination control

Problem. The primary responsibility of the scheduling and coordination control functions is to exercise a central control on case actions to ensure their timely completion. The scheduling and coordination functions should provide means for data collection on workload and case activity monitoring.

The scheduling log must be revised constantly to accommodate the daily influx of requests for same-day and rescheduled studies, changes, and cancelled examinations. This initial entry reporting method is seriously deficient as a rapid and accurate source of patient data. Coordination difficulties result in the formation of queues of patients awaiting diagnostic x-ray procedures.

Scheduling and coordination problems include the following:
1. Failure of floor personnel to have the patient ready on time
2. X-ray equipment failure
3. Work assignment coverage
4. Presence of STAT or emergency patients
5. Incomplete knowledge of the patient's condition
6. Variability of lengths of examination times
7. Necessity for retakes
8. Loss of escort slips from the examination rooms to the central film processing department and to the front desk
9. Notification of patient's arrival for examination
10. Notification of completion of each patient's examination, signaling room availability
11. Notification of patient's departure from the radiology department

SOLUTION. The application of automated techniques to resolve vexatious scheduling concerns presupposes a carefully orchestrated interface with the patient escort, the patient, the technician performing the x-ray examination, and the quality control technician. The success of this function would be dependent on the ability of the coordinator to manage, assign, and control the activities of the several individuals involved in the process.

An automated, dynamic computer system would provide a current scheduling log to support the management control functions by updating revisions because of additional requests, changes in examination, time or type, cancellations of examinations, delays in completion of studies, and no-shows. The scheduling function would forecast the expected variability of the work load. It would account for the daily varying work load of the fixed, nonphysician, processing staff. An improved data flow would ameliorate personnel handling, room assignment, and control of patient coordination activities.

Future and previous appointments can be produced for CRT display. Automated monitoring would regulate patient traffic in controlled stages throughout the radiologic processing. Instead of queues of inpatients at certain peak hours, there would be a steady flow of inpatients to be processed. An advantage is that scheduling conflicts or duplicate examinations would be avoided. Moreover, automated devices will reject specified conflicts such as assigning an intravenous pyelogram the day after a gastrointestinal series.

Communication control

Problem. Incoming telephone calls require time-consuming routing, checking, and responding.

SOLUTION. Because automated coordination and scheduling techniques supervise departmental control activities, telephone inquiries volume can be reduced. Timely delivery of wet readings and finished diagnostic reports would eliminate repetitive inquiries. Information displayed on a terminal could reduce the length of patient status calls from an average of 5 minutes to less than 1 minute. Entering request and diagnostic results calls can be similarly reduced in duration.

Film library control

Problem. Tasks involved in the film-handling function are hampered by the need for improved monitoring control and accountability procedures, the lack of appropriate and timely information flow, and the need for improved storage in situ and retrieval methods.

An analysis of a number of film requests received in the film-filing area revealed that approximately 40% of desired films were unavailable on the first search because they were on loan or for other reasons. Of these, only 15% to 20% could be located after further search and retrieved in about a week. Films could not be located for a variety of reasons:

1. Failure of outside borrowers to return films after the length of time necessary to record their findings
2. Misfiling
3. Failure of film unit personnel to check off film requests that had been handled
4. Failure to take action on overdue film loans
5. Duplicate patient numbers
6. Failure to update master film folder number

SOLUTION. A support system dependent on continuous, accurate, and carefully controlled inputs can be successful when the library staff is dedicated to quality performance. Management information furnished by automation should provide orderly assistance to the librarians for their manual tasks. By responding to these new outputs in a positive manner, automation would become a useful and willing tool.

A rapid access and retrieval information system could monitor and control film library activities with greater effectiveness. Location and contents of a patient folder could be readily provided. Accountability controls could ensure greater return of "lost" or borrowed films. Patient records would be cross-referenced for film retrieval, and the correct number would be assigned for updating.

A library management control system would fill requests for previous films on demand, thus minimizing diagnostic reporting delays attributable to the absence of supportive film studies.

Coordination control

Problem. Present reporting methods do not provide the radiology coordinator with a high reliability control on room availability nor positively guarantee that the patient will be examined for the study requested.

SOLUTION. The technician performing the x-ray examination and the technician performing film quality control must respond to an automated system by providing appropriate data inputs. Control data elements, including notification of patient entry into the examination room, type of examination performed, and notification of room availability on completion of examination, are received by the coordinator to control ongoing activities. Performance data, including number of and reason for film retakes, additional views taken, and poor visualization, may be collected for research and evaluation reporting.

Equipment dependability

Problem. Equipment maintenance and repair require room assignment changes. Equipment failure also results in the problems of increased patient waiting time, patient reexamination, prolonged examinations and reduced room utilization, and room downtime.

SOLUTION. An automated scheduling system can improve x-ray room utilization by the use of dynamic update techniques. The system can reassign patients when rooms are blocked. By monitoring room availability, the coordinator can adjust and reschedule room use; a demonstrated savings on x-ray room useage can be derived. Through production of a maintenance report, scheduled and unscheduled downtime for equipment in each room can be observed.

Management decision making

Problem. In the face of inflation and demands for increased services and volume of work, the department must make decisions that will optimize the utilization of available resources and increase the efficiency of each operating unit.

SOLUTION. An automated system can effectively produce savings in time and labor costs by monitoring work loads, providing data to analyze costs, detecting ways to evaluate and improve operational procedures, and furnishing information to predict undesirable outcomes so that positive actions may be taken before they occur.

Management information reporting

Problem. The production of monthly reports is an exacting, manual data compilation. Ancillary data are not readily available for administrative use in a manual operation.

The radiology department produces weekly and monthly summary reports, which indicate the number of studies performed according to category and type of patient service. Financial summaries reporting the total number of dollars that should have been billed are also produced. Uncoordinated procedures for reporting cancelled and rescheduled studies result in inaccurate and redundant data descriptions. The exclusive use of hard copy documents in the filing system makes it extremely difficult to respond to special information or statistical requests. Even when a response is made to these requests, the accuracy of it is questionable.

SOLUTION. An automated system can provide data to assist in administrative decision making—data for unit costing, exception reporting, timing and volume studies, financial and accounting reporting, expansion projections, and statistical analysis. An automated system can maintain short-term daily work load files, which include data on patients who are late or who fail to appear for examination. The central order entry control system should reduce the no-shows caused by conflicting inpatient scheduling among ancillary departments.

Automation can provide statistical summaries and cumulative reports. The data generated during daily operations will be used for measuring station performance, work leveling, personnel scheduling, predicting future work loads, and general monitoring functions. The reports will also perform the following functions:

1. Measure personnel productivity
2. Provide data to forecast future personnel, facilities, and equipment requirements fot specific time periods under varying demand stimuli
3. Provide statistics to forecast direct costs under varying volumes and productivity rates
4. Perform cost-effectiveness analyses for management planning
5. Provide statistics to forecast patient loads that can be handled with specific time constraints
6. Detect critical factors such as capacity of personnel, equipment, and facilities
7. Provide data to forecast the resource requirements and costs to meet a given objective

By automation, virtually all forms are generated and printed within the radiology department.

Radiology department management control

Problem. Without adequate management reporting mechanisms, it is difficult to establish priority of assignments in advance and to effectively allocate time to various areas of concern.

SOLUTION. A management reporting system would increase operational efficiency for the several units within the department. It would help in predicting future needs at various stages in time. Evaluating personnel performance and assessing techniques of planning, scheduling, estimating, and budgeting would be facilitated. It would aid management in judging the quality of the product. Attention would be focused on problems in time to take remedial action.

Billing

Problem. The present manual outpatient billing system contains the faults of any clerical system in that it is tedious, time-consuming, and slow. The use of Opscan forms for inpatient billing produces an unacceptable margin of error.

SOLUTION. Automation offers an opportunity to improve billing procedures by sending outpatient charge data on-line to a central location or to generate professional fee billing within the department. Inpatient charges could be made available to the central hospital accounting system (Shared Hospital Accounting System or SHAS).

Space utilization considerations

Problem. The department has been able to process increased patient examination volume within the confines of its allocated space. In the future a point will be reached where additional volume will require more working space.

SOLUTION. An automated system can direct the allocation of resources and assignment of facilties and improve patient scheduling to maximize utilization and constrain space demands. If additional work details are assigned to the automated system, requirements for additional personnel and staff space should be minimized.

Service to physicians, staff, and patients

A fourth objective is to optimize service to physicians, staff, and patients and to improve liaison and sharing of resources among professional staff and other personnel.

Need for prompt delivery of diagnosis

Problem. The major complaint of all referring physicians is the delay in the receipt of diagnostic reports.

SOLUTION. The unique capabilities of an automated system purposefully designed for radiologic diagnostic reporting can provide rapid study results, but cooperation is needed in several areas. Because the capability of this salient innovation is dependent on the support of the radiologist, he must be available to dictate the report by the consultation sessions following the examination and be present to verify and sign the completed report. To coordinate patient scheduling for x-ray examination, the radiology department must be able to control escort assignments. To expedite pickup of study requests and delivery of diagnostic reports, the department must be able to assign and control messengers. With such cooperation, delay in delivery of diagnostic reports should be significantly reduced.

Film retrieval

Problem. The referring physician is frustrated when a required film is lost or not readily available for study.

SOLUTION. Automated control of the film library will reduce film loss by effi-

ciently monitoring the access to and retrieval of films and providing rapid availability to the physician.

Need for liaison between x-ray department and nursing units

Problem 1. The nursing units have not been given ample advance notice for
patient x-ray examination.

SOLUTION. An automated system can produce and deliver a patient census activity log by 7 AM to effectively serve the nursing unit requirements. Lead time
will allow the units to provide appropriate conveyances for patient movement to
the x-ray area. Accurate scheduling of patients will also permit the units
to prepare patient activities without the possibility of time conflicts with the
radiology department.

Problem 2. The nursing units require information on patient department and
patient examination status on return to the unit.

SOLUTION. The new system will automatically print notices with the appropriate information to be delivered to the nursing unit by the escort—patient departure for the x-ray department, appointment time, and type of study. On the patient's return to the floor, the notice will indicate departure time from the x-ray
department and examination status (study completed or cancelled and rescheduled and the reschedule date).

Delayed diagnostic results

Problem. Patient stays may be prolonged for as long as a week in instances
of delayed receipt of radiologic reports.

SOLUTION. In most instances an automated system could provide diagnostic
results for inclusion on the patient chart within a 24-hour period.

Deficient work flow synchronization

Problem. Present scheduling and monitoring methods create disruptions in
operational work flow.

SOLUTION. An automated system to support sound management practices
should synchronize and level the valleys and peaks of the operational work flow.
By equalizing personnel work loads, staff efficiency will be improved. Energies
may be devoted to proficiency in assigned tasks, thereby optimizing patient service. Reduced work tensions would create a more relaxed atmosphere necessary
to establish rapport between staff and patient.

A noteworthy feature of an automated system is the ability to respond to
involved data inputs as readily as they occur. When each operating unit is furnished with pertinent data on command, measurable efficiencies that exceed present imprecise methods may be obtained. The automated system can produce the
following:

1. Daily schedules for each radiographic room
2. Patient census activity logs produced immediately on completion of request

data would be made available for the consulting diagnostician and/or the technologist.

Economics

Problem. The operation of the radiology department is a complex mix of several economic factors. Future examination volume, the need for competent health care personnel in all units, space and facility limitations, allocation of resources, compliance with changing procedures and additional regulatory agencies requirements are all factors that must be considered in allocating the department budget during a period of apparently unabated inflation.

SOLUTION. A computer system devised during the first half of the decade would be ready to meet the anticipated needs of the department during the next decade and provide the economic benefits and controls that appear necessary in an environment of social and economic turbulence.

An automated system would control billing, reduce future demands for personnel, contain the growth of the present work force, systematize and upgrade clerical procedures, monitor and control utilization of present facilities and resources, and prepare data for statistical analysis and management decision making and forcasting. These improvements will contain or lower the average unit cost of the product.

Following are the department expenses involved in computing the unit cost for each examination:

1. Examination supplies. These are summarized and priced by the purchasing department from logs maintained by the technicians in each room.
2. Film. Periodic inventory of each size is multiplied by the unit cost of each (Purchasing).
3. Fixed expenses. Rent plus nonexamination room equipment costs (determined once a year from an inventory) are added to the total nonidentifiable supply expense determined by purchasing.
4. Salaries of technologists, students, staff support, radiologists, and residents. A report now prepared by the department's timekeeper shows these expenses, which are reported to the Business Office.
5. Fringe expenses. These are calculated by multiplying the monthly regular hours expense for technologists by twelve (Business Office).
6. Equipment. Once a year all equipment is inventoried and an annual cost determined. The total cost for all equipment used in examination rooms is divided by the number of periods in the year. Thus equipment expense would be the same each period (Purchasing).
7. Physics. This expense is obtained from the operating expense report each month (Purchasing).

Table 1-1 indicates the percentage of return on a theoretical investment to develop an automated system over a 7-year period. Fig. 1-1 indicates the costs of operation of a manual operation versus a computer-supported system based on a projected 6% annual growth in volume, 8% inflation, and 14% increase in

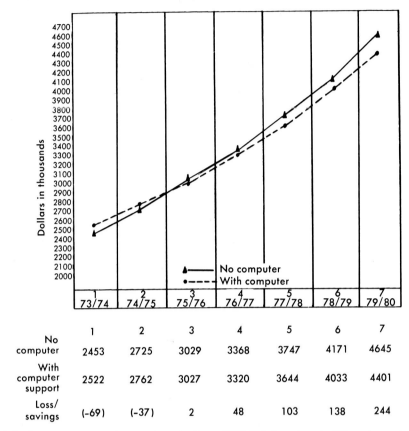

Fig. 1-1. Seven-year operating cost projection—$360,000 investment, 6% volume increase, 3% ROI.

Table 1-1. Seven-year projection for percent return on investment

Volume increase/year	Total radiology investment: $360,000
10%	27%
9%	22%
8%	16%
7%	10%
6%	3%
5%	Break even
4%	Loss
3%	
2%	
1%	
0%	

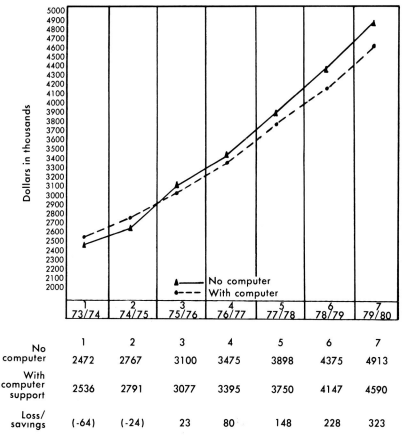

	1	2	3	4	5	6	7
No computer	2472	2767	3100	3475	3898	4375	4913
With computer support	2536	2791	3077	3395	3750	4147	4590
Loss/ savings	(-64)	(-24)	23	80	148	228	323

Fig. 1-2. Seven-year operating cost projection—$360,000 investment, 7% volume increase, 10% ROI.

fringe benefits and overhead expenses. Fig. 1-2 indicates 7% annual growth in volume.

AUTOMATED SYSTEM VERSUS MANUAL SYSTEM
Discounted cash flow and yearly dollar comparisons

A theoretical investment cost of $360,000 is calculated as the bottom-line figure for development of an automated system. To illustrate, 6% increase in volume will project a 3% return on investment at the end of 7 years (Fig. 1-1).

A model projection covering a 7-year estimation discounts the $360,000 development expenditure at the outset. It assumes that development is completed, and the analysis of costs is predicated on a fully operational system. In fact, development model expenditures are budgeted for the first year at $94,000, second year at $131,900, and third year at $134,000. Based on the model expenditure of $360,000, operational costs show an increase of $69,140 for the first year of operation. In fact, since an expenditure of $94,000 is anticipated, operational costs would probably show a minimal increase, if any.

At the seventh model year operational milestone, a manual system cost is projected at $4,644,960 versus a computer system cost at $4,400,870—an operational cost saving of $244,090.

The model indicates a minus turnaround to a savings of $2,360 at the third year of operation. This could in fact happen sooner, since total budget expenditures have been appropriated in increments during this 3-year period.

The model assumes a 6% a year volume increase. Three percent of gross revenue is assumed as an accurate value in the projection of an actual hospital cash flow.

RETURN ON INVESTMENT
Discounted cash flow analysis

The theoretical model assumes an initial investment of $360,000. Depending on market conditions and prevailing interest rates at the time of investment, how

Table 1-2. 3% return on $360,000 investment

Year	Transfer cash (cash flow in thousands)	Interest rate Divisor* $(1 + i)^n$	Interest rate Present value
0	$ 0.00	1.00	−360.00
1	0.00	1.02	− 69.64
2	0.00	1.06	− 36.64
3	0.20	1.09	2.16
4	5.23	1.12	43.54
5	13.53	1.15	90.16
6	26.88	1.19	141.46
7	44.02	1.22	200.07
Total present value = 11.61			

*Divisor—classical interest rate based on power of year.

Table 1-3. 10% return on $360,000 investment

Year	Transfer cash (cash flow in thousands)	Interest rate Divisor $(1 + i)^n$	Interest rate Present value
0	$ 0.00	1.00	−360.00
1	0.00	1.09	− 63.70
2	0.00	1.20	− 24.36
3	5.74	1.33	17.39
4	25.23	1.46	54.83
5	56.03	1.61	91.83
6	99.26	1.77	128.90
7	156.45	1.94	166.42
Total present value = 11.31			

does the percentage return on investment in a security compare to an investment in a department and the savings (hence increased income) generated? With a volume increase of 6% a total annual savings yield of more than 3% will be returned on investment (Table 1-2).* An annual savings yield of more than 10% will be returned on investment at a 7% volume increase (Table 1-3). Determination of interest rates and computing the value of the cash flows are necessary. When the value is zero, the interest rate is obtained.†

The model assumes benefits for the extent of a 7-year projection, but, in fact, benefits are derived during the entire life of the system and on a conservative estimate of investment return.

---

*If $360,000 were invested in a security, the interest it would have to pay to equal the value of the savings projected by the radiology department automated system would be $465,780.

Formula: $C = \dfrac{A}{B}$ (A = cash flow, B = interest rate divisor, C = present value.)

†-360,000	2,160
- 69,140	43,540
- 36,640	90,460
	141,460
	200,070
-465,780	477,690
	- 11,610 Total present value
	465,780

Table 1-4. Labor projections

	Current volume		Double volume	
	No computer	Computer support	No computer	Computer support
Professional staff	12	12	21	19
Residents	19	19	19	19
Administrative	1	1	1	1
Operations manager	—	—	—	1
Technical staff	22	22	52	39
Receptionists	8	8	15	5
Librarians	11	11	18	10
Business office	9	9	17	1
Secretarial	13	13	19	9
Nurse	1	1	3	2
Service (aids, maids, porters)	6	6	9	9
Miscellaneous (dark room)	6	6	9	9
Total staff	108	108	183	124
Annual personnel cost	$1,255	$1,255	$2,064	$1,643

- Day shift only—8 AM to 5 PM
- Includes vacation, overtime hours
- Overhead and fringe benefits not included
- Assume current dollar rate for personnel—dollars in thousands

COST ANALYSIS

The objective of cost analysis was to quantitatively assess the effect of a theoretical computerized system in a radiology department. Only department and computer personnel staffing were considered when estimates were gathered for staffing requirements under current and double volume operation (Table 1-4). However, resources are not doubled when volume doubles in a manual or computer-supported system.

The current staffing pattern shows a manpower profile close to the limits of AUR and SCARD[1] standards:

Current system personnel

Technicians	22
Total number of examinations	76,000
AUR and SCARD standards	29 technicians/75,000 examinations
Professional staff	12
Total number of examinations	76,000
AUR and SCARD standards	15 professional staff/75,000 examinations

To compute operating costs, assuming an annual growth rate, inflation factor, overhead and fringe benefits, for any given year, see the following calculation of personnel costs:

Return on investment procedure (ROI)

Model

The ROI model used here measures the discounted cash flow and allows for yearly dollar comparison between the new and present systems.

Model parameters

Pv = Fractional increase in volume/year (estimated productivity)
Ps = Fractional increase in salaries (estimated average increase)
Pf = Fringe benefits (fractional estimate of salaries)
A   = Current salary expenditure in thousands
B   = Salary expenditure in thousands when present volume is double, assuming no wage increase
n   = Number of years for which ROI is projected
SFC = Personnel and expense cost/year as a function of volume increase
CE = Current expenses in thousands
ED = Expenses (volume double) in thousands
FI   = Projected average inflation rate (fractional)

Formula

$$SFC\,[((B - A)\,(1 + Pv)^n + (2A - B))\,(1 + Pf)\,(1 + Ps)^n]$$
$$+\,((ED - CE)\,(1 + Pv)^n + (2CE - ED))\,(1 + FI)^n$$

Results

No computer	A = 1255	B = 2064
With computer (on-line)	A = 1255	B = 1643

PROJECT SCHEDULE

To evolve a forecast of scheduled events, a mix of standardized data and empirical judgements can at best create approximate time frames. As plans develop into events and are set in motion, time frames may alter and be revised.

The tasks to be considered in creating an automated system will be considered in the following pages.

Development and implementation of an automated system for the radiology department

In preparing for the installation of an automated system one must produce a project plan and budget justification. Then it is necessary to establish priorities and estimate requirements.

Design, development, and implementation of a data management system for the Word Processing Center

1. Analyze and evaluate alternative equipment and make a selection.
2. Organize supervisor training classes (two weeks).
3. Develop procedures for the operation of the Word Process Center.
4. Coordinate installation and develop an implementation schedule.
5. Coordinate instructional sessions.

Hardware and software evaluation and selection

In selecting hardware and software one must analyze and evaluate alternatives and then select EDP equipment. Other tasks include coordinating installation of equipment and developing an implementation schedule.

Development of a data management system for data base data communications

To develop a system for data communication a structural data base for the total radiology system must be established, including a communications software interface in line with the applications considered.

A scheduling algorithm based on scheduling requirements and power considerations must be designed.

Development of a data base management system

A major objective is to establish a communication network with a capability for storage and dissemination of appropriate patient information. An automated hospital data communication system could track and monitor patient progress from initial contact at admission to discharge. Pertinent data controls could enable report information on patient name, location, medical condition, attending physician, tests and therapy data, treatment and medications, and billing charges. For quality assurance, other related patient information such as estimated duration of stay and special diets and treatment plans could be reported. The system allows access to this information continuously at whatever area or time it is needed within the institution. In serving administrative and medical management functions, control and receipt of timely patient information will enhance patient care.

By means of a network of on-line terminals strategically located throughout the hospital, medical staff personnel may at any time enter patient-related transaction data into the system. This updated information may also be retrieved immediately on the terminal screen. The control and storage for this information flow is provided by the central processing unit.

Data base concept. A data base is defined as "a nonredundant collection of interrelated data items processable by one or more applications." All application data is stored in one or more data bases in a hierarchical manner. The most significant data reside on higher levels while less significant but related, dependent data appear on subordinate levels. Using a concept called "sensitivity," each application program views only that data in the structure which it uses.

Central patient data base. The *patient data base* is a compendium of factual information directly relating to the automated processing of patient activities (Fig. 1-3). The structure comprising the logical data base record contains a set of hierarchically related, fixed-length segments of one or more types. Each segment type has a unique length and format. Segments are fixed-length elements containing one or more logically related data fields. It is the basic data element that interfaces between the application program and the file.

The keystone of the hierarchical structure is the *root segment,* which contains patient biographic and demographic information. The salient feature is a unique, internal, computer-generated patient identification number containing hospital code, date of entry and time in tenths of seconds.

The *clinical history segment* contains information about the physical and mental status of the patient appropriate for facilitating patient care during the x-ray examination. Entry is also available for ad hoc comment.

An application program will control assignment of a sequential number from the *number assignment data base* and insert this patient unit number in the *file locator segment.* As a system requirement, the patient must have at least one file locator segment. Every patient must have a permanent, immutable unit number; however, additional numbers may be assigned by other hospital units. A user option allows the entry and continuance of a previously assigned unit number to the file locator segment. In this case, the application program will bypass the number assignment data base to negate the issuance of a new number.

The *case segment* maintains a file description of appropriate source type patient encounters within the hospital. The number assignment data base conveys a billing number for case segment hospital charges. The physician number is a pointer to the *physician data base* to access pertinent physician identification information.

For the type or types of insurance coverage carried by the patient, separate insurance segments are provided.

Prescribed requests relative to patient examination are stored in the *order segment.* The patient examination code is a pointer to the *services data base,* which contains specific information relating to the examination.

Finally, the *result segment* will contain the diagnosis relating to the order request. When automated diagnostic reporting is implemented, diagnostic data will be stored within this segment is encoded format.

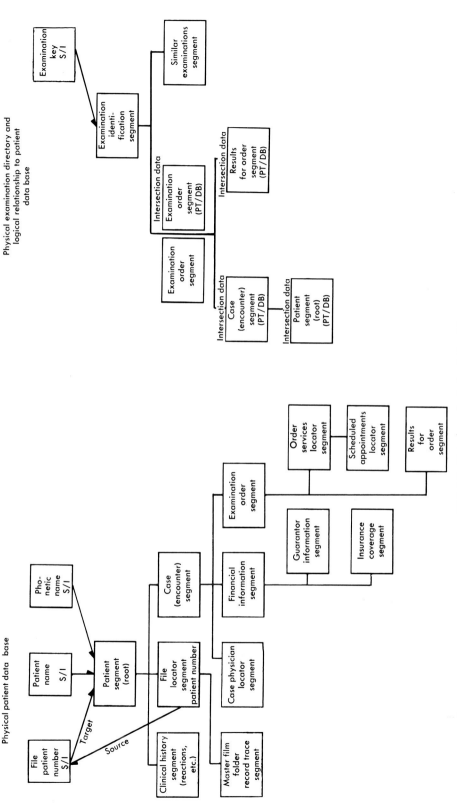

Fig. 1-3. Data base logical relationships.

Patient name secondary index data base. The *name secondary index* is an alphabetic cross-index to the patient data base. For each patient record there is an entry in the cross-index, keyed by the patient's name. This provides additional flexibility for retrieving data from the patient data base. The secondary index, sequenced by name, allows for rapid retrieval of data from the patient data base in a sequence other than that in which the data is stored. The secondary index containing the relative byte address acts as a pointer to the root segment of the patient data base.

The *secondary index data base* has a hierarchical sequential structure (root segment only). In addition to serving as an alternate access path to the patient data base, it may be independently processed as a data base.

Number assignment data base. The *number assignment data base* is a single-segment sequential file organized by department code and record type. The integer is incremented to assign a new unit number.

Service data base. The *examination directory* contains descriptive, clinical, and financial data relative to the examination process only; it is not involved with the individual patient. The examination code from the order segment of the patient data base functions as intersection data for record retrieval.

Examination schedule data base. The *radiology scheduling data base*, when keyed to the *patient unit record number*, provides effective utilization of resources by designating room group, date, room number, and time slot for patient examination assignments.

Film location data base. The film location data base monitors and provides film location source for effective library supervision and control. An application program provides parameters for a variety of situations relating to removal and return of films.

Patient tracking data base. The *patient location data base* monitors the patient in transit within the department during the examination process. An application program provides continual updating of ephemeral control data.

Scheduling features

1. Patient examination appointments will be scheduled by operators using a CRT keyboard terminal.
2. The system will supply correct appointments on request. It will screen and avoid examination conflicts, detect and question duplicate or similar examination orders, request physician approval when necessary, and monitor examination room availability.
3. The system will allow overbooking on user command.
4. The system will permit the schedule for any particular room to be blocked, and it can also free previously blocked space.
5. Patients who have been scheduled in a room that has been blocked will be identified and rescheduled.
6. The schedule will be updated dynamically; multiple scheduling terminals may operate simultaneously without conflict.
7. The system will record cancelled appointments.

8. The computer will generate the patient census activity log ("call-down list") and an alphabetized outpatient reception list.
9. It will print escort transportation notices for patient convoy service as well as a notification card to advise the nursing unit of patient departure to the radiology department.
10. The computer will print flash cards for marking films.
11. The computer will print film retrieval vouchers to notify the file room of each pending examination.
12. The system will print dispatch notices for the technicians using portable equipment.
13. The system can respond to inquiries by patient or room. It can print or display the radiology schedule for any specific time frame for any room.
14. The system can generate weekly room assignments for the staff.
15. Weekly and monthly management information reports can be generated by the computer system.

Emergency room procedures. Installation of a terminal in the emergency room will provide for inquiry to the patient file for retrieval of information. On completion of the examination, patients status data are entered into the system through the terminal.

Patient charges. Computer file storage of all patient examination data provides access for direct SHAS billing of inpatient charges. Outpatient charges will be automatically billed from the radiology department files.

Development of a data management system for the film library

File room notification from the patient scheduling system. The file room will receive notification of every scheduled examination. Data will include the date of the last examination, as this will be the best guide to the present master folder location. In the case of an examination cancellation or the addition of an examination, a second advisory notice will be printed.

Examination display. An examination for any specific date can be recalled, or the entire file of examinations can be displayed. Information on all cancelled examinations will be available from the central patient data base.

Film library window log-in procedure. The film clerk will receive newly taken radiographs accompanied by the consultation request. A terminal entry will log in receipt of the study to the computer. The notice of the appointment, which was received earlier, will have initiated the search for the master film folder, and a terminal entry will log in its arrival. The clerk will match new and comparison films for transmission to the interpretation area.

Film movement after reporting. When the interpretation has been completed, the master film folders are returned to the file room, logged in, and returned to the active shelves.

Film and teaching material loan.
1. A file of approved borrowers can be created and stored on disk. Film requests entered through a CRT will be checked against this file. If a re-

quested film folder has been previously signed out, the system will signal "unavailable," and display current location.

2. Log-outs, film returns, and cancellation requests will be entered on a terminal.

3. Overdue film folders will be automatically detected, and notices to borrowers prepared by the computer on self-mailer forms.

4. Library staff will be instructed and automatically guided through the transactions by messages displayed on the terminal guidance panel.

5. The computer will print a monthly library listing to inform the staff of the status of films on loan or location of teaching material temporarily removed from the stacks.

Library maintenance. To maintain accurate information in the library, the computer will print a list of master film folders to be relocated to the less active file and a list of those requiring number updating or correction.

Development of a data management system for patient tracking and monitoring

Automatic patient traffic monitoring. The computer will assist in regulating patient traffic by identifying rooms available for emergency procedures and walk-in outpatient examinations. In addition, a CRT entry will signal the patient's arrival in the radiology department and his departure for the care unit. Coordination of arrivals and departures at the radiology department will be possible.

Examination room monitoring. The technician will signal the arrival of the patient in the examination room by means of a CRT. After the examination and film quality control approval, the technician will enter the code indicating the type of examination completed, if retakes were made, or examination cancellation. In the gastrointestinal or genitourinary areas, the technician could also enter the code for poor visualization, which would initiate automatic rescheduling of the patient. The CRT entry will signal availability of the room.

Reporting patient status. A telephone "wet-reading" reporting and answering service will be introduced to report patient status. The operator will key patient number or name, and the CRT will display the study result information and patient status.

Plans based on film and patient tracking operations include locating a hard copy terminal outside the file room for use by clinicians. The CRT display will indicate immediately the future or past schedules of patients, whether a scheduled examination has been completed or is in progress, the location of current studies and master film folders, or the present location of patients. If the master folder is in the file room, the slip can be presented to the file room clerk.

Management reporting. The matrix for the average time span for each type of examination together with the appropriate examination room for each type of study should be developed for use by the computer system. Inputs of empirical data collected in daily operation will aid in refinement of the matrix. Weekly and monthly management information reports will be generated by the computer system.

Development of a unit cost system

The unit cost system will provide determinants to effectively manage the department's labor and material resources through the following:

1. Development of staffing guidelines in response to the actual demand for service
2. Control of film and related supplies used in examinations
3. Preparation of personnel and material budgets
4. Preplanning future departmental requirements 2 to 5 years in advance
5. Evaluation of equipment alternatives
6. Standardization of materials and procedures
7. Evaluation of staff performance
8. Balancing posted examination charges to the actual costs incurred
9. Determination of third-party hospital reimbursement

The maintenance and basis of a unit cost system includes consideration of the standards of performance for cost items that vary with the type of examination and prorated costs for items that do not vary with the type or number of examinations. Three major control mechanisms, reviewed on a monthly basis, will provide insights for effective managerial policies:

1. *Standard costs* should be calculated each month by multiplying the volume of each examination by standard cost of each expense item of each examination. When costs of each expense item for all examinations for that month are summarized, management may review what should have been expanded for each expense item. Calculated expenses would be based on preset unit or standard costs for the expense item components of each examination.
2. *Budgeted costs* are the second component of the unit cost system. Each year the department should predict examination volumes for the ensuing fiscal year and on that basis calculate the monthly costs for each component.
3. *Actual costs* data will come from payroll figures, internal reports developed for the department, and existing hospital reports costs.

Development and installation of advanced automated systems for the radiology department

The radiology department must evaluate, synthesize, and futurize the state-of-the-art possibilities of advanced radiologic systems in light of technical feasibility, worth, and acceptability. Several areas should be considered for future development.

1. Automated diagnostic reporting—Modify existing applications for advanced concepts in automated diagnostic reporting.

2. Statistics and management reporting—Design and develop management reporting systems that emphasize exception reporting, simulation, and forecasting techniques to aid in advanced administrative decision making.

3. Teaching and research—Design a flexible system to allow ready access to the data base.

4. Quality assurrance—Design systems to determine type of examination required based on preliminary patient diagnosis, information from previous examinations, and other data from patient medical history.

5. Advanced text management systems—Design an interactive, conversational, time-sharing system that enables the user to enter, edit, store, format, proofread, and display textual information in an efficient manner.

LONG-RANGE IMPLICATIONS

Structuring of a system containing the proper computer configuration, programming language, and data base will assure provision for growth and future development. Considering present state-of-the-art development and predicted outcomes for the next decade and beyond, the system design should be adequate to include the following future long-range goals:

1. On-line patient census data from the admissions department.

2. Centralized hospital billing for inpatient and outpatient charges.

3. Quality assurance—provision of complete, accurate, and timely information for a thorough medical audit program.

4. Advanced diagnostic aids—the development of an on-line computer reporting system that interfaces the radiologist, via a CRT, to the computer to produce instant, automated, diagnostic reporting.

5. Recording of MRAD exposure factors for calculating exposure and dose. Reduction of unnecessary radiation dose is likely through the knowledge of film location, for if a physician does not have access to the report or cannot locate the radiographs, he may order a repeat study.

6. A central hospital order entry system comprising a network of display terminals at the admissions desk, nursing stations, and support areas. Operating and responding instantaneously, the terminals will accept requests for radiologic examinations, receive diagnostic results, and minimize data-handling errors.

7. Expansion projects—interface the radiology department to future Hospital Information System support to the new Clinical Teaching Facility, which will provide approximately eighteen radiologic examination rooms, separating inpatients from outpatients, and two rooms in the emergency area to provide operating room support.

The introduction of electronic data-processing methods to dynamically reorganize the radiology department is a radical but necessary step into the future. It is, however, but a preliminary involvement with a process that demands acceptance as a condition of progress.

HOSPITAL AND RADIOLOGY DEPARTMENT AUTOMATION SUPPORT

The radiology department functions as a service arm for the general hospital health care delivery system. The design of a radiologic system requires that automation benefits be requisite to and in a configuration appropriate to hospital information and communication structures. The effective delivery of radiographic service supported by automated techniques envisions a communication-information system eventually comprising the total hospital complex. Optimum benefits will accrue when the several branches of a health care delivery institution may store, transmit, and retrieve shared data from a central source.

Reference

1. Report of the Advisory Committee on Academic Radiology of the Association of University Radiologists and Society of Chairmen of Academic Radiology Departments: The needs of academic radiology in the seventies, Radiology **111**:223, 1974.

2 Image quality of computed tomography

David J. Goodenough

The recent success of computed tomography (CT) systems has once again raised the question of the complexity of relating physical measurements of diagnostic imaging systems to the diagnostic efficacy afforded by such systems. Thus a CT system with spatial resolution and noise amplitude inferior to many diagnostic screen-film combinations is found in certain situations to be a considerable improvement over such diagnostic systems. This fact should point out the intrinsic danger of evaluating a system on the basis of isolated physical measurements.

Evaluation of image quality, especially as it depends on a human observer detection performance, is a complex task involving analysis of several physical and psychophysical variables. This can be seen in the following outline of experimental parameters to be controlled and specified in evaluating human detection performance.[15]

A. Image parameters
  1. Signal to be detected
    a. Size
    b. Shape
    c. Inherent contrast
  2. Number of possible signals
  3. Image system
    a. Spatial resolution (MTF)
    b. Sensitivity
    c. Linearity
    d. Noise (amplitude and character)
    e. Speed (dose)
  4. Nonsignal structure
  5. Field size
B. Observational parameters
  1. Display system
    a. Brightness scale
    b. Gain
    c. Offset
    d. Any nonlinearity
    e. Magnification/minification

Supported in part by the Himmelfarb Foundation.

2. Viewing condition
    a. Viewing distance
    b. Ambient room brightness
3. Detection task
4. Number of observations
C. Psychophysical parameters
    1. A priori information given observer
    2. Feedback given observer (if any)
    3. Observer experience for *other* given parameters
        a. Clinical vs. nonclinical experience
        b. Familiarity with signal, display, and especially with type of noise artifacts to be expected

As the outline indicates, one needs to know more than just spatial resolution and noise amplitude and character.[18] One must also consider system sensitivity, system speed (especially as it relates to patient motion), and any other image-degrading characteristics that may enter into the final image, such as scattered radiation and image artifacts. Then, too, there is the extremely complicated task of evaluating the influence of overlapping structure (e.g., anatomic detail or grid lines), an excellent image of which may actually be a problem. This is sometimes called "structure noise."

Until a way is found whereby the physical variables describing image quality can be combined with other factors such as financial costs, time utilization, patient dose, and, of course, diagnostic yield to give a general equation of diagnostic efficacy, one must basically approach the problem of system evaluation by adopting independent measures of each of these factors, realizing that it is their mutual effect which must be ultimately considered.

For convenience, let us consider the diagnostic process to be composed of at least three basic steps: (1) the "detection step," in which a decision is made as to whether some (as yet unspecified) abnormality is present in the image; (2) the "classification step," in which decisions are made as to the attributes (size, shape, etc.) of any detected abnormalities; and (3) the "recognition step," in which decisions are made as to likely disease patterns that correspond to the classified, detected abnormalities.

In this chapter I will attempt to show how certain basic physical measurements of images obtained from CT systems may be related to the detection and classification steps of the diagnostic process. The extremely important recognition step, which involves the training of the individual physician and his ability to incorporate the patient's history with the diagnostic information from the image, must remain for later investigation.[9]

In considering the detection step, first note that it has long been recognized that several factors influence human perception of a diagnostic signal.[2,7] These factors include the contrast between the suspected abnormality and non-suspected areas (background) of the image, the rate of change of the boundary of the suspected abnormality (this is often discussed as sharpness, edge gradient, acutance, etc. and is important because of the known human perceptual preference for sharp edges), and the amplitude and character (standard deviation and spatial frequency content) of any image noise that may tend to diminish the perception of the abnormality.

To illustrate the improvement that is yet to be realized in CT scanning, one can use Fig. 2-1 to compare typical head and body scans obtained from present generation scanning units with similar accompanying radiographic cadaver slices.[20] It is clear that when considerations of patient dose and overlapping anatomic structure and patient motion do not limit technique factors, one may use combinations of kVp, mAs, and nonscreen films to yield superb images that show radiographic contrast with excellent resolution and virtually noiseless images. Unfortunately, the latter procedure is slightly invasive.

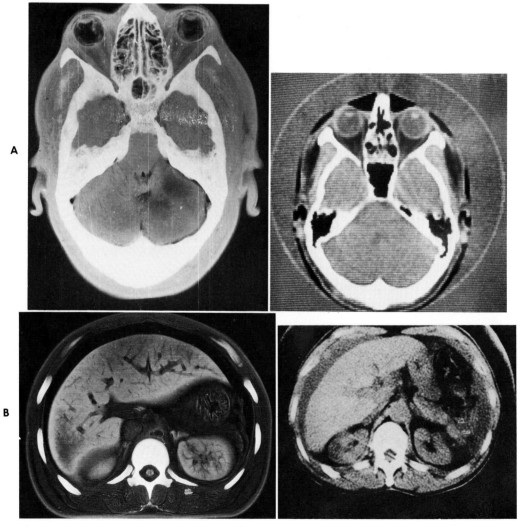

Fig. 2-1. Comparisons of current EMI head scan and body scan with radiographs of similar cadaver slices: **A,** head; **B,** body.

EMI HEAD SCANNER

In this chapter the EMI head scanner will be considered as an example of CT scanners. This type of scanner uses two adjacent scintillation crystals on one side of the head to monitor the intensity variations of the x-ray beam as a single source scans linearly across the subject. Each linear pass is repeated at 1° intervals around the subject until the system has rotated through 180° (or 225°), as illustrated schematically in Fig. 2-2. The data acquired by these two basic motions of linear scans and angular rotation are then used to estimate the relative x-ray attenuation coefficients characterizing different regions of the head. It is noted parenthetically that such information is useful to the physician only in as much as changes in the relative x-ray attenuation coefficient carry meaningful diagnostic information. Therefore not only must the system detect the changes in chemical composition (such as density and effective atomic number) that will affect the x-ray attenuation coefficient, but also the physician must have some feeling for the physiologic implications of such chemical changes. Thus one must first establish the sensitivity of the EMI system in detecting differences in inherent contrast (chemical composition). It has been stated that over a wide range of attenuation coefficients, the output of the EMI system (i.e., the EMI number) is linearly related to the linear attenuation coefficient (μ) determined at the effective energy of the emerging beam.[13]

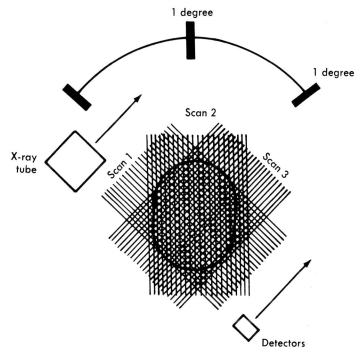

Fig. 2-2. Schematic illustration of combination of linear and rotational motions used in EMI head scanner.

It is important to realize, however, that this "linear" relationship was tested and is strictly valid only for the EMI number that results from homogeneous sampled volume elements, $\Delta V = \Delta x \Delta y \Delta z$ (e.g., $\Delta x = \Delta y = 1.5$ mm, $\Delta z = 13$ mm), where Δx and Δy represent the matrix size in terms of the axial plane variables (x,y) and Δz represents the EMI average slice thickness in the vertical (z) dimension. That is to say, the effective μ does not vary over the volume element. For objects that have a varying composition (μ) within the volume element, the EMI number will represent an average attenuation coefficient that results from the attenuation of the local x-ray intensity by the particular chemical composition and density found in each region of the volume element. Thus statements of system linearity must be carefully restricted to the EMI number that results from the "average" attenuation coefficient resulting from the volume element under consideration. (Note that system input-output intensity linearity should not be confused with geometric linearity— that is, the question of whether a straight-line input is imaged as a straight-line output.) Knowledge of the EMI number does not give information as to the regional variations within the volume element, which, indeed, may happen to cancel one another and thus obscure diagnostic information. The real potential of CT systems will not be realized until the sample volume element is small enough to represent fairly homogeneous regions of the objects of interest. This is the principal reason that smaller slice thicknesses (Δz) are sought.

This question of system linearity is important not only because of the diagnostic usefulness of the CT output but also because most tools of system analysis, such as modulation transfer function (MTF), are practically useful only when applied to linear systems. Nonlinear systems can be very difficult to analyze and often must be broken down into pseudolinear regions of the system. In fact, those systems which can be described most successfully by an MTF analysis are those which are linear and which have point spread functions that are isoplanatic (position invariant). In such cases, in the absence of noise a complete description of the relationship between the output intensity and input intensity pattern can theoretically be obtained by knowledge of the MTF (which is, of course, just the modulus of the Fourier transform of the point spread function). In addition, for such systems the relationship between the input and output noise power (variance and spatial frequency characteristics) can often be obtained from knowledge of the MTF.

Unfortunately, the EMI system is neither strictly linear nor isoplanatic. The point source response function (PSRF)—the resulting image of an effective "point" object—is dependent on the relative position (x,y,z) of the object within the scan slice. This nonlinearity and nonisoplanacity result from variations within the local x-ray intensity field as well as the discrete sampling nature of the EMI scanner. Thus to fully describe the imaging characteristics of the EMI scanner, one would need information on the PSRF at each position within the three-dimensional scan field for each possible chemical composition of the point. This information could then be used in a complicated convolution operation to predict the output that would result from attenuation of the x-ray beam spectrum by a three-dimensional object. Such a procedure would be tedious at best, and therefore, with the preceding caveats in mind, let us restrict our analysis of the EMI system to pseudolinear regions or situations where analytic measurements should afford a reasonable prediction of image quality.

Measurements of sensitivity

As mentioned previously, for homogeneously composed volume elements, the EMI output does seem to be related linearly to the linear attenuation coefficient (μ), characterizing the volume element. In fact, it has been reported that:

$$\text{EMI number} = 2.63 \times 10^3 \, [\mu(\text{E} = 73 \text{ keV}) - .190] \tag{1}$$

This relationship states that for homogeneous substances, differences in μ from .190 (the approximate linear attenuation coefficient of water at E=73 keV) are *linearly* amplified by a factor of 2630 to establish the EMI number, which can then be displayed as some relative light intensity on a CRT screen. This relationship is shown in functional form in Fig. 2-3. The exact relationship between EMI number and attenuation coefficient is complicated by the fact that the EMI system uses a polychromatic spectrum of x-ray energies from an x-ray tube operating at 100, 120, or 140 kVp. Because the x-ray photons

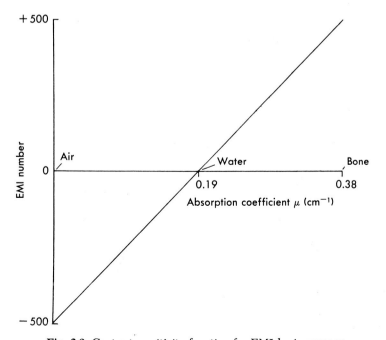

Fig. 2-3. Contrast sensitivity function for EMI brain scanner.

in this energy spectrum are subject to both photoelectric ($\mu_{p\varepsilon}$) and compton (μ_c) interactions, the total attenuation coefficient will be given by:

$$\mu = \mu_{p\varepsilon} + \mu_c \qquad (2)$$

Then since $\mu_{p\varepsilon}$ is strongly dependent on atomic number (e.g., Z^3) and μ is primarily dependent on electron density (N_ε), it is implied that the determined values of EMI number (i.e., μ) will represent a complicated dependence on both the atomic number and the electron density of the material attenuating the beam. This subject has been discussed in a recent article[16] in which the EMI values were examined for correlation with physical density, electron density, and atomic number cubed (Z^3).

Another consideration in the applicability of this linear relationship is that the x-ray intensity distribution may vary over the object volume, and therefore one needs to know the relative x-ray intensity distribution at each point within the object volume before one can predict the (weighted average) attenuation coefficent that will be assigned to the particular volume element. An example of this position-dependent effect can be seen in Fig. 2-4 by the differences in the images of the same nominal beads, which differ in their depth (z) within their own relative volume elements.

Measurements of resolution

It was stated earlier that for effectively homogeneous volume elements, the EMI system can be considered essentially linear. Thus for this special case one may consider the resolving ability of the EMI system by looking at the MTF obtained by Fourier in transforming the average data resulting from several EMI scans of a thin wire object (0.35 mm diameter) aligned with the vertical axis (z) of a centrally located volume element. This wire object then constitutes a point source input in the axial scan (x-y) plane of the EMI system. This and all other test objects were mounted in the head phantom (water-filled) shown in Fig. 2-5. The two-dimensional MTF describing the transfer character-

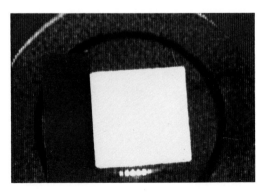

Fig. 2-4. EMI scan of beads placed at different depths within the slice. Dependence of bead image on coordinate position can be seen. Beads at top and bottom of slice are less intense. (See also Figs. 2-21 and 2-22.)

istics found with the EMI system operating at 120 kVp and using a 160 by 160 scanning matrix (i.e., a 1.5 mm by 1.5 mm pixel size) is shown in Fig. 2-6. It is found that there is at least a 10% modulation transfer of frequencies below three cycles per centimeter. In addition, there appears to be a slight gain in low-frequency modulation, probably giving rise to the edge enhancement often seen in EMI scans.

As stated previously, because of questions of linearity and isoplanacity, such MTF data will be dependent on the relative spatial position of the point source and will not necessarily be generally useful in predicting output data from known input data (unless the positional dependence and volumetric averaging are taken into account). Moreover, it should be noted that because the EMI system presently uses a square matrix element, the point spread function and

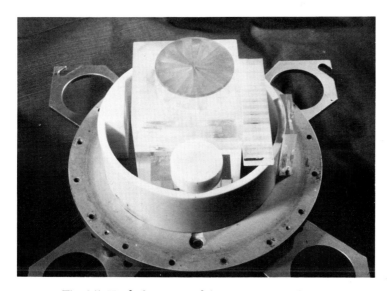

Fig. 2-5. Head phantom used for scanning test objects.

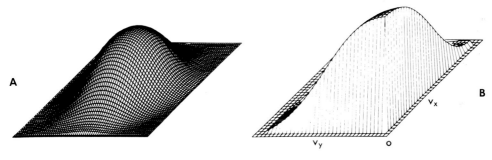

Fig. 2-6. A, Two-dimensional MTF resulting from Fourier transform of EMI scan of effective point source, normalized to unit height at zero spatial frequency. (See also **B** for scale.) **B, A** sliced through v_x and v_y spatial frequency axes. Scaling is $\Delta v_x = \Delta v_y = 0.10$ cycle/cm.

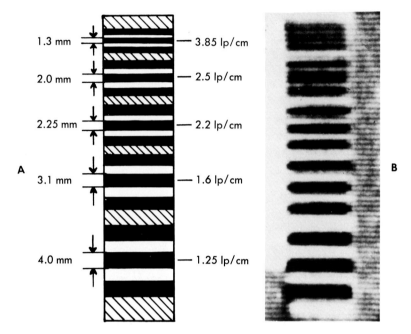

Fig. 2-7. A, Schematic illustration of an air-Lucite resolution gauge. **B,** EMI scan of **A.** (Interfering fine structure lines appear to be CRT scan lines.)

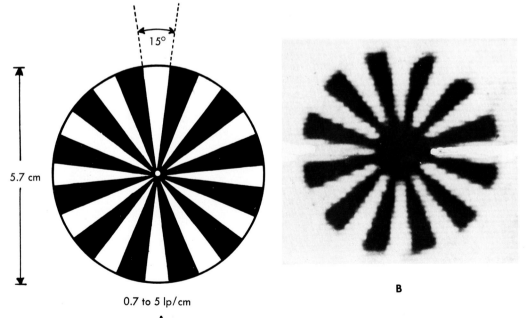

Fig. 2-8. A, Schematic illustration of an air-Lucite star pattern. **B,** EMI scan of **A.**

the MTF will be asymmetric. Therefore attempts to describe the MTF of the system by a one-dimensional Fourier transform of a line spread function will be dependent on the relative orientation of the line source within the scan plane and thus not generally valid, unless the line spread function and corresponding Fourier transform are obtained for each possible orientation of the line source.

In a more classical sense, the ability of the EMI system to resolve between steps in an air-Lucite resolution step gauge can be seen in Fig. 2-7. The result agrees quite well with the MTF prediction in that one can visually resolve about 2.5 line pairs per centimeter on this particular resolution gauge. This value may of course vary with position and orientation of the resolution gauge as well as with the intrinsic contrast provided by the materials used in the step gauge. Good correlation is also found between the MTF data and the EMI display of an air-Lucite star pattern shown in Fig. 2-8. The cutoff frequency can be seen to occur at about 3 line pairs per centimeter.

Measurements of noise

Fig. 2-9 shows an example of how well the EMI system can resolve small air holes of various diameters drilled to various depths in a bone-approximate phantom (thus assuring maximum subject contrast). The smallest hole that can be clearly visualized on the display is of 0.5 mm diameter and 10 mm depth. There is some question as to whether the 0.5 mm diameter by 6 mm depth hole is visualized. The ability to visually resolve such small holes in this phantom raises the question not only of the physical resolution characteristics and contrast sensitivity of the EMI system but also of the effect of noise, which is seen in the water-bath scan in Fig. 2-10. The noise is seen in the fluctuating nonuniform pattern of this figure. It is important to try to estimate the limits imposed by such sources of noise to the detection of low-contrast objects.

In considering noise in a diagnostic image, one should really consider not only its amplitude or standard deviation from the mean value (i.e., σ) but also its character or appearance (spatial frequency composition or power spectrum) as well as any positional dependence the noise may assume. However, the complexity of generating the noise-power spectrum of such a system and serious questions about its applicability and utility in nonlinear, position-dependent (nonstationary) systems reserve this important area for future study. In the meantime we will investigate changes in the standard deviation (σ) of EMI values resulting from scanning a uniformly composed object—a water bath.

Scanning geometry. In considering the schematic representation (Fig. 2-11) of x-ray source, detectors, and respective collimators, one can see how the EMI system is actually scanning two adjacent (A and B) slices of the head. These slices are of some mean thickness ($\overline{\Delta z}$).

For a uniform object the A and B slices would be expected to have the same mean image characteristics. However, the collimation on the A and B slices must be precisely balanced, or the x-ray intensity distribution reaching the respective crystals will be unequal, and different noise levels may be found in these slices.

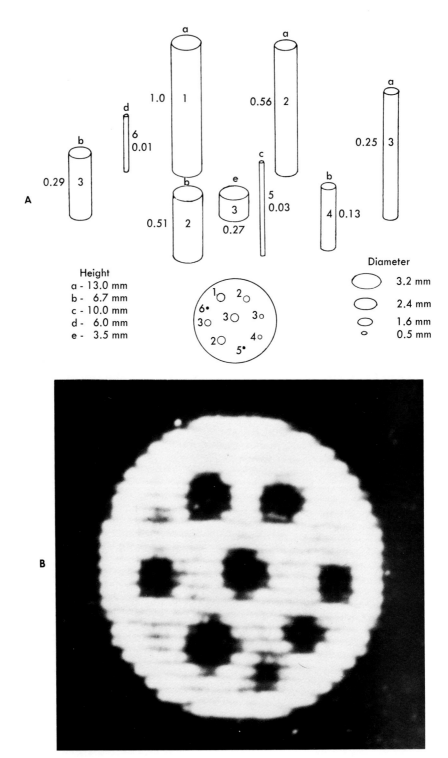

Fig. 2-9. A, Schematic illustration of an air-bone (calcium carbonate mixture) contrast detail phantom. Relative volumes (scaled to $1.0 = 103$ mm^3) are shown along with corresponding numerical volume ranking. **B,** EMI scan of **A.**

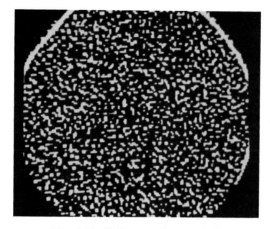

Fig. 2-10. EMI scan of water bath.

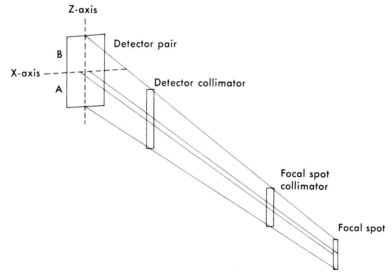

Fig. 2-11. Scanning geometry. Schematic illustration of EMI scanner tube and detector collimation system.

Such misalignment and its subsequent correction are illustrated in Fig. 2-12. With the A and B scans balanced, the statistical noise levels (σ) can be examined as certain physical and geometrical factors of the EMI scanning system are varied independently. These factors include peak kilovoltage (kVp), tube current (mA), scan speed (s), and mean slice thickness ($\overline{\Delta z}$). The values of σ were determined by using the EMI diagnostic disc program to analyze some 2000 centrally located EMI values.

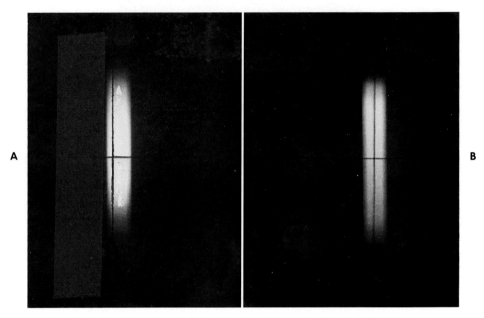

Fig. 2-12. A, Misalignment of x-ray beam found at detector collimator. **B,** Subsequent correction.

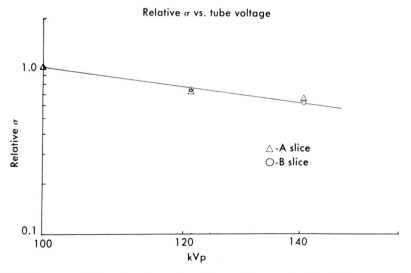

Fig. 2-13. Experimental data describing dependence of σ on tube kVp. Values normalized to 2.6 EMI units at 100 kVp.

Dependence of σ on kVp. The experimental data describing the dependence of σ on the x-ray tube kVp are seen in Fig. 2-13. These data points were found to fit a power function relationship whereby

$$\sigma \propto (\text{kVp})^M \tag{3}$$

with M = −1.27 ± .12, with a correlation coefficient of 98%.

This dependence seems reasonable in that the narrow beam of x rays is highly filtered, and the increased x-ray intensity with increased kVp that would result in the decreased noise level is consistent with previously published studies.[19]

Dependence of σ on tube current (mA). The experimental data describing the dependence of σ on the tube current can be seen in Fig. 2-14; σ was found to vary as

$$\sigma \propto (\text{mA})^N \tag{4}$$

where N = −.58 ± .03. This relationship held for three different mean slice thicknesses as can be seen from the illustration. Because the patient dose will be expected to change at the same rate as tube current, it is obvious that values of σ reported for various CT devices should be carefully examined in light of the patient dose that would result from the techniques used to establish the appropriate value of σ.

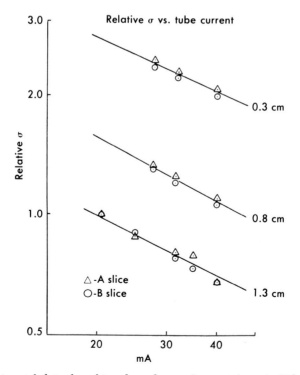

Fig. 2-14. Experimental data describing dependence of σ on tube mA. Values normalized to 2.13 EMI units at 20.5 mA (13 mm slice).

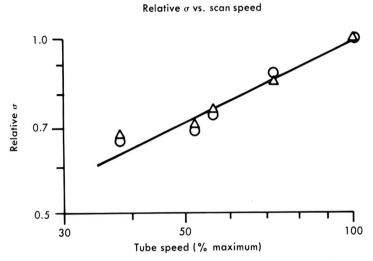

Fig. 2-15. Experimental data describing dependence of σ on scan speed (S). Values normalized to 1.93 EMI units at 100% speed.

Dependence of σ on mean slice thickness ($\overline{\Delta z}$). The dependence of σ on the mean slice thickness as shown in Fig. 2-14 is more complicated than generally appreciated. The dependence is given by

$$\sigma \propto (\overline{\Delta z})^P \tag{5}$$

where $P = P(L,l)$ is a complicated function of the detector (L) and source (l) collimators influencing the x-ray intensity distribution. As $\overline{\Delta z}$ is decreased, the value of σ will be seen to increase more rapidly than the expected $(\overline{\Delta z})$ to the $-.5$ power whenever the detector collimator controlling the x-ray intensity distribution reaching the crystal is decreasing at a faster rate than $\overline{\Delta z}$.

Dependence of σ on scan speed(s). The experimental data describing the dependence of σ on scan speed (S) are shown in Fig. 2-15. Over a limited set of speeds available for analysis, it was found that

$$\sigma \propto S^Q \tag{6}$$

where $Q \approx .45$.

Noise stationarity. One other consideration of noise values in CT scanning is the degree of stationarity or positional independence of σ. The mean σ of eight independent readings of each of the five designated areas of the scan field as shown in Fig. 2-16 were found to agree within 2.5%–the values ranged from $\sigma = 1.90 \pm 0.8$ to $1.95 \pm .09$.

Choice of operating parameters. The experimental data seem consistent with a general predictive dependence of σ on the following parameters:

$$\sigma \propto (kVp)^M \ (mA)^N \ (\Delta z)^P \ (S)^Q \tag{7}$$

If one now considers the preceding results of the independent effect of each

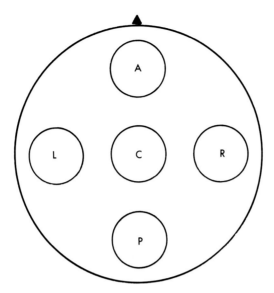

Fig. 2-16. Illustration of five areas (*A, R, P, L, C*) of scan field of head (large circle) tested for noise amplitude.

factor on σ, in the realistic situation of a finite heat loading, on the x-ray tube, it may be seen from Fig. 2-17 that for a tube heat loading of 4 kw, there is very little advantage to operating at 140 kVp and 28 mA, as compared to 120 kVp and 33 mA within a water-bath object.

Of course, other factors will be expected to affect the noise found in a CT scan. These factors include noise intrinsic to the photomultiplier tubes (e.g., dark current noise). Moreover, the CT algorithm itself will tend to enhance or diminish the physical sources of variation, depending on the choice of reconstruction algorithm and beam hardening effects within the skull.

Potential artifacts in CT scanning

In addition to considering noise in CT scanning, possible artifacts encountered in this scanning should be studied because they also can obscure or diminish the possibility of correct diagnosis.

Probably the most commonly encountered artifact in CT scanning is the streak artifact, which can result from either patient motion or system misalignment. In both cases the reconstruction algorithm is thwarted by data that appear to have been obtained from a moving frame of reference. The data are essentially out of registration during different times within the scan. In some cases patient motion can be reduced by head restraints. The problem of misalignment can often be corrected by adjustment of the timing graticule.

Another type of artifact results from the basic geometric and physical factors involved with simultaneous monitoring of a single x-ray focal spot by two detectors, as illustrated in Fig. 2-18. It can be noted from Fig. 2-18, *A* and *B*, that on any single linear scan pass, the field of view of the focal spot by one detector

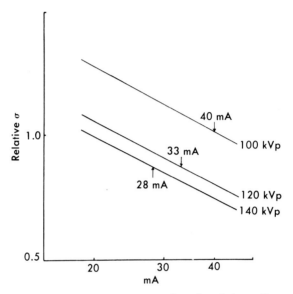

Fig. 2-17. Arrows indicate comparison of noise values found for a finite tube heat loading of 4 kw. Values normalized to 2.13 EMI units at 20.5 mA, 140 kVp.

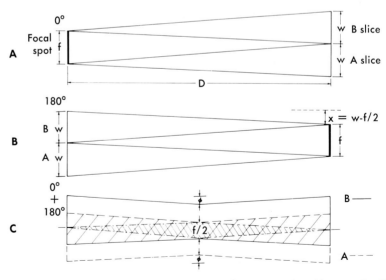

Fig. 2-18. A, Basic geometrical factors in any single linear (e.g., 0°) pass. **B,** Opposing field (180°) pass. **C,** Superposition of 0° and 180° linear passes. (From Goodenough, D. J., et al.: Radiology **117:**615, 1975.)

will overlap the field of view of the adjacent detector. The superposition of the 180° rotations of the linear scan passes will cause the overall scan slice to have a position-dependent thickness and to show a rather unusual shape, as illustrated in Fig. 2-18, *C*. Here we see the expected A and B slice patterns found in a plane cut through the center of the overall scan, normal to the 0° to 180° linear scans. One can notice several interesting facts about this particular plane cut through the scan slice. The slices are clearly not contiguous, contrary to encountered information. The region of overlap has a thickness of f/2 at the center of the scan and will increase uniformly as it moves radially outward from the center. Moreover, there is a depression of $\phi(r)$ in the top of the B slice and elevation of $\phi(r)$ in the bottom of the A slice, compared to the "expected" top of the B slice and "expected" bottom of the A slice, respectively:

$$\phi(r) = (\tfrac{1}{2} - r/D),(w - f/2) \tag{8}$$

where r is the distance from the center of the scan and D equals the distance between the focal spot of effective length (f) and the positions where each pair of detectors would assume effective width (w). Thus at the center of the scan (r = 0), one finds a void in the top of the B slice and the bottom of the A slice given by

$$\phi = w/2 - f/4 \tag{9}$$

which is a function of the assumed detector width (w) and the effective focal spot length (f), after appropriate collimation factors are included. One can note that $\phi = 0$ only when w = f/2, and thus in this geometric configuration, by minimizing the depression and elevation, A and B are found to overlap 50% at the center.

The complete description of the A and B scan slices is only obtained by considering the combination of linear and rotational motions of the scanner and is shown in the computer-generated plot of the effective slice shape in Fig. 2-19.

Each time the operator increments his system so that the extreme bottom of the A slice coincides with the extreme top of the B slice, one would find a missing region (void) in the potential scan field. The void results from the superposition of the top of the B slice and the bottom of the A slice. Such a void might also be found in single-slice tomographic imaging systems whenever the sampled slice assumes other than a rectangular cross section on which the incrementation is based.

Now consider the size of the missing region at the central point within the EMI scan fields. It should be noted that the EMI scanning system does not have its center of rotation located midway between the focal spot and the detectors; rather, it is located about three fifths of the way from the focal spot to the detectors. Therefore in using equation 9 to predict the void, the detector width (w) that is used is not the physical detector width but rather the width the detector could be assumed to subtend if removed to a distance from the center of rotation equal to that distance of the focal spot from the center of rotation. In addition, for an assumed slice width (N) in the center of the scan field, the void (V) will be given by:

$$V = N - w + \emptyset \qquad (10)$$

Similar considerations of the location of the center of rotation lead to the prediction that the overlap at the center of the EMI scan will be given by f/2.5.

These predictions have been tested experimentally for the nominal 1.3 cm slice by the following procedure. A phantom was designed wherein small beads were placed at constant distances on a straight line oriented at an angle of 23° with respect to an axial (x-y) plane of the head. In this fashion, a missing region

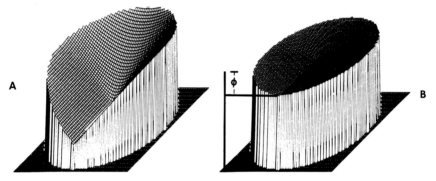

Fig. 2-19. **A,** Computer generated plot of top of CT slice. **B,** Scaled version of **A** to amplify shape of depression in top of scan. (Elevation in bottom of scan is not shown.) (From Goodenough, D. J., et al.: Radiology **117:**615, 1975.)

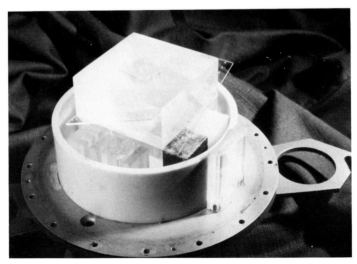

Fig. 2-20. Modified EMI head phantom designed to test scan slice geometry. (From Goodenough, D. J., et al.: Radiology **117:**615, 1975.)

of the head would manifest itself as a number of missing beads from the projection of the line, which would be seen in the EMI axial scans. The phantom is shown in Fig. 2-20 and illustrated schematically in Fig. 2-21. The missing region of the head is clearly demonstrated by the space in the line in the superimposed EMI scans shown in Fig. 2-22, in which the nominal distance between bead centers in the x-y plane represents 2 mm in the z plane. The results agree well with the theory that predicts that following incrementation by 1.3 cm, there should be a void of approximately 2 mm (corresponding to a missing bead) at points at the center and on the 90° radius line of the scan. There should be a somewhat smaller void at other points in the scan, depending on the particular values of f and w, which in this case are given by $f = 12$ mm and $w = 17.9$ mm.[10]

The problem of overlap of the A and B slices can result in spurious dual-imaging situations. An isolated object situated within a region of overlapping fields of view will modulate both detectors simultaneously and could be displayed in both slices simultaneously, giving incorrect diagnostic information as to the number and position of small objects truly present.

This dual-imaging problem has been verified using the nominal 0.8 cm slice width. Fig. 2-23 shows how an isolated object actually located within only one of the nominal slices appears to occur in both nominal slices simultaneously. This dual imaging may be troublesome in any attempted subtraction techniques of nominal scan slices.

In any linear scan, the A and B slices have the greatest geometric overlapping at the tube side of the scan. However, when one considers the combination of linear and rotational motions, it becomes clear that the time spent in mutual modulation will affect the intensity of the spurious image seen in the overall scan. Thus one would expect objects within the f/2.5 region of overlap at the center

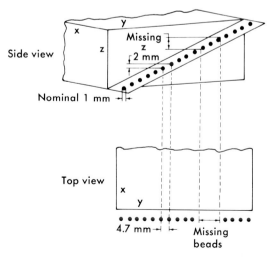

Fig. 2-21. Schematic illustration of arrangement of beads designed to test scan slice geometry. (From Goodenough, D. J., et al.: Radiology 117:615, 1975.)

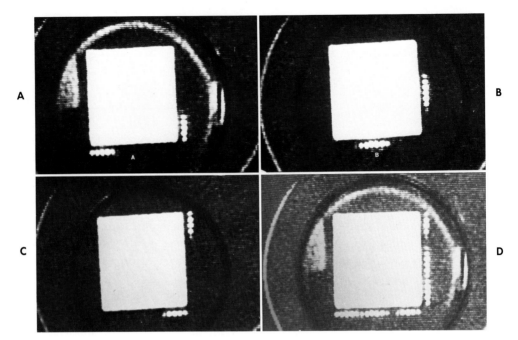

Fig. 2-22. **A,** A slice of EMI bead phantom. **B,** B slice of EMI bead phantom. **C,** Incremented A slice of EMI bead phantom. **D,** Superimposed EMI scans (**A** to **C**) showing missing region. (From Goodenough, D. J., et al.: Radiology **117**:615, 1975.)

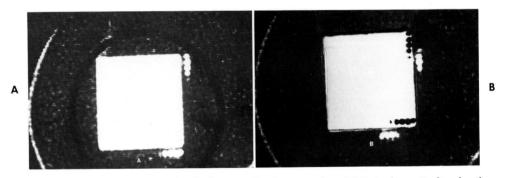

Fig. 2-23. **A,** EMI B slice of bead phantom. **B,** Corresponding EMI A slice—B slice beads indicated in black ink to illustrate overlap of slices. (From Goodenough, D. J., et al.: Radiology **117**:615, 1975.)

of the scan to show the most intense dual image. Figs. 2-22 and 2-23 also show that beads near the top and bottom of the EMI slice width show lower contrast than those near the center, raising important questions concerning the system response of the EMI scan. This differing contrast probably results from the nonuniformity of the total x-ray intensity, as viewed across the detector width during the combination of linear and rotational motions.

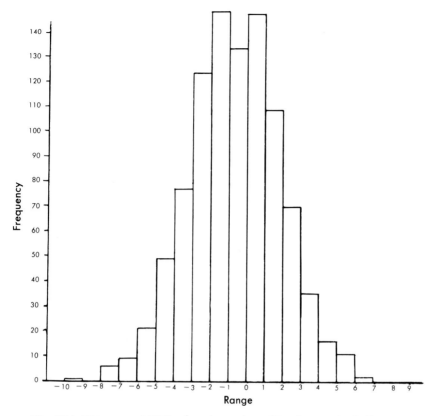

Fig. 2-24. Histogram of EMI values (range) resulting from water-bath scan.

SIGNAL DETECTION THEORY APPLIED TO CT SCANNING

The previous measurements of contrast sensitivity, resolution, and noise were by design essentially independent. However, as stated, the possible detection of a signal will depend on the mutual interplay of the signal's contrast, sharpness, and noise background. One must therefore seek to examine not only the independent magnitude of signal and noise variables but also the magnitude of the signal-to-noise ratio.[1, 5, 7, 17]

It is clear that the magnitude of the noise (σ) may be easily suppressed by well-known noise-smoothing algorithms. Of course, such a smoothing operation will also tend to reduce the contrast and sharpness of the signal. Therefore independent examination of one σ value compared to another may be very misleading as to the actual detectability of the signal.[11, 12, 14]

If Fig. 2-24 is examined, where the distribution of EMI values that results from scanning a water bath is shown, it is noted, that the distribution is approximately normal with a mean of about –1 EMI unit and a standard deviation of about 2.5 units. For attenuation coefficients close to that of water, this standard

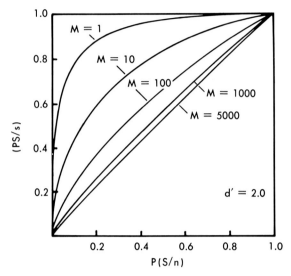

Fig. 2-25. Receiver operating characteristic (ROC) curves as a function of number of matrix elements (M) that must be searched.

deviation corresponds to about ±0.5% uncertainty in the x-ray attenuation reading in any one matrix element.

It is of interest to consider the implications of such a distribution of EMI readings in light of signal detection theory.[4, 8] Now consider a hypothetical signal detection task wherein an EMI scan (water) of a region of an object is to be searched for the possible presence of a signal having an intrinsic attenuation contrast of about 1% compared to water (corresponding to a difference of about 5 EMI units). In this example the presence of one or more matrix elements with an EMI number of +5 or more will then be used as an indicator that a signal (e.g., lesion) is present. Using the distribution of EMI values shown in Fig. 2-24, one can now predict the conditional probabilities of true positive P(S/s) and false positive P(S/n) signal detection. These probabilities are shown in receiver operating characteristic (ROC) form in Fig. 2-25.[3, 8] It is learned from this illustration that performance will be expected to decrease as the number of matrix elements (M) that must be searched increases. Thus in this example where the intrinsic signal to noise ratio (d) in any one matrix element is d = 2, note that for M = 1, one can operate at P(S/s) = 0.88, P(S/n) = 0.20; whereas for M = 1000, one's detection could drop to P(S/s) = 0.24, P(S/n) = 0.20—for the same false positive level.

Fig. 2-26 shows the d values that would be needed for the indicated true and false conditional probabilities of detection as a function of the number of matrix areas (M) that must be searched.[22] It can be seen that if one wishes to operate with at least P(S/s) = 0.50 and P(S/n) = 0.20 for M = 1000, then one really needs about ± 1/6% uncertainty in the attenuation coefficient (i.e., less than ± 1 EMI unit) to detect a 0.5% signal at the previously stated probability levels. It

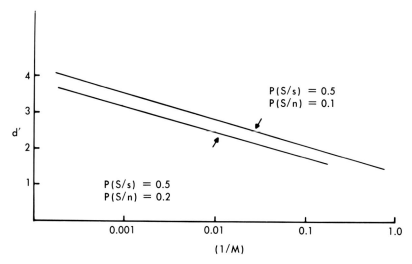

Fig. 2-26. Signal to noise ratio *(d')* necessary for indicated performance levels as a function of *(1/M)*.

should be clearly recognized that this hypothetical example is based on the (limiting) case of inspection of single uncorrelated matrix elements. The more complicated case of inspecting several matrix elements in the presence of correlated noise must remain for future investigation.[3, 5, 6, 14]

FUTURE OF CT SCANNING

As CT systems become capable of scanning and reconstructing data at higher speeds in systems that do not need water baths, one can look for their successful use in other parts of the body where patient motion might otherwise have mitigated against CT scanning. However, such systems may be expected to become more and more complex, and much attention will have to be paid to questions of quality assurance in CT scanning. Tests of mechanical and electrical stability as well as of image quality obtained from multiple detector, fan-beam CT systems will need to be perfected. In addition, the high cost of such complex systems will probably demand increased attention to the need for assessing diagnostic efficacy in light of finite medical financial resources.

References

1. Coltman, J. W., and Anderson, A. E.: Noise limitations to resolving power in electronic imaging, Proc. I. R. E. **48:** 858, 1960.
2. Cornsweet, T. N.: Visual perception, New York, 1970, Academic Press, Inc.
3. Goodenough, D. J.: Radiographic applications of signal detection, doctoral dissertation, University of Chicago, 1972.

4. Goodenough, D. J.: The need for physical and psychophysical measures of system performance. In Proceedings of Medical X-Ray Photo-Optical Systems Evaluation Symposium, Columbia, Md., 1974.
5. Goodenough, D. J.: Objective measures related to ROC curves. In Proceedings of the Society of Photo-Optical Instrumen-

tation Engineers Symposium, Kansas City, 1974.

6. Goodenough, D. J., and Metz, C. E.: Effect of listening interval on auditory detection performance, J. Acoust. Soc. Am. **55**:111, Jan., 1974.

7. Goodenough, D. J., Rossmann, K., and Lusted, L. B.: Factors affecting the detectability of a simulated radiographic signal, Invest. Radiol. **8**:339, 1974.

8. Goodenough, D. J., Rossmann, K., and Lusted, L. B.: Radiographic applications of receiver operating characteristic curves, Radiology **110**:89, 1974.

9. Goodenough, D. J., Weaver, K. E., and Davis, D. O.: Physical measurements of the EMI imaging system. In Proceedings of the Workshop on Reconstruction Tomography in Diagnostic Radiology and Nuclear Medicine, San Juan, P.R., April 17-19, 1975.

10. Goodenough, D. J., Weaver, K. E., and Davis, D. O.: Potential artifacts associated with the scanning pattern of the EMI scanner, Radiology **117**:615, 1975.

11. Kohlenstein, L. C.: Observer performance in detecting lesions in radionuclide scans, The Johns Hopkins Applied Physics Laboratory report, CP 028, Aug., 1973.

12. Kuhl, D. E., et al.: Failure to improve observer performance with scan smoothing, J. Nucl. Med. **13**:752, 1972.

13. McCullough, E. C., Baker, H. I., Hauser, O. W., and Reese, D. F.: An evaluation of the quantitative and radiation features of a scanning x-ray transverse axial Tomograph: the EMI scanner, Radiology **111**:709, 1974.

14. Metz, C. E., and Goodenough, D. J.: On failure to improve observer performance with scan smoothing: a rebuttal (letter to the editor), J. Nucl. Med. **14**:873, 1973.

15. Metz, C. E., and Goodenough, D. J.: Quantitative evaluation of human visual detection performance using empirical receiver operating characteristic curves. In Proceedings of the Third International Conference on Data Handling and Image Processing in Scintigraphy, Boston, 1973.

16. Phelps, M. E., Gado, M. H., and Hoff-

man, E. J.: Correlation of effective atomic number and electron density with attenuation coefficients measured with polychromatic x-rays, Radiology **117**: 585, 1975.

17. Rose, A.: The sensitivity performance of the human eye on an absolute scale, J. Opt. Soc. Am. **38**:196, 1948.

18. Rossmann, K.: Spatial fluctuations of x-rays quanta and the recording of radiograph mottle, Am. J. Roentgenol. Radium Ther. Nucl. Med. **90**:863, 1963.

19. Trout, E. D., Kelley, J. P., and Gross, R. E.: beam quality measurements in diagnostic roentgenology, Am. J. Roentgenol. Radium Ther. Nucl. Med. **103**: 681, 1968.

20. Weaver, K. E.: Personal communication.

Suggested readings

Brooks, R. A.: Theory of image reconstruction in computed tomography, Radiology **117**:561, 1975.

Davis, D. O., Marden, D., and Staples, S.: A head-holding device for computed tomography, Radiology **117**:480, 1975.

Gado, M. H., Phelps, M. E., and Coleman, R. E.: An extravascular component of contrast enhancement in cranial computed tomography, Radiology **117**:589, 1975.

Gordon, R., and Herman, G. T.: Three-dimensional reconstruction from projections: a review of algorithms, Int. Rev. Cytol. **38**:111, 1974.

Phelps, M. E., Hoffman, E. J., and Ter-Pogossian, M. M.: Attenuation coefficients of various body tissues, fluids, and lesions at photon energies of 18 to 136 keV[1], Radiology **117**:573, 1975.

Ter-Pogossian, M. M., Phelps, M. E., Hoffman, E. J., and Eichling, J. O.: The extraction of the yet unused wealth of information in diagnostic radiology, Radiology **113**:515, 1974.

Weaver, K. E., Goodenough, D. J., and Davis, D. O.: Physical measurements of the EMI computerized axial tomographic system. In Proceedings of the Joint SPIE and SPSE meeting on Application of Optical Instrumentation in Medicine IV, Atlanta, Sept., 1975.

3 Computed tomography and its application to nuclear medical imaging

Gerald C. Huth and Ernest L. Hall

In the past three years an entirely new concept in imaging has been developed that is now being generically called "computed tomography." In diagnostic radiology this term refers to systems that use transmitted x rays as the information-gathering source. Because a transverse-axial motion is used, this development initially was rather ponderously termed "computerized transverse-axial tomography" (CTAT or CAT, for short). We propose and will use the simpler "transmission computed tomography" to encompass any situation in which transmitted radiation is used as the information-gathering source. Computed tomography has more recently been applied in nuclear medicine to image positron-emitting isotopes. We will term this "emission computed tomography."

The aim of this chapter is to give the potential user of computed tomography systems an understanding of their fundamental principles of operation. We will discuss in nonmathematical terms the current state of the art as well as some newer developments and their potential applications in nuclear medicine. It is hoped that this brief review will provide a greater appreciation of the advantages and limitations of computed tomography and help in the proper application and interpretation of this exciting new tool.

Computed tomography began with the introduction to diagnostic radiology of the now famous x-ray transmission scanning systems for the brain developed by EMI, Ltd., in England. Subsequently, Ter-Pogossian[8] and Phelps[7] applied the principles of computed tomography to nuclear medical imaging with their development of tomographic systems for use with isotopes that decay by positron emission. More recently Budinger et al.[2] have used the principles of computed tomography in conjunction with very high-energy, accelerator-produced, heavy ions in reconstructing tomographic images of the ventricles. Each of these three concepts is discussed in more detail later.

BASIC ASPECTS OF COMPUTED TOMOGRAPHY

The essence of computed tomography is that the image produced is totally a product of the computer; that is, the computer plays an integral or fundamental part in the process of forming the image. This is in contrast to, for example, computer "enhancement" of images, which has found some use in radiology and nuclear medicine. In the enhancement application, the computer is used following the image-formation process, and its use might be termed "peripheral."

In discussing the principles of computed tomography, a logical place to begin is where it began—with the x-ray transmission embodiment. Fig. 3-1 indicates the basic elements of that system. In conventional radiography, as illustrated here with a cerebral angiogram, information from the three-dimensional object is superimposed in two-dimensional form on film. In some instances, contrast-enhancing agents (generally iodinated) are required to regain contrast and obtain diagnostically useful information. Computed tomography is "tomography" in the sense that the image is obtained from a transverse section, or cut, of the object. In reality, then, computed tomography "unravels" a section of the radiographic image, as we attempt to show in the figure. Within this section, an imaginary image matrix composed of square elements of predetermined size is constructed (also indicated in the illustration). In the x-ray brain-imaging system the element size is 1 to 3 mm square. The matrix must be made large enough to generally encompass the target to be imaged. Therefore, in the case of the head, approximately 160 elements are typically used to span approximately 25 cm.

To obtain the transmission data from which to form the image, an aligned x-ray source-detector arrangement is used. This assembly is highly collimated to the width of one image element. The initial transverse part of the scanning motion is a linear motion in which each of the 160 or more rows (each containing 160 or more elements) is interrogated. This motion can be accomplished in approximately 1½ seconds. Thus 160 or more separate data points are entered into the computer during this traverse. One should think of each data point as representing a "line being drawn" from which, ultimately, the image can be reconstructed. These lines can also be termed "projections." After each single traverse, the entire source-detector geometry is rotated a preset angular increment (e.g., 1°), and the linear, transverse scan motion commences again. If 180 angular projections are used, the result is 180 times 160, or 28,800, separate projections entered into the computer. The total time required to accomplish this is 180×1½ seconds, or 4½ minutes. Data in digital form is stored in the computer as the scan is in progress.

A very important aspect of x-ray transmission computed tomography is that the "information density" of the final image is controllable at this point. The EMI scanner has aptly demonstrated that variations in x-ray absorption coefficients can be measured to the accuracy of a few percent; this corresponds to the small differences between fat, muscle, and other tissue. But radiation statistics must be satisfied to achieve this, which means that each data point must contain 40,000 to 50,000 counts. This number of x-ray photons must therefore exit from the object being scanned and be counted by the x-ray detector.

We mentioned the concept of information density of an image. Radiographic film has a very high information density, whereas the gamma camera or scanner in nuclear medicine produces an image with a relatively low value. This is readily apparent to the eye. The computed tomographic image lies midway between the two but possesses an additional peculiar characteristic. It is composed of relatively coarse blocks (the "elements" already discussed), but the information contained in each block is very well determined, as indicated by the preceding statistical argument. This information is related to the concept of a "gray scale" and can be displayed in discrete steps of gray. The initial computed reconstruction does not allow the blocks to ineract, so there is no "spill-over" from one block to another, as is introduced in the gamma camera image through the mechanism of photon scatter. The image therefore is at first glance deceptive because the unparalleled accuracy of determinations computed within each block is masked by a coarse overall appearance. However, this coarseness can be and is being artificially obscured in newer computed tomography image displays. There is an interesting analogy between computed tomographic images and the images returned from the planet Mars in the Mariner program conducted by NASA. Those images are similar in that they have a relatively low number of picture elements (pixels), but the gray scale of each element is repeatedly determined to a very high accuracy.

While the computed tomography scan is underway, the digital data (representing projections) is being entered into the computer for processing into the final image. We will attempt to give some insight into how the computer accomplishes this task. Comparison with traditional radiographic film tomography is helpful.[6] In that technique the transverse motion and the x-ray detector of the computed tomography system are replaced by a film cassette. The film plane must obviously be placed at an angle through the object to accept the x-ray beam, whereas computed tomography is directly "end-on," but this makes no difference in our argument here. The point is that film possesses only the ability to integrate what it sees. Thus adjacent components of the image are superimposed (a prin-

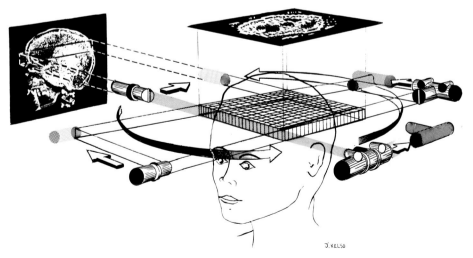

Fig. 3-1. Elements of an x-ray transmission computed tomography system.

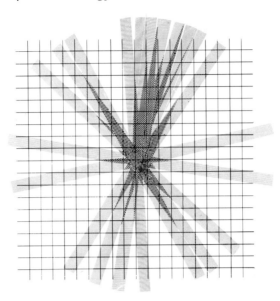

Fig. 3-2. Star pattern formed by finite beam width.

ciple of "superposition"), resulting in the blurred quality characteristic of film tomography. If a beam of finite width is rotated, as in the axial tomographic motions, the additive intensity over one hypothetical image element "blurs" to form a star pattern as shown in Fig. 3-2. The more projections used, the wider the blur circle, but the denser the central point becomes. This is exactly the superposition effect described.

So far we have been considering only one element of an image. The situation is made worse by the overlapping of the blur circles from adjacent elements in an actual large matrix image. If film were used as the detector, it would simply integrate or superimpose each component line image or projection, including the blurring. However, when the information is digitized, as in computed tomography, it is possible to apply corrections to each element to reduce blurring and regain much of the original image.

There are a large number of approaches to applying this deblurring correction in the computer image reconstruction process. This process, incidentally, is not new, having been generically termed "image reconstruction from projections." It has been applied in such diverse fields as optics, electron microscopy, and radioastronomy. Image reconstruction techniques have been based on algebraic methods, Fourier or frequency domain methods, and what are termed spatial domain methods. We will use the latter in the following discussion because it is the easiest to visualize.

In Fig. 3-3 we show in the backround the hypothetical image matrix of computed tomography intersected by a beam of finite width. Note that the beam intersects each element of the matrix to a different degree and thus has the ability to interrogate that element only to that amount. A correction can be applied to

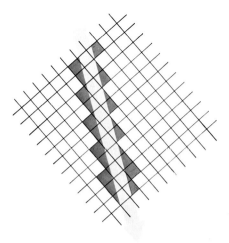

Fig. 3-3. Image matrix of computed tomography.

account for the differing amount of each element covered by each beam. These "weighting factors"[3] can be precalculated for the entire matrix and stored in the computer memory. In solving each element the computed then corrects the recorded value by an appropriate amount in what might be termed a "first correction" toward obtaining the more accurate approach to the true value. The weighting factors are presented as an example of a correction procedure and may not be used in a practical machine because of the large storage and computation time required.

The next correction is the general deblurring correction for the "halo" effect illustrated in Fig. 3-2. In an actual image the information (e.g., brain structure) in each element effectively adds to the halo blur and is spread into adjacent elements. Thus a deblurring function of the type shown at the left of Fig. 3-4 must next be applied. The shape of the deblurring function is typical of several functions used in practical machines. The largest value is located at the center for correcting the projection from the central element. Usually, the next elements from the center are negative to produce the largest cancellation from the spreading. The remaining elements may be both positive and negative. The particular shape on this function is based on a trade-off of, for example, the sharpness of an edge and the width of the blur in reconstructing it. This deblurring function, shown in Fig. 3-4, usually produces the sharpest edges, whereas a function with all negative values will produce a wider edge width but will eliminate a multiple-edge presentation. The deblurring function is applied to the set of projections from each angle by the process of convolution. This process simply consists of multiplying each projection by the corresponding deblurring function value where the deblurring function is centered on the image element being corrected, as shown by the lightly shaded point in Fig. 3-4. The results of these multiplications are added together and then added to the image element. The darker-shaded

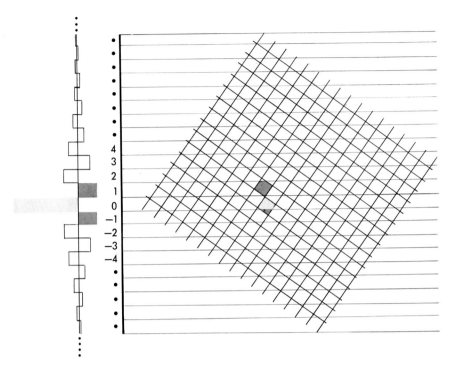

Fig. 3-4. Deblurring function applied to image matrix.

noncentral points illustrate that the entire set of projections is used in the multiplications, since the blur from a single element can extend over a great distance in the matrix. In fact, in practice the deblurring function shown in Fig. 3-4 must extend to the ends of the matrix for each element to provide an accurate correction. It is important to point out that different deblurring function shapes may be encountered in different machine designs because of the compromises required. No particular shape has yet been shown to be optimum. Also, we have discussed the practical situation in which the finite beam width produces the blurring shown in Fig. 3-2; however, it is interesting to note that the convolution deblurring correction would be required even if the beam were infinitely narrow. The weighting factor would not be required for the very narrow beam, since element would then be correctly interrogated by the ray.

The results of these corrections may be illustrated by a computer simulation.[4] A phantom object image was designed with varying absorption coefficient values (Fig. 3-5, *A*). The concentric ring values were selected to be 20%, 2%, and 50% above the background. A computer program was used to generate the projections; in an x-ray transmission system these projections would be experimentally generated. A set of such projections was produced for each angle from 0° to 180°. The results were first superimposed to simulate integration. The resulting image is shown in the isometric plot of Fig. 3-5, *B*. Note that the 50% variation and background are visible, but the 2% and 20% rings are barely distinguishable.

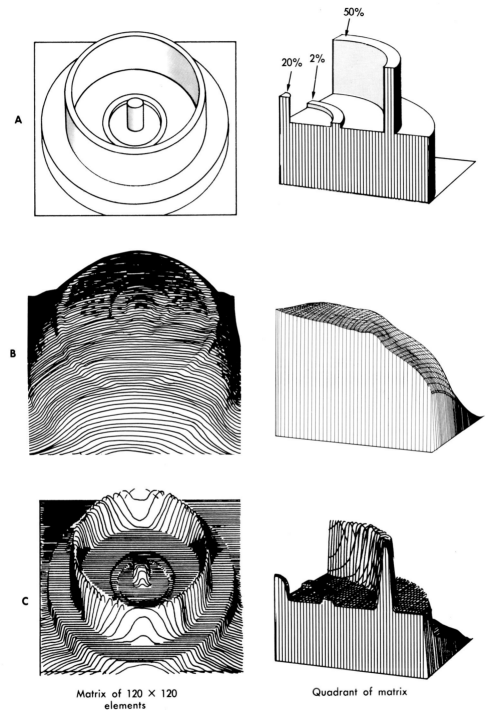

Matrix of 120 × 120
elements

Quadrant of matrix

Fig. 3-5. A, Phantom image with varying absorption coefficients. **B,** Image resulting from superposition. **C,** Image resulting from deblurring.

The simple addition of the ray lines produces a barely recognizable and inaccurate representation of the cross-section image.

The result of the corrections on this phantom image is shown in Fig. 3-5, *C*. Both weighting factors as well as the general deblurring function were implemented. Note the increased sharpness of the edges and the ease of visualization of not only the 20% but also the 2% object.

The previous techniques are applicable to transmission systems with rectangular or fan beam geometries or emission systems with rectangular or ring detectors. It is easily shown that a projection data point collected on one system could also have been collected on a system with a different geometry. Thus the computer's ability to "unravel" the data can be used to accommodate different geometries.

This is admittedly a far too simple presentation of a rather complex problem. The concepts presented were intended to give some idea of the types of manipulations possible in the *digital world*, which make computed tomographic image reconstructions clinically useful.

APPLICATION OF COMPUTED TOMOGRAPHY TO IMAGING POSITRON-EMITTING ISOTOPES

The potential usefulness of positron-emitting isotopes in nuclear medicine has been recognized for many years. Much has been written concerning the significance of carbon 11, oxygen 15, and nitrogen 13 (half-lives of 20, 2, and 10 minutes, respectively) to medical and physiologic measurements. However, except for the limited use of fluorine 18 in bone scanning, positron-emitting isotopes have not so far been utilized extensively in nuclear medicine.

Positron decay results in the annihilation of the positron and emission of two 0.511 mev gamma rays at a 180° angle to each other (back to back). Gamma ray scatter and absorption is minimized at this high energy level. One obstacle to positron emitter usage has been the lack of an imaging system with adequate sensitivity at the required 0.511 mev energy. The Anger gamma ray camera imaging system is only a few percent efficient at this energy, transmitting and thus losing precious photons and negating the potential advantage of the high specific activity of these isotopes. Brownell et al.[1] have perhaps contributed most to the area of positron imaging with development of a conceptually unique but complex positron imaging system. Ter-Pogossian and Phelps have more recently applied the principles of computed tomography to imaging positron-emitting isotopes in a progression of systems to which they give the name "positron emission transaxial tomography," or PETT.

In the PETT concept, gamma ray detectors are arranged around the object to be measured, as shown in Fig. 3-6. The shape of the array could take the form of a circle, as proposed by Eriksson et al.[5] and Thompson et al.,[9] or of a hexagon, as preferred by Ter-Pogossian. In both configurations, opposing detectors are placed in coincidence to detect the back to back gamma rays from positron annihilation. With the detection of each coincidence event, a line or projection is effectively drawn to be applied to the image eventually reconstructed by the

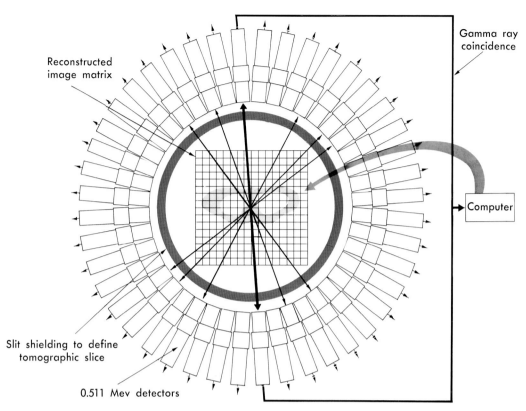

Fig. 3-6. Schematic representation of gamma ray detectors used in positron emission tomography.

computer. It is possible to increase the sensitivity of the system by placing each detector in coincidence with a number of opposing detectors—in effect, increasing the number of projections.

Fig. 3-7 presents a side-looking view of two opposing detectors of the array. Shielding can be used to define the tomographic plane to be imaged and helps to reject detection of unwanted annihilation events that occur out of this plane. As indicated in Fig. 3-6, coincidence events representing projections enter and are stored in the computer, and the image reconstruction proceeds. The computer solution or algorithm used for reconstruction can be very similar to the one used in the x-ray transmission systems. One such approach rearranges the projections to simulate the transverse-axial geometry of the x-ray systems. Solution is then identical.

An important aspect of positron emission tomography derives from the penetration and lower scatter of the 0.511 mev annihilation gamma rays as compared to the 0.140 mev energy of technitium so widely used in nuclear medicine. The higher energy level, as mentioned earlier, has traditionally been a disadvantage primarily because of the insensitivity of the imaging systems available for use with it. In positron emission tomography the total distance traveled by both

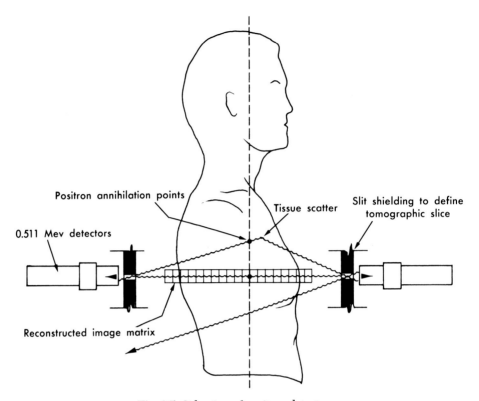

Positron annihilation points

Tissue scatter

Slit shielding to define tomographic slice

0.511 Mev detectors

Reconstructed image matrix

Fig. 3-7. Side view of positron detectors.

gamma rays is independent of the location of the annihilation. This factor, in conjunction with lower scatter and absorption, results in a "purer" image that is, one more independent of depth. Ter-Pogossian has brilliantly demonstrated this point (Fig. 3-8). Images of the same deep water phantom are compared using a traditional gamma camera and a 0.140 mev gamma emitter and his PETT emission tomography system in connection with a 0.511 mev positron emitter. The depth-independent quality of the 0.511 mev image is obvious.

The most fully engineered emission tomography system at this time is the PETT III system developed and put into operation by Ter-Pogossian and his group at Washington University in St. Louis. This system with its control console is shown in Fig. 3-9. The computational facility for reconstructing the image and the image display unit are located in an adjacent room. The PETT III system utilizes 48 sodium iodide gamma ray detectors solving 192 coincidence pairs (each detector is in coincidence with 8 detectors opposing it). Some transverse motion is used, with each bank of 8 detectors being shifted through 3° increments twenty times to obtain more projections. The system produces high-quality images with integration times of 2 to 3 minutes in the human head, thorax, and abdomen with 10 to 20 mCi of positron activity introduced.

The image reconstructed in the PETT III system is a 50 by 50 element matrix.

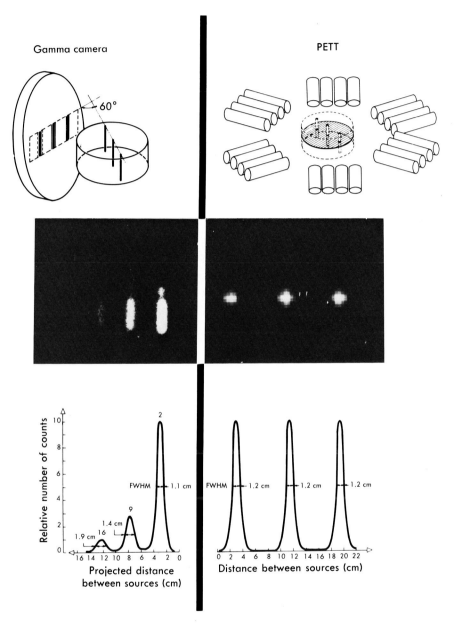

Fig. 3-8. Comparison of images obtained by conventional gamma camera and new positron camera. (From Ter-Pogossian, M. M., Phelps, M. E., Hoffman, E. J., and Mullani, N. A.: Radiology **114**:93, 1975.)

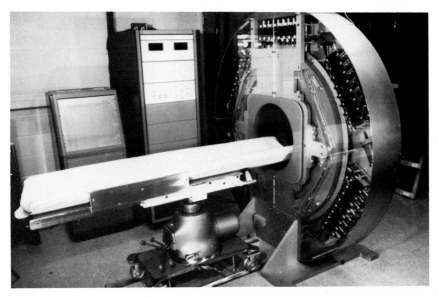

Fig. 3-9. Positron emission transaxial tomography system. (From Phelps, M. E., et al.: I.E.E.E. Trans. Nucl. Sci. [n.s.] **23**:516, 1976.)

Nominal resolution of this system and most other emission tomography systems under development is in the 0.8 to 1.0 cm range. Although the image is somewhat coarser than the x-ray transmission images (160 by 160), this element size is consistent with 0.511 mev scatter and detection considerations. The image has the same quality as the x-ray images discussed earlier in which each picture element is coarse but statistically well determined. It is simple, as illustrated by the PETT III scans shown in Fig. 3-10, to eliminate the coarse steps in the image display. A gamma camera image possessing an equal number of events appears smeared by comparison because of scatter–in this case, into adjacent, hypothetical picture elements. This tends to mask the fact that the resolutions for both are roughly comparable.

A group of representative images obtained with the PETT III system by the Washington University group are shown in Fig. 3-10. The series of tomographic cuts in the top row were taken at the level of the fourth intercostal space. In the "transmission" image (the method of obtaining this is discussed later) the myocardium and rib structure are imaged. The series at the bottom was taken 2 to 3 cm lower, imaging a part of the liver in a transmission view. Fifteen millicurie (± 20%) activity levels were utilized to obtain the emission images. The lower series is particularly interesting. In the $^{13}NH_3$ experiment the myocardial wall is well defined on the right, and with liver uptake appears at the left in the image. In the ^{11}CO image the four chambers of the heart are shown; the left ventricle just appears on the lower right.

The "transmission" images shown in Fig. 3-10 are obtained by placing a uniform (solution) ring source inside the detector array and around the patient to

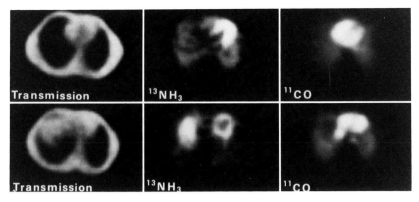

Fig. 3-10. Positron images obtained both in transmission and emission modes of PETT. (From Phelps, M. E., et al.: I.E.E.E. Trans. Nucl. Sci. [n.s.] **23**:520, 1976.)

be imaged. Operation of the system is identical to that described earlier, except that one of the coincidence gammas travels the entire distance through the patient ("transmission"), and the other is detected very close to the point of annihilation. In addition to having a potential diagnostic significance, this mode of operation is used to correct the emission image for differential absorption within the object and in standardizing the entire detector array.

COMPUTED TOMOGRAPHIC IMAGING WITH HEAVY CHARGED PARTICLES

Budinger et al.[2] have used the principles of computed tomography in connection with beams of heavy charged particles obtained from the Berkeley 184-inch cyclotron to obtain reconstructed images of sections of the brain. These images have an interesting and potentially important character. The use of such singular or esoteric sources of radiation should not deter one from gaining an understanding of the new capability that this experiment could portend.

Heavy charged particles such as protons, helium ions, and even heavier nuclei can be accelerated so that they penetrate through the body. In Budinger's experiment 910 mev helium ions with a range of 30 cm of tissue were used in transmission through the human head. The fascinating properties of heavy ions that make them attractive as information-gathering probes are minimum scatter and an extremely well-defined stopping point in tissue. These properties allow highly accurate determinations of the thickness and electron density of the tissue traversed. In heavy ion "radiography" or computed tomography this is translated into high-contrast and high-depth resolution. Information is thus obtained by measurement of the stopping point or residual energy of each ion rather than the attenuation or elimination of photons from a beam as is characteristic of x-ray tomography.

The Berkeley experimental situation is depicted in Fig. 3-11. The patient is rotated to obtain the axial motion. The residual range of each ion can be de-

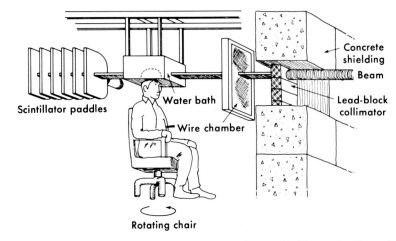

Fig. 3-11. Heavy ion tomography systems. (From Budinger, T. F., et al.: Trans. Nucl. Sci. [n.s.] **22**:1752, 1975.)

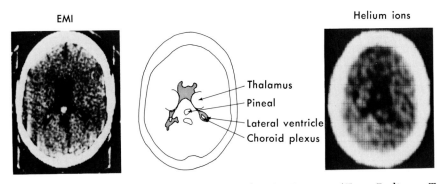

Fig. 3-12. Helium ion transmission image compared to EMI image. (From Budinger, T. F., et al.: Trans. Nucl. Sci. [n.s.] **22**:1752, 1975.)

termined by a succession of scintillator "paddles" with the x-ray position (or specific projection coordinate) determined by a multiwire, proportional gas-counting chamber. This information along with the angular coordinate is fed into the computer and image reconstruction performed.

Fig. 3-12 is the helium ion transmission image of a section of the brain. One hundred twenty-eight discrete angular projections of 5000 counts each were determined. In the figure the resultant image is compared with an EMI x-ray transmission image of the same subject. The interesting point is that even in this preliminary helium ion image the expected high definition of the ventricular structure is readily apparent.

Table 3-1. Characteristics of computed tomography systems

Radiation/source energy	Mode of operation	Information-gathering principle	Primary attributes
X rays 0.04 to 0.10 mev	Transmission	Removal of x-ray photons from transmitted beam by photoelectric and Compton absorption	Noninvasive organ visualization of unparalleled sensitivity
Positrons/radio-isotopes-cyclotron-0.511 mev.	Emission	Detection of back to back annihilation gamma rays from positron decay	Ability to utilize organ specificity of agents labelled with positron-emitting isotopes
Heavy ions/accelerator cyclotron-910 mev	Transmission	Measurement of stopping point or residual energy of each ion	Potential ability to visualize abrupt density differences such as tissue-air interfaces; large dose reduction

SUMMARY

The basic principles of operation of computed tomography systems have been presented. While technology in this field is rapidly evolving, these systems have the common feature that the resultant images are entirely a product of the computer. In the three concepts that have been considered here, images are reconstructed from multiple projections obtained by (1) transmitted x rays, (2) positron-emitting isotopes, or (3) heavy ions. The bases of operation and primary attributes of each system are summarized in Table 3-1.

There is one profound lesson, we believe, in the discovery and evolution of computed tomography in diagnostic radiology and, more recently, in nuclear medicine. It was easy to think of radiology as a saturated or "completed" discipline (as indeed it was) and that the probability of any new "turning-point" development was remote. Yet one *did* occur, and an entirely new dimension in extracting increased information from the x-ray image was revealed. Perhaps the lesson is that we should search for more such developments in what have been assumed to be mature areas of technology.

References

1. Brownell, G. L., et al.: New developments in positron scintigraphy and the application of positron emitting isotopes. In IAEA Medical Isotope Scintigraphy, vol. HD 9697, p. 163, 1968.
2. Budinger, T. F., et al.: Transverse section imaging with heavy charged particles: theory and application. In Proceedings of Conference on Image Processing for 2-D and 3-D Reconstruction from Projections, Stanford University, Aug., 1975.
3. Cho, Z. H., Ahn, I., Bohm, C., and Huth,

G. C.: Computerized image reconstruction methods with multiple photon/x-ray transmission scanning, Phys. Med. Biol. **19:** 511, 1974.

4. Cho, Z. H., et al.: A comparison of 3-D reconstruction algorithm with reference to number of projections and noise filtering, IEEE Trans. Nucl. Sci. **14:** March, 1975.

5. Ericksson, L., Chan, J. K., and Cho, Z. H.: Emission tomography with a circular ring transverse axial positron camera. In Proceedings of Conference on Image Processing for 2-D and 3-D Reconstructions from Projections, Stanford University, Aug., 1975.

6. Farr, R. F., Scott, A. C. H., Ollerenshar, R., Everard, G. J. H.: Monograph on transverse axial tomography, Oxford, England, 1966, Blackwell Scientific Publications.

7. Phelps, M. E., Hoffman, E. J., and Ter-Pogossian, M. M.: The application of annihilation coincidence detection to transaxial reconstruction tomography, J. Nucl. Med. 16:1, 1975.

8. Ter-Pogossian, M. M., Phelps, M. E., Hoffman, E. G., and Mullani, N. A.: A positron-emission transaxial tomography for nuclear imaging (PETT), Radiology **114:**89, 1975.

9. Thompson, C. J., Yamamoto, Y. L., and Meyer, E.: Reconstruction of images from a multiple detector ring. In Proceedings of Conference on Image Processing for 2-D and 3-D Reconstructions from Projections, Stanford University, Aug., 1975.

4 Computed tomography of the abdomen and aorta

John Haaga and Ralph J. Alfidi

Computed tomography of the abdomen is a promising diagnostic tool for demonstrating intra-abdominal pathology. Experience with in vivo[3] in vitro[2, 9] work indicates that many abnormalities have differences in attenuation values that can be detected with the CT scanner. The purpose of this chapter is to relate our initial experience at the Cleveland Clinic with abnormalities of abdominal organs and to make preliminary comparisons with other conventional diagnostic modalities when possible.

The CT scan used to accumulate this information was the Delta whole-body scanner manufactured by the Ohio Nuclear Corporation. The scanner employs a Macklett tube operating at 120 kv and 30 mA with 6 calcium fluoride scintillation of detectors. The detectors and x-ray tube move in a linear translating motion with rotation of the gantry at thirty increments through a total arc of 180°. The thickness of each slice is 13 mm; two contiguous slices are examined simultaneously. The scanner completes these two slices during a 2¼-minute interval. The CRT and digital display consist of 256 by 256 matrix points. The range of densities varies from –1000 to +1000 (the delta numbers equal EMI numbers times 2).

Because of rapid technologic advances in the field of CT scanning, a comment concerning the state of the art is appropriate. Up to this date our experience with CT scanning has been with the first-generation scanner just described and also a second-generation 18-second scanner. Our experience has shown that motion resulting from respiratory excursions and peristalsis degrades the image of the CT scan.[4] Despite those limitations, the data and information accumulated by the early scanners should remain valid in basic principles. Shorter scan times of future scanners should lessen the effect of motion and improve resolution and diagnostic accuracy.

In this discussion a range of numbers, not absolute numbers, is provided for several reasons. When images are obtained by a 2-minute scanner, respiratory motion can move a lesion in and out of the scan, yielding an averaged value. Even with shorter scans of 20-second duration, the attenuation value can vary greatly from patient to patient because different patient diameters produce a nonlinear attenuation of the x-ray beam and partial volume effect.[8] In spite of these factors the range of attenuation numbers has been of value for distinguishing different abnormalities in the abdomen.

LIVER

The normal liver, except for the biliary system, has a uniform attenuation. Without contrast material the liver parenchyma measures 40 to 70 delta attenuation numbers, and following the administration of intravenous iodinated contrast material, the attenuation value of the parenchyma increases to the range of 50 to 90. This enhancement typically improves visualization of abnormalities, which present as nonuniformity of attenuation numbers. Optimally, however, the liver should be scanned with and without contrast material because some lesions may be obscured by contrast enhancement.

Mass lesions of the liver can be detected because of differences in attenuation numbers or, occasionally, atypical contour. The hepatomas we have encountered have had lower attenuation numbers than normal parenchyma, despite the fact that they appeared highly vascular on hepatic angiograms (Fig. 4-1). All the hepatomas we have encountered have had attenuation numbers approximately 10 to 15 numbers lower than that of normal hepatic parenchyma, with one exception. In this patient with a hepatoma, the scan demonstrated some areas with attenuation numbers as low as 10 units. Metastatic lesions of the liver also show differences in attenuation, and the CT· scan in virtually all cases of noncalcified metastatic disease showed areas of decreased attenuation throughout (Fig. 4-2). In the vast majority of cases the differences between neoplasms and normal parenchyma were definitely enhanced by the administration of contrast material. However, in some patients with metastatic disease, lesions could be better visualized on scans without contrast material. Specifically, in several cases of metastases from carcinoid and renal carcinoma, the mass lesions were identified on

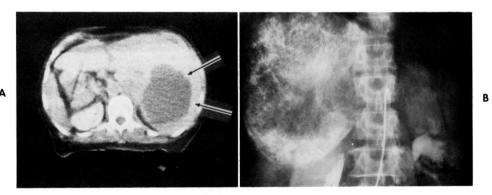

A

B

Fig. 4-1. A, Hepatoma appears as area of decreased attenuation in posterior portion of right lobe of liver (arrows). B, Angiogram of patient with hepatoma demonstrates hypervascularity in region of large mass. (From Alfidi, R. J., Haaga, J. R., and Havrilla, T. R.: Am. J. Roentgenol. Radium Ther. Nucl. Med. **127**:69, 1976.)

the noncontrast scans but were invisible following the administration of contrast material. In those cases in which contrast material enhances the normal parenchyma and not the metastasis, the metastases are 10 to 20 attenuation numbers less than the normal parenchyma. Calcified metastatic lesions such as mucinous carcinomas of the ovary have higher attenuation numbers, which produce a striking appearance on CT scan (Fig. 4-3). Another group of patients with metastatic disease demonstrated no abnormalities on the CT scan, either in configuration or attenuation. One can speculate that perhaps this is due to diffuse infiltration of the neoplasm or simply to lack of attenuation differences.

A

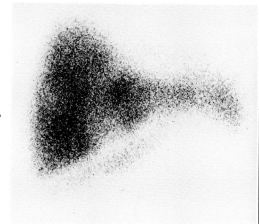

B

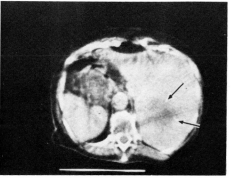

Fig. 4-2. A, Technetium 99m sulfur colloid isotope scan demonstrates multiple areas of low activity, which represent metastases. **B,** CT scan through liver of same patient as Fig. 4-1, *A*. Note area of decreased attenuation (arrows) in midportion of right lobe of liver, which represents metastases. (From Alfidi, R. J., Haaga, J. R., and Havrilla, T. R.: Am. J. Roentgenol. Radium Ther. Nucl. Med. **127**:69, 1976.)

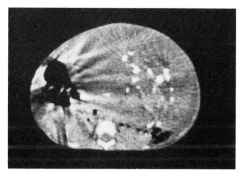

Fig. 4-3. CT scan of child with mucinous teratoma of ovary. White areas represent multiple calcifications within liver.

In benign mass lesions of the liver the normal morphology and attenuation numbers are again altered. In several benign adenomas that were scanned the attenuation numbers appeared normal, but an abnormal contour was noted. In these patients the right lobe of the liver appeared atypically bulbous. The unusual configuration of the lobe of each was noted on the preoperative scans; however, the significance was not appreciated. Benign cysts, abscesses, and hemorrhage into the liver were consistently demonstrated with the CT scan. Hepatic cysts were typically multiple in number and scattered throughout the liver (Fig. 4-4). We have seen a single case of a cystic adenoma of the liver. Hemorrhage into the liver can produce attenuation numbers ranging from 10 to as high as 50; the value of the numbers varies inversely with the age of the hematoma in the liver. The blood in a hematoma gradually breaks down, and there is an influx of body fluid, so that the attenuation numbers of a hemorrhage decrease over a period of time. Abscesses within or around the liver were typically in the range of 5 to 20 attenuation units; these will be discussed in detail later.

In one of our initial investigations we made a study of the CT scan and the technetium sulfur colloid radioisotope scan to directly compare their efficacy in mass lesion detection. The patients in the study[3] were selected at random. Each examination was interpreted without knowledge of the results of the other. CT scans in each case were performed both with and without intravenous contrast material. The patient was scanned in the right decubitus position with the gantry straight. The technetium sulfur colloid examinations were performed with a Searle gamma camera following the injection of 4 millicuries of technetium 99m sulfur colloid. In the final analysis of the data the accuracy rates of the CT scan and the radioisotope scan were equal in the detection of mass lesions (Table 4-1). The CT scan proved to be deficient in the detection of hepatic cirrhosis, discovering abnormalities in 8 of 11 cases of cirrhosis compared to the nuclear scans, which were positive in 10 of 11 cases. Those cases with fatty infiltration

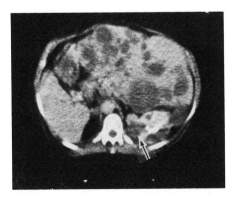

Fig. 4-4. Multiple hepatic cysts in patients with polycystic disease. Note that mass lesions are well circumscribed and low in attenuation. There are also several cysts on right kidney (arrow).

Table 4-1. Comparison of CT and nuclear medicine in detecting mass lesions of the liver in 61 patients

Liver diagnosis	Number of patients	CT−	NM−
Normal	10	9	8
"Normal"*	10	8	9
Total	20	17	17

		CT+	NM+
Tumor I° or II° Bx†	10	9	9
Tumor I° or II° Cl	9	7	7
Tumor I° or II° SO	3	1	1
Abscess	2	1	1
Cirrhosis Bx	11	8	10
Toxic hepatitis	2	0	2
"Triaditis"	2	0	2
Regenerating nodule	1	1	1
Polycystic renal and liver disease	1	1	1
Total	41	28	34
Mass lesions of liver—tumors, abscesses, nodules, and cysts (from above)	26	20	20

*In this category were 10 patients who had a proved disorder that could produce an imaging abnormality in the liver. However, based on final clinical diagnosis, the liver was not believed to be involved. Because of the equivocal nature of this group and the fact that there were more "false positives" indicated by CT than by nuclear medicine, it was decided that these should be placed in a special "normal" category.

†Bx = biopsy proved; Cl = clinical and laboratory evidence of hepatic involvement; SO = surgical observation of tumor in liver.

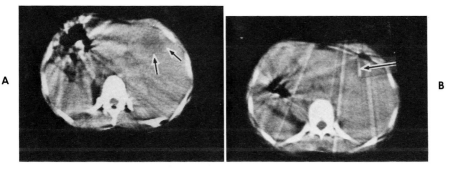

Fig. 4-5. A, CT scan through area of liver in patient with known metastatic disease. Metastasis is lower in attenuation than normal liver (arrows). **B,** CT scan through liver in same patient as **A** during a CT-guided biopsy. Arrow points to needle in place within metastasis.

demonstrated low attenuation numbers on the CT scan. These results indicate great promise for future CT scanners with shorter scan times. They should theoretically have better resolution and be more effective in detecting mass lesions.

CT-guided biopsy has been used for biopsy and aspiration of mass lesions of the liver, including neoplasms, cysts, and abscesses.[5] In any abnormal CT scan, the biopsy instrument can be guided to obtain a histologic specimen. The chief advantage over the blind biopsy technique is that a specific focus can be selected and a specimen obtained from that area (Fig. 4-5). This allows recovery of a histologic specimen so that proper therapeutic or additional diagnostic measures can be initiated.

BILIARY SYSTEMS

In our initial study of the biliary system, the CT scanner imaged not only the normal biliary system but also detected several abnormalities.[3] The normal gallbladder appears as a pear-shaped area of decreased attenuation surrounded by the denser hepatic parenchyma (Fig. 4-6). The biliary ducts can be seen in the portal area; they become enlarged in cases of obstructive jaundice. Because of this, we successfully detected obstructive jaundice in 4 out of 5 patients with common duct obstruction.[3] In many patients we have visualized both calcified and uncalcified biliary calculi (Fig. 4-7).

An additional use for the scanners is CT guidance of percutaneous transhepatic cholangiograms (Fig. 4-8). Previously these procedures were performed under fluoroscopic guidance—an essentially blind procedure. With the CT scan the needle can be inserted into the abdominal wall and guided into the area of the main biliary radicles. This can provide either a diagnostic cholangiogram or drainage for an obstructive biliary tree.

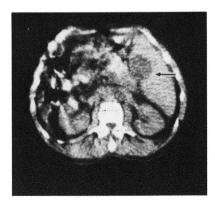

Fig. 4-6. Gallbladder appears as a pear-shaped density of lower attenuation than liver (arrow). Normal gallbladder can typically be seen in the normal patient.

PANCREAS

The pancreas, which has been a difficult organ to image, can now be visualized almost routinely with the CT scan. The normal as well as the diseased gland states can be directly visualized.[7]

Our technique for pancreas examination follows. The patient is first examined lying in the supine position with the top of the gantry angled 10°. Angulation emphasizes the fat plane around the SMA artery, which serves as a reliable landmark for the normal pancreas. In approximately 50% of patients the normal pancreatic head is not clearly seen by this technique, and so certain modifications are made during the examination. The patient is given 5 ounces of a 10% Renografin solution orally and rescanned in the right decubitus position. With the

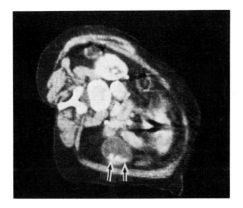

Fig. 4-7. Scan of patient on right side. Gallbladder is somewhat large and extends inferiorly below liver, obscuring it from view on this scan. Gallbladder itself appears as somewhat lower attenuation numbers, 5 to 20. Within gallbladder are several calcified gallstones (arrows). These stones were not visible on a radiograph. (From Alfidi, R. J., Haaga, J. R., and Havrilla, T. R.: Am. J. Roentgenol. Radium Ther. Nucl. Med. **127:**69, 1976.)

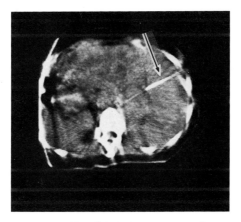

Fig. 4-8. CT scan of patient with dilated bile ducts. Arrow designates needle being placed within a major biliary radicle.

gantry straight the pancreatic area is now scanned. This maneuver permits the abdominal viscera to shift away from the pancreas, making the head more visible (Fig. 4-9). It also produces partial mobilization of the right diaphragm, which improves resolution.

The normal head and body of the pancreas are surrounded by a fat plane and lie anterior to the aorta and the SMA artery. The tail of the pancreas is immediately anterior to the left kidney and lies close to the hilum of the spleen. According to a previous study,[7] the AP diameter of the tail and body of the pancreas should measure at least one third, but no greater than two thirds, the transverse diameter of the vertebral body. The AP diameter of the head of the pancreas should be at least one half the diameter, but no greater than the full transverse diameter, of the vertebral body.

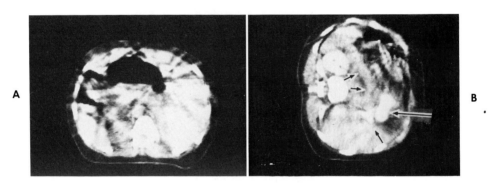

Fig. 4-9. **A,** Scan of pancreatic area in a patient does not clearly demonstrate pancreas because of scattered artifact from the gas and because of overlying soft tissues. **B,** Scan of same patient as **A,** taken in right decubitus position. Pancreas is now better defined (small arrows). Note contrast material within gastric antrum (larger arrow) and duodenal bulb (single small arrow).

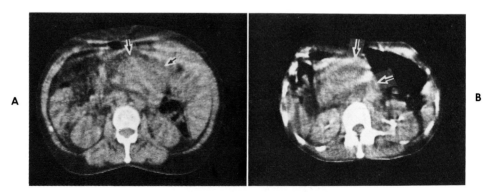

Fig. 4-10. **A,** Large mass in area of head of pancreas, which later proved to be adenocarcinoma (arrows). **B,** Another scan on a different patient demonstrates a mass in area of body of pancreas (arrows). Fat plane around aorta is lost in addition to large mass. This also was an adenocarcinoma. (From Haaga, J. R., Alfidi, R. J., and Zelch, M.: Radiology **120:**589, 1976.)

Neoplasms of the pancreatic area produce alterations of the normal anatomy. The most consistent finding is enlargement of the pancreatic contour beyond the normal dimensions just described (Fig. 4-10). Also the fat planes surrounding the pancreas and the SMA artery may be obliterated, apparently due to infiltration of the neoplasm. These changes can be produced by a variety of neoplasms and are nonspecific. We have encountered these positive findings with a variety of neoplasms, including pancreatic adenocarcinoma, metastatic adenocarcinoma, lymphoma, cholangiocarcinoma, and mesenchymoma. Thus far we have been unable to detect any attenuation number difference among the various neoplasms.

Cystic areas in the pancreas can be easily detected and appear as decreased attenuation on the image. Pseudocysts as well as cystic dilatation of the pancreatic ducts have been visualized (Fig. 4-11).

Several abnormalities of the pancreatic duct have been demonstrated by CT scan. In our first study group there were 3 patients in which an apparent dilatation of the duct was demonstrated. Since then we have examined a patient with a calculus in the pancreatic duct; the calculus was imaged on the CT scan and appeared as a single area of calcium in the center of the pancreas. The diagnosis was made correctly preoperatively (Fig. 4-12).

We have discerned several distinct appearances of inflammatory disease of the pancreas. In our initial series there were cases of biopsy-proved pancreatitis that did not appear abnormal on the CT scan. Another group of cases of both acute and chronic pancreatitis showed enlargement of a portion of the gland. In those patients with chronic calcific pancreatitis there is a distinctive appearance characterized by multiple calcium deposits of varying size throughout the pancreas (Fig. 4-13). This is in contrast to the single calcification noted in the pancreatic duct calculus. Chronic atrophic pancreatitis, in which the gland has been reduced in size from scarring and atrophy, demonstrates a diminished anteroposterior dimension on the CT scan (Fig. 4-14). With the exception of calcific pancreatitis

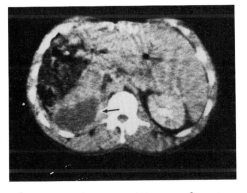

Fig. 4-11. This patient has traumatic pancreatitis secondary to surgery. Note increased diameter of pancreatic tail. Pseudocyst appears as area of decreased attenuation adjacent to tail (arrow). (From Haaga, J. R., Alfidi, R. J., and Zelch, M.: Radiology **120:**589, 1976.)

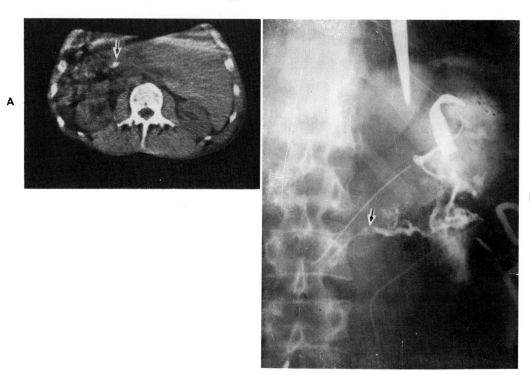

Fig. 4-12. A, Scan of patient with suspected pancreatic disease demonstrates a single high-density calcium deposit within area of pancreas (arrow). On the basis of this isolated calcification the diagnosis of pancreatic duct calculus was made on the CT scan preoperatively. B, Radiograph of an antegrade pancreatogram in which contrast material was injected from tail of duct toward head. Pancreatic calculus (arrow) obstructs flow of contrast material. The CT scan was the only diagnostic modality that made the correct diagnosis preoperatively.

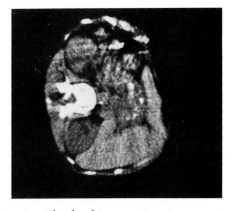

Fig. 4-13. Scan of patient in right decubitus position. Pancreas is somewhat enlarged, and there are multiple calcifications of varying size throughout gland. This is characteristic of chronic calcific pancreatitis. (From Haaga, J. R., Alfidi, R. J., and Zelch, M.: Radiology **120:** 589, 1976.)

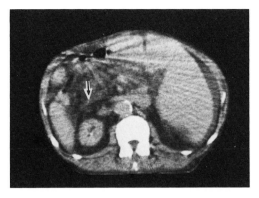

Fig. 4-14. CT scan of patient with uremia and chronic atrophic pancreatitis. Pancreas body and tail are reduced in size (arrow). (From Haaga, J. R., Alfidi, R. J., and Zelch, M.: Radiology **120:**589, 1976.)

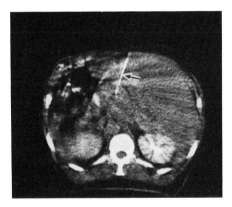

Fig. 4-15. Percutaneous aspiration biopsy of pancreas. Arrow points to fine needle guided into mass in head of pancreas. Aspiration specimen yielded adenocarcinoma.

and pseudocysts, attenuation numbers for the various types of pancreatitis were not distinctive from those of a normal pancreas.

Distinguishing pancreatitis from neoplasm in the pancreas has been only partially successful. Attenuation numbers of normal, inflammatory, and neoplastic states have not varied significantly. When there is focal enlargement of the gland it is not possible as yet to distinguish an area of focal pancreatitis from a localized neoplastic process. In our study, differentiation of pancreatitis and neoplasm required correlation with clinical and laboratory information.

In patients who are considered inoperable, percutaneous aspiration biopsy of the pancreas can be achieved under CT guidance (Fig. 4-15). We believe that CT guidance is the most accurate means of performing such a biopsy.[5]

KIDNEY

For kidney examination the patient is placed in the supine position and given an intravenous bolus injection of 50 ml of 60% Renografin. The gantry is straight and the scans are initiated at the iliac crest and continued at 2 cm increments until the kidneys have been covered. To date, most evaluations of kidneys have involved examination of mass lesions. Mass lesions are evident on the CT scan because of the mass effect and also because of the variation in attenuation numbers. The lesions can produce an abnormal contour of the kidney and effacement of the collecting systems. Cystic lesions appear darker than the normal kidney and measure in the range of –5 to +20 attenuation numbers (Fig. 4-16). Attenuation of solid neoplasm has measured in the range of +20 to +80 units—greater than that of cystic lesions, and yet less than that of a normal renal parenchyma (Fig. 4-17).

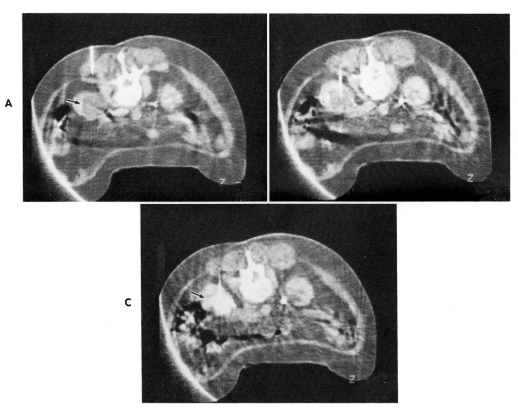

Fig. 4-16. **A,** Scan of patient in prone position. Area of decreased attenuation within right kidney represents a renal cyst (arrow). A percutaneous puncture is being performed, and there is a needle in place within the abdominal wall for an initial localization scan. **B,** Needle has been guided into area of cyst cavity. Note that proximal end of needle from the skin is not visible because needle was angulated slightly and proximal portion was outside scan diameter. **C,** Needle is in place within cyst cavity. Contrast material has been injected into cyst (arrow).

Because of the excellent density discrimination, in the CT scanners, hydronephrosis can be easily seen even though there is no excretion of the contrast material into the collecting system. The dilated renal pelvis can be seen as a "water-density" structure within the central portion of the kidney even without contrast enhancement (Fig. 4-18, *A*).

Because the scanner directly visualizes the perinephric area even without contrast, the cross-sectional image is valuable in detection of perinephric abnormalities. Perinephric abscesses, lipomatosis, lymphoma, and metastasis are among the various entities we have encountered in the perinephric area.

CT-guided biopsy has been extremely useful in kidney evaluation. Cyst aspirations can be accurately performed (Fig. 4-16). Even small cysts that could not be localized fluoroscopically have been properly drained by CT-guided aspiration. In a similar manner, inoperable neoplasm can be biopsied percutaneously because accurate localization of the instruments into the chosen area of the neoplasm is possible.[5] Finally, antegrade pyelography and temporary percutaneous nephrostomy can be performed in nonfunctioning kidneys (Fig. 4-18). Because

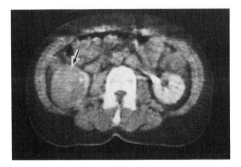

Fig. 4-17. Mass lesion in left kidney is distorting renal cortex (arrow). Mass is higher in attenuation than a renal cyst and lower than a normal kidney. Mass is a renal cell carcinoma.

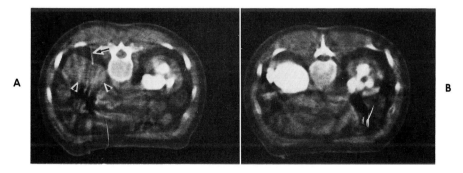

Fig. 4-18. A, This patient had a nonfunctioning right kidney demonstrated on urogram. Small arrows demonstrate "water-density" pelvis, which does not contain any contrast material. Single arrow points to needle being guided into hydronephrotic collecting system. **B,** Same patient as **A.** Hydronephrotic pelvis has been injected with contrast material.

of the extreme sensitivity of CT scanners in detecting density variations, the renal pelvis and kidney can be visualized as "water-density" structures, despite the fact that there is no concentration of the contrast material. By this means, those procedures which would have been difficult with a blind or fluoroscopic technique can now be performed with CT guidance.

DETECTION OF INTRA-ABDOMINAL ABSCESS

Intra-abdominal abscess is discussed in this chapter because there are characteristics common to all the organ systems.

One of the most valuable indicators of abscess is the presence of air outside the gastrointestinal tract. The CT scan is very useful in this case because localization of gas is simplified. Extraluminal gas typically will be demonstrated on the scan even when on a radiograph the gas pattern is ill defined and resembles intestinal gas (Fig. 4-19).

Intrahepatic abscesses appear as areas of lower attenuation when compared to the normal hepatic parenchyma (Fig. 4-20, *A*). The cross-sectional image displays the abscess in relation to the costal margin, the diaphragmatic sulcus, and intraperitoneal structures. The importance of such accurate localization has been emphasized by authors such as Whalen, who has discussed anatomic guidelines to serve as criteria for various surgical approaches.

In addition to its utility in diagnosing abscess collections, the CT scanner is very useful for guidance of needle aspiration and drainage procedures. We have performed three types of aspiration procedures using instruments of varying sizes, depending on the purpose of the aspiration. To obtain a small specimen for culture without drainage, a 22-gauge needle can be inserted into the abscess cavity. For limited drainage and also a specimen for culture, a 17-gauge Teflon-sheath needle can be guided into the abscess cavity and the catheter left for a small drainage tube (Fig. 4-20, *B* and *C*). In certain instances in which the purulent material is quite thin, the small catheter may suffice for drainage, producing cure.

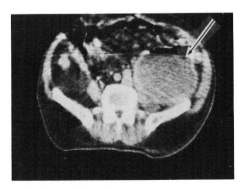

Fig. 4-19. Large mass adjacent to right iliac crest. Mass contains fluid and has a thick capsule surrounding it. Arrow points to air-fluid level at superior portion of mass. From the CT scan the diagnosis of abscess was made, which was confirmed at surgery.

Finally, for individuals who are not operative candidates, a primary drainage by a percutaneous procedure may be performed. We have drained a hepatic abscess with a 14F balloon catheter inserted percutaneously.[6]

There are several distinct advantages in using the CT scanner for detection of intra-abdominal abscesses. Because the image displays attenuation numbers, purulent fluid collections in inflammatory tissue can be detected. In addition, we have seen several cases in which small extraluminal gas collections were discernible on the CT scan but were invisible on a plain radiograph. Finally, the aspiration procedures mentioned can guide specific antibiotic therapy or planned surgical procedures.

AORTA

The aorta is surrounded by a fat plane, which makes it routinely visible in the CT scan. With aneurysmal dilatation the diameter of an aneurysm can be measured, whether or not the walls are calcified (Fig. 4-21). The relationship to the renal artery, superior mesenteric artery, and iliac arteries can be demonstrated without the injection of contrast material, providing valuable information for possible surgical repair.

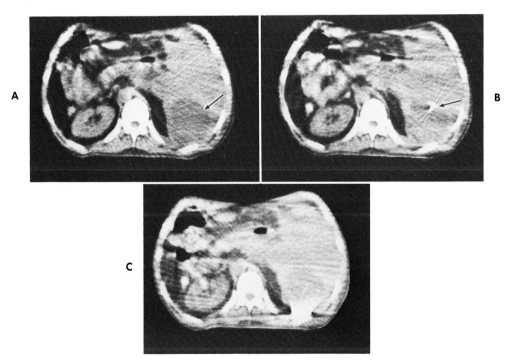

Fig. 4-20. A, Intrahepatic abscess in posterior portion of right lobe of liver appears as area of decreased attenuation (arrow). B, Same abscess cavity with point of needle (arrow) in place within it. Proximal portion of needle from skin to lesion cannot be seen because needle has been angulated to avoid a diaphragmatic insertion. C, Contrast material fills abscess cavity and is gravitated posteriorly.

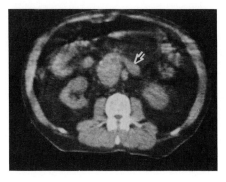

Fig. 4-21. Scan of aneurysm of abdominal aorta. Note that proximal renal artery on right side is also involved with the aneurysm (arrow).

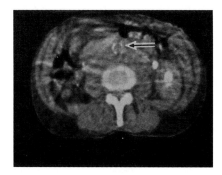

Fig. 4-22. Scan of a large retroperitoneal mass, which has displaced the calcified aorta anteriorly (arrow). Patient had metastatic prostate carcinoma to the retroperitoneal lymph nodes.

If calcium is present within the wall, the aorta can be discerned even if the fat plane is absent. In those cases in which tumor obliterates the fat plane, the calcified aorta can be visualized—at times displaced by the adjacent tumor (Fig. 4-22).

SUMMARY

The CT scan can detect various abnormalities in the abdomen. In the liver, mass lesions can definitely be detected as accurately as with isotopic scans. In the pancreas, inflammatory disease and neoplasm have specific characteristics that can be demonstrated on the CT scan. In the genitourinary tract, mass lesions of the kidneys as well as hydronephrosis can be accurately diagnosed. Finally, guidance of percutaneous aspiration and biopsy procedures are possible in all the organ systems we have discussed.

References

1. Alfidi, R. J., et al.: Computed tomography of the thorax and abdomen; a preliminary report, Radiology **117:**257, 1975.

2. Alfidi, R. J., et al.: Experimental studies to determine application of CAT scanning to the human body, Am. J. Roent-

genol. Radium Ther. Nucl. Med. **124**:199, 1975.

3. Alfidi, R. J., Haaga, J. R., and Havrilla, T. R.: Computed tomography of the liver, Am. J. Roentgenol. Radium Ther. Nucl. Med. **127**:69, 1976.

4. Alfidi, R. J., MacIntyre, W. J., and Haaga, J. R.: The effects of biological motion on CT resolution, Am. J. Roentgenol. Radium Ther. Nucl. Med. **127**:11, 1976.

5. Haaga, J. R., and Alfidi, R. J.: Precise biopsy localization by computed tomography, Radiology **118**:3, 1976.

6. Haaga, J. R., Alfidi, R. J., and Cooper-man, A.: CT detection and aspiration of abscesses, Am. J. Roentgenol. Radium Ther. Nucl. Med., 1977.

7. Haaga, J. R., Alfidi, R. J., and Zelch, M.: In vivo CT scanning of the pancreas, Radiology **120**:589, 1976.

8. McCullough, E., et al.: Performance evaluation and quality assurance of computed tomography scanners with illustrations from EMI, ACTA, and Delta scanners, Radiology **120**:173, 1976.

9. Philips, R. L., and Stephens, D. H.: Computed tomography of liver specimens, Radiology **115**:43, 1975.

5 Alternative display formats for computed tomography (CT) data

William V. Glenn, Jr., Kenneth R. Davis, Gregory N. Larsen, and Samuel J. Dwyer, III

In view of the prominent role computed tomography (CT) systems are attaining in the evaluation of various neurologic problems,* it is increasingly important to demonstrate some of the additional image manipulation and display capabilities that present scanning systems might provide[25-28]:

1. Interpolation of thin transverse sections
2. Reconstruction of coronal, sagittal, and oblique sections
3. Production of shaded pseudo–three-dimensional images
4. Production of stereo pairs (of no. 3)
5. Rapid framing for walkthrough or rotational effect (nos. 1 to 4)
6. Production of absorption value histograms of local areas
7. Image subtraction
8. Volume determination of tumors, ventricles, hemorrhages, etc.

Access to these additional capabilities has important quantitative and qualitative implications. This is particularly true when the potential clinical benefits are extended beyond the impact of CT head scanners to include CT body scanners† and other forms of cross-sectional imaging, such as those based on positron emission‡ or ultrasound.

From a quantitative standpoint, over 500 first-generation CT head scanners will soon be operational. This represents a total equipment expenditure of $200 to $300 million in a market (both foreign and domestic) predicted to exceed $2 billion in cumulative sales by 1985.[1, 49] Even though development of these systems will continue to advance rapidly, the present scanners will be performing the majority of CT examinations for the next several years. Therefore it is important that CT suppliers extract the full latent potential of such huge investments by finding ways of keeping the earlier systems as up-to-date as possible, thus delaying obsolescence.

From the qualitative or clinical aspect, patients can now be given a more sophisticated and accurate level of evaluation with the existing noninvasive CT

---

*References 3-10, 18-21, 24, 31, 35, 36, 39-47, 52, 53.
†References 2, 22, 37, 51, 54, 56.
‡References 11-13, 17, 33, 34, 48, 55.

system. A number of situations discussed by Kramer, Janetos, and Perlstein[32] warrant the special anatomic detail gained by the use of intravenous contrast material. Other indications for special detail include the need for a more thorough evaluation of the ventricular system, triangulation of lesions (e.g., for surgery, biopsy, or radiation therapy), and more definition of difficult basal areas such as the parasellar region, subtemporal areas, orbits, and posterior fossa. The remainder of the chapter is divided into sections that will provide examples of capabilities satisfying the needs just listed and discuss future developments in computed tomography.

INTERPOLATED THIN TRANSVERSE CT IMAGES

Fig. 5-1 illustrates that when viewing a conventional transverse CT image, one is in effect looking along the z axis at a plane parallel to the x and y axes. The apparent resolution of the square 1.5 by 1.5 mm picture elements in such an x-y plane is misleading, since the slice thickness or depth of each picture element is 8 to 13 mm, depending on beam collimation. This means that the z-axis resolution, as manifest by picture element dimensions, is considerably less than resolution along the x or y axes. When the data of adjacent 8.0 mm transverse planes are rearranged into a coronal projection, as in the top of Fig. 5-2, the resulting x-z image plane is of poor quality because such a reconstructed plane is composed of rectangular picture elements. However, in the absence of de novo thin 2.0 mm sections from CT scanning systems, good quality coronal and sagittal images can be obtained by interpolating from overlapped thick to adjacent thin transverse planes. This is illustrated at the bottom of Fig.

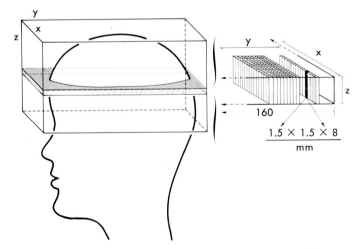

Fig. 5-1. Conventional transverse CT scan. Depending on x-ray beam collimation, routine CT sections or planes are 8 to 13 mm thick. This schematic drawing represents an 8.0 mm tissue section composed of 25,600 picture elements (160×160 array), each measuring 1.5 by 1.5 by 8.0 mm.

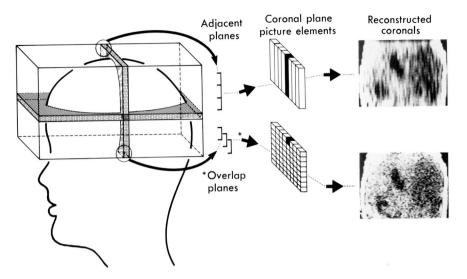

Fig. 5-2. Alternative schemes for reconstructing a coronal CT plane. In top method no attempt is made to improve z-axis resolution beyond that obtained by 8.0 mm beam collimation. Coronal plane picture elements appear rectangular (top) as opposed to square (bottom) when z-axis resolution is enhanced fivefold to eightfold by an interpolation procedure (°) from thick overlapped 8.0 mm transverse planes to thin adjacent 1.0 mm transverse planes.

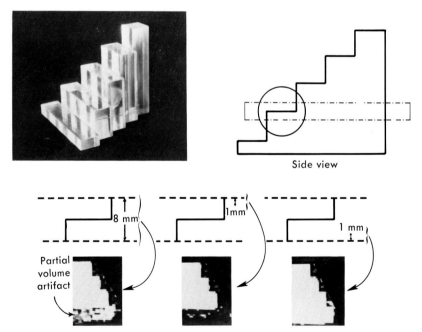

Fig. 5-3. Phantom experiment showing increased accuracy in transverse CT sections. In this phantom experiment one step in the Lucite step wedge was only partially "seen" by the 8.0 mm collimated x-ray beam. Averaging artifact (i.e., fuzzy area) in initial CT image can be removed by an interpolation procedure (see text) that produces very thin sections.

5-2. The resulting fivefold to eightfold increase in z-axis resolution essentially equalizes picture element dimensions along the x, y, and z axes. This is true because after the interpolation procedure, individual picture elements are roughly cubic. Details for gathering a series of overlapped CT sections are given later.

An illustration of how interpolation can minimize thick-section partial-volume artifact is provided by an early phantom experiment[26] with Lucite step wedges (Fig. 5-3). The results show that the process of fractionating one 8.0 mm plane into eight 1.0 mm planes did not compromise the original x-y resolution. More important, resolution in the z axis was considerably improved. The increase in resolution is demonstrated in Fig. 5-3 by the removal of a fuzzy area of partial volume artifact. This artifact occurred because one step in the Lucite wedge was just grazed by the plane of the section; specifically, only the lower half of the 8.0 mm plane of the section "saw" this particular step. The upper half of the slice was water and the lower half Lucite. Note that the thin sections in Fig. 5-3 show no evidence of the partial volume problem.

RECONSTRUCTED CT IMAGES: CORONALS, SAGITTALS, AND OBLIQUES

CT data from the following detailed clinical example are used to illustrate the image manipulation and display capabilities of reconstructed coronal, sagittal, and oblique images as well as of interactive graphics and three-dimensional displays, which are discussed later.

Example case

A. L., a 19-year-old woman, was admitted for evaluation of right-sided headaches of variable frequency and intensity that had been occurring for 2 years. She presented with droop of the right eyelid, horizontal diplopia, and numbness and tingling of the right forehead, cheek, and eyelid. Her past history was remarkable in that she had documented Ollier's disease and had undergone nineteen previous operations for lower extremity deformities. A detailed eye examination showed good visual acuity, an upper right temporal quadrantic field defect, right ptosis, and slight right exophthalmus. The right fourth nerve was intact. Fifth nerve testing showed moderately dense hypesthesia involving V1 and V2, with a slightly decreased corneal sensitivity on the right. The patient also had a complete right sixth nerve palsy.

Radiographic evaluation of this partial cavernous sinus syndrome began with plain films (Fig. 5-4) and polytome laminograms (Fig. 5-5), which showed right parasellar amorphous calcification and minimal erosion of the right superior lateral aspect of the dorsum sellae. The angiogram (Fig. 5-6) demonstrated an avascular mass effect in the right parasellar region, extending below the edge of the tentorial incisura. The CT findings following injection of intravenous contrast material (Fig. 5-7) showed elevation of absorption values over a larger area than that seen on the noncontrast study (not shown). This provided a relatively good estimate of the size and shape of the entire tumor.

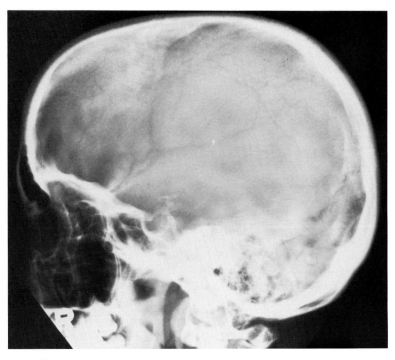

Fig. 5-4. Lateral skull film. This plain film shows abnormal calcification projecting above and somewhat anterior to dorsum. This 19-year-old white woman presented with a partial right cavernous sinus syndrome.

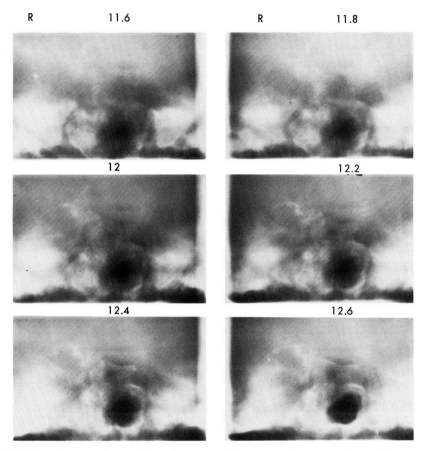

Fig. 5-5. AP polytomes of sella. These laminographic sections show amorphous right parasellar calcification and erosion of right side of dorsum sellae.

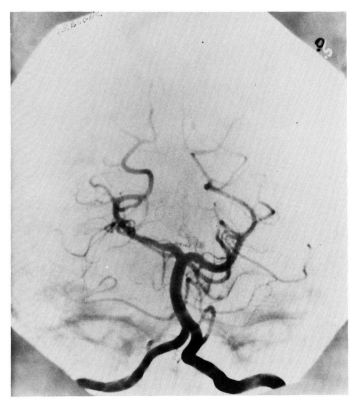

Fig. 5-6. Left vertebral angiogram. This AP projection (subtraction image) shows an avascular mass effect in right cerebellopontine angle. There is elevation of right posterior cerebral and right superior cerebellar arteries. Lesion was histologically a right parasellar chondrosarcoma.

Involvement of the right parasellar region with extension through the tentorial incisura is noted on the horizontal sections. The method by which the overlapped series of 8.0 mm transverse CT sections (Fig. 5-7) were obtained is shown schematically in Fig. 5-8. With slow scanners requiring 6½ minutes per scan, an attempt has been made to optimize factors of patient exposure, patient cooperation, resolution of reconstructed images, and vertical territory covered. Four sets of scan levels separated by 2.0 mm are obtained by withdrawing the patient couch in 2.0 mm increments. As noted in Fig. 5-8, there is a 1.0 cm gap between each group of four scan levels. The detailed overlap sequence (bottom of Fig. 5-8) accounts for each pair of adjacent 8.0 mm slices at all scan levels. With such a continuous overlapped series, the next step in the process is simply to interpolate for thin sections represented by the shaded areas. This approach increases patient exposure by a factor of four, meaning that the published range of 1 to 2.5 rads to the skin is now 4 to 10 rads.[27, 36, 46] The eight overlapped levels usually obtained require approximately 50 minutes, or twice the normal CT examination time. The vertical distance of 3 to 3.5 cm covered by this technique is sufficient to provide reconstructed images of

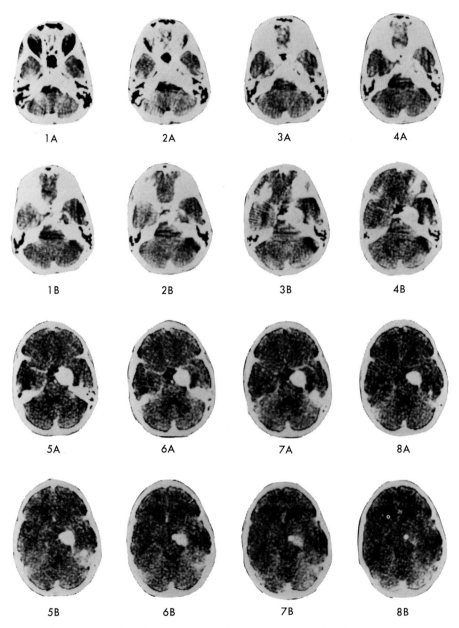

1A   2A   3A   4A

1B   2B   3B   4B

5A   6A   7A   8A

5B   6B   7B   8B

Fig. 5-7. Right parasellar chondrosarcoma (transverse images). These images constitute original overlapped sequence of 8.0 mm horizontal sections. The sixteen images represent the A and B slices at eight scan levels. Arranged here in ascending order, they demonstrate contrast enhancement (following 300 ml of 30% methylglucamine diatrizoate) of a large right parasellar abnormality, which extends posteriorly and inferiorly through the tentorial incisura. Superior extension of this lesion is noted on higher sections, well above dorsum sellae. Reconstructed coronal and sagittal images are shown in Figs. 5-9 and 5-10, respectively.

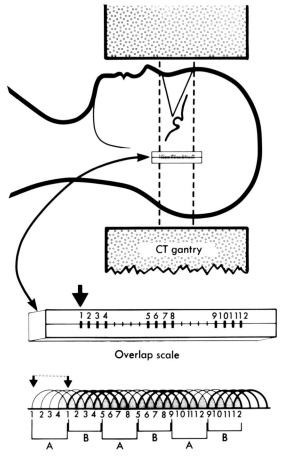

Fig. 5-8. Overlap technique. Eight or twelve scan levels are used clinically. Within each group of four scan levels the offset is 2.0 mm. Between each group of four scan levels the offset is 1.0 cm. The anatomic region covered is limited but sufficient to encompass difficult basal areas. (See text.)

areas such as the parasellar region, subtemporal areas, orbits, and posterior fossa (particularly cerebellopontine angles).

Once the interpolation procedure has provided a cubic array of roughly cubic picture elements, coronal, sagittal, and oblique reconstructed images perpendicular to the original transverse sections can be easily created. Figs. 5-9 and 5-10 complement the horizontal sections of Fig. 5-7 by showing the tumor's anterior extension almost to the right anterior clinoid process (Fig. 5-9, *C*), asymmetry of the chiasmatic cistern (Fig. 5-9, *D*), the vertical dimension of the lesion with respect to the sellar floor and dorsum (Figs. 5-9, *D* and *E*), and growth through the tentorial incisura into the right cerebellopontine angle cistern (Figs. 5-10, *E* and *F*). Central low absorption values in the tumor (Figs. 5-9, *D*, and 5-10, *C* and *D*) were identified only on the 1.5 mm coronal and sagittal sections, indicating a partially necrotic or cystic central component of the lesion.

Coronal

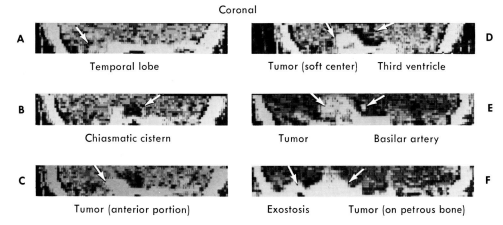

A Temporal lobe

D Tumor (soft center) Third ventricle

B Chiasmatic cistern

E Tumor Basilar artery

C Tumor (anterior portion)

F Exostosis Tumor (on petrous bone)

Fig. 5-9. Right parasellar chondrosarcoma (coronal images). These six images are representative 1.5 mm coronal sections obtained from original overlap series in Fig. 5-7.

Sagittal

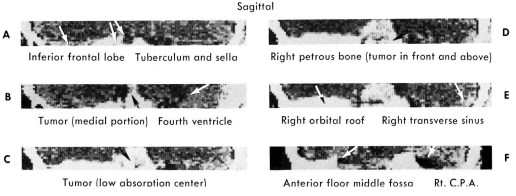

A Inferior frontal lobe Tuberculum and sella

D Right petrous bone (tumor in front and above)

B Tumor (medial portion) Fourth ventricle

E Right orbital roof Right transverse sinus

C Tumor (low absorption center)

F Anterior floor middle fossa Rt. C.P.A.

Fig. 5-10. Right parasellar chondrosarcoma (sagittal images). These six images are representative sagittal images obtained from original overlap series in Fig. 5-7.

A subsequent overlap study during this patient's course of radiation therapy was obtained for consideration of possible therapy port adjustments relating to her supravoltage boost. Figs. 5-11 to 5-14 represent selected coronal, saggital, and oblique reconstructed CT planes. These reconstructions were requested to correlate the treatment ports (lateral, posterior oblique, and anterior oblique) with CT planes parallel and perpendicular to these ports.

An important factor illustrated by this case is the increased geometric detail and triangulation provided by the combination of multiple image formats. Prior to surgery, the neurosurgeons carefully inspected the adjacent 1.5 mm coronal and sagittal images on a stand-alone interactive video display device.[16] During this review session the lesion's low absorption center was noted and believed to be due to either a cystic component or malignant transformation because of the patient's history of Ollier's disease. This knowledge prompted a more exten-

Text continued on p. 102.

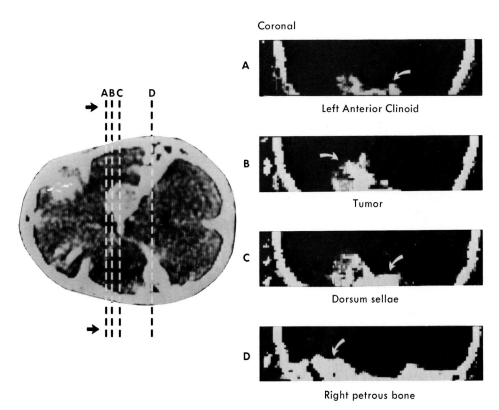

Fig. 5-11. Right parasellar chondrosarcoma (coronal images). A second overlapped series of transverse images was obtained midway in this patient's course of radiation therapy and yielded these coronal reconstructions and also sagittal and oblique sections in Figs. 5-12 to 5-14. These images were used by the radiation therapists to assess tissue densities in planes both parallel and perpendicular to the three radiation fields.

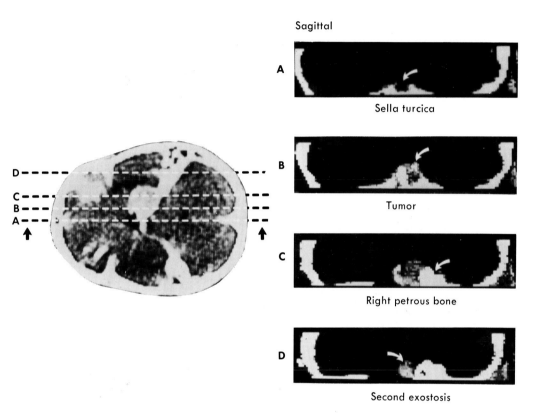

Fig. 5-12. Right parasellar chondrosarcoma (sagittal images). Here again bulk of this tumor mass is situated anterior and slightly superior to right petrous bone. *D* shows second exostosis located further laterally and anterior to right petrous bone.

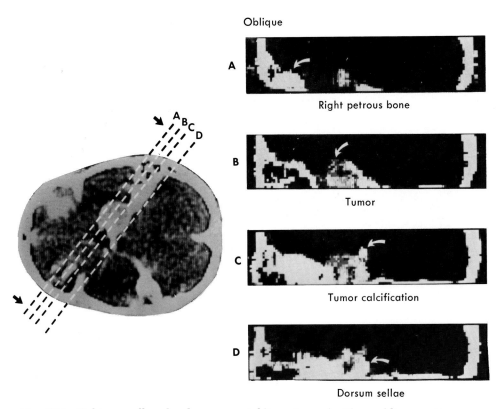

Oblique

A

Right petrous bone

B

Tumor

C

Tumor calcification

D

Dorsum sellae

Fig. 5-13. Right parasellar chondrosarcoma (oblique images). These oblique sections pass through tumor mass and right petrous bone.

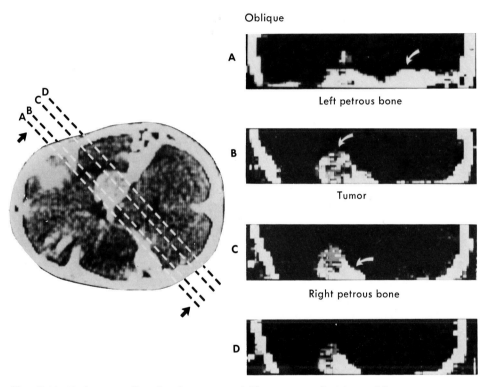

Fig. 5-14. Right parasellar chondrosarcoma (oblique images). These oblique sections pass through tumor mass and left petrous bone.

sive surgical decompression rather than a simple biopsy. The main reasons for this decision were the anticipation of subsequent radiation therapy and the need to surgically reduce the tumor's volume as much as possible. The opportunity to preview the multiplanar CT images provided the surgeons with a better sense of geometry and detail as well as a basis for more aggressive surgery on the lesion, which proved to be a malignant chondrosarcoma.

Another important aspect of this case was the fact that after surgery the combined multiplanar CT images were of prime importance in devising this patient's radiation therapy treatment plan. The advent of CT scanning has provided a far clearer spatial evaluation of intracranial tumors than radio-therapists have previously been able to obtain from the integration of other types of diagnostic studies. Accurate high-dose radiation therapy is only feasible with this kind of information, as the ceiling on dose is dependent on knowledge of the tumor's full extent and the anatomic relations of normal and, in particular, vulnerable tissues. This case of right parasellar chondrosarcoma presented a difficult clinical situation. The tumor is relatively radioresistant and would usually require doses of about 6,000 to 7,000 rads delivered over 6 to 8 weeks to offer a chance of tumor control. Furthermore, the brain stem, the most radiosensitive of normal central nervous system structures, was in close approximation to the tumor site and would therefore represent the limiting factors in such high-dose administrations. The availability of multiplanar CT images in helping to determine this patient's three-field megavoltage treatment plan provided both greater accuracy and a greater sense of security in tumor localization and sparing of normal tissue.

From our limited experience in combining CT with radiation therapy planning, there is reason to believe that further studies are mandatory and may well offer significant advances in patient management. If care is taken to accurately relate external landmarks to tumor during the diagnostic studies themselves, it may be possible to eliminate the time-consuming and inconvenient simulation procedures currently needed for treatment planning. This would decrease the time and cost of arriving at a treatment plan while increasing tumor localization accuracy at the same time. It is also likely that CT scanning can provide radiation therapists with a more accurate appreciation of the complex density relationships of intracranial structures necessary for compensation techniques in both photon and proton therapy. The aim, once again, would be to maximize high-dose potential.

INTERACTIVE GRAPHICS: HISTOGRAMS, VOLUME ESTIMATES

Data from the preceding case provided an opportunity to isolate a selected portion of a CT image and generate a histogram of the absorption values within that selected area.[40] Fig. 5-15 shows an early example of a contrast enhancement profile of this patient's tumor. The approach was to prepare CT absorption value histograms from the tumor area of CT scans obtained before administration of contrast material as well as 5 and 15 minutes, respectively, after ad-

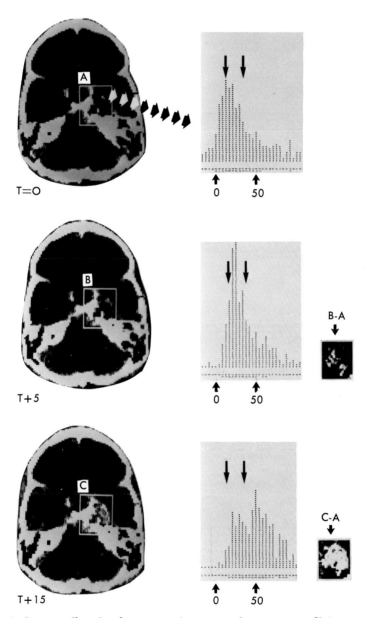

Fig. 5-15. Right parasellar chondrosarcoma (contrast enhancement profile). Using an interactive graphics capability, the same area has been isolated from the three CT scans obtained before contrast enhancement and at 5 and 15 minutes following infusion of 300 ml of 30% methylglucamine diatrizoate. Second column contains computer-generated histograms of absorption values within this selected region. With this capability it is possible to study the time course of contrast enhancement and correlate it with the histology of the tumor. Third column demonstrates an ability to subtract images or portions of images.

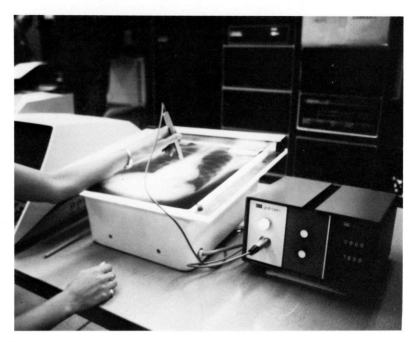

Fig. 5-16. Tracing device for interactive graphics work. Instrument shown is a sonic digitizer known as a Graf pen and is used for transferring x-y edge coordinates of a traced object into the computer. These digital data can then be used for area and volume measurements.

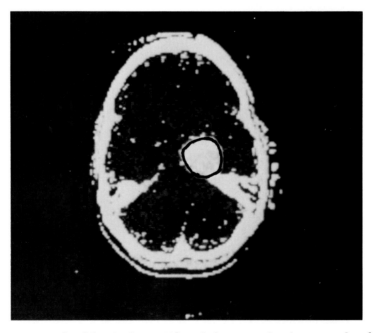

Fig. 5-17. Tumor outlined by Graf pen. Edge of this tumor has been traced and resulting series of x-y coordinates transferred to the computer in digital form for area and volume calculations. Since tracing device allows an irregular object to be isolated, it is superior to the capability that isolated rectangular area in Fig. 5-15.

STUDY NUMBER; 1 - CHRONDROSARCOMA

CT SECTION 1
    AREA OF CURVE 1= 1.81 SQ. CM.   SLICE DEPTH= 0.20 CM.   VOLUME= 0.36 CC.

CT SECTION 2
    AREA OF CURVE 1= 2.97 SQ. CM.   SLICE DEPTH= 0.20 CM.   VOLUME= 0.59 CC.

CT SECTION 3
    AREA OF CURVE 1= 2.78 SQ. CM.   SLICE DEPTH= 0.20 CM.   VOLUME= 0.56 CC.

CT SECTION 4
    AREA OF CURVE 1= 4.18 SQ. CM.   SLICE DEPTH= 0.20 CM.   VOLUME= 0.84 CC.

CT SECTION 5
    AREA OF CURVE 1= 4.25 SQ. CM.   SLICE DEPTH= 0.20 CM.   VOLUME= 0.85 CC.

CT SECTION 6
    AREA OF CURVE 1= 3.90 SQ. CM.   SLICE DEPTH= 0.20 CM.   VOLUME= 0.78 CC.

• • • • • • •

CT SECTION 12
    AREA OF CURVE 1= 0.33 SQ. CM.   SLICE DEPTH= 0.20 CM.   VOLUME= 0.07 CC.
CT SECTION 12
    AREA OF CURVE 2= 1.09 SQ. CM.   SLICE DEPTH= 0.20 CM.   VOLUME= 0.22 CC.

• • • • • • •

CT SECTION 15
    AREA OF CURVE 1= 2.01 SQ. CM.   SLICE DEPTH= 0.20 CM.   VOLUME= 0.40 CC.

CT SECTION 16
    AREA OF CURVE 1= 1.83 Sq. CM.   SLICE DEPTH= 0.20 CM.   VOLUME= 0.37 CC.

STUDY NUMBER: 1-CHRONDROSARCOMA | 16 IMAGES   TOTAL VOLUME= 8.91 CC. OR 8,910 CU. ML. |

Fig. 5-18. Interactive volume estimation. Computer printout of area and volume calculations from a series of horizontal CT sections of tumor. Total volume estimate was 8.91 cc or 8910 cu ml (see box at bottom). Note that on CT section 12 (middle) it is possible to trace more than one area in a single CT section.

ministration of contrast material. The histograms changed over time, indicating acquisition of iodonated contrast material by the tumor (Fig. 5-15). Faster scanners will provide more precise contrast enhancement profiles and therefore a better correlation between these characteristics and the histology of various tumors. Fig. 5-15 also illustrates the ability to subtract images or portions of images from one another.

Another form of interactive graphics is illustrated by the use of a tracing device (Fig. 5-16). With this instrument the boundaries of an object such as a tumor (Fig. 5-17) can be traced. The computer can then compute a surface area, which, when coupled with the CT section's thickness, provides a sectional volume determination. This approach can be repeated on a series of adjacent CT images to determine the total volume of a tumor (Fig. 5-18), ventricle, hemorrhage, or other structure.

THREE-DIMENSIONAL DISPLAYS

Special computer programs that "look through" the three-dimensional data array from arbitrary angular perspectives have been able to provide shaded three-dimensional images. Our initial report of this capability illustrated the three-dimensional visualization of a ventricular system with a series of postmortem CT scans.[25] The images in Fig. 5-19 represent our first attempt to apply these techniques to patient data. This example is from the chondrosarcoma case presented previously.

A series of shaded three-dimensional images (Fig. 5-19) have been generated at 5° intervals from 0° to 360°. When these images are viewed rapidly on a tape-driven CT viewer,[16] the effect is a shaded and rotating visualization of this tumor. The same data can be combined as stereo pairs (Fig. 5-20). Work is continuing on alternative ways of generating three-dimensional displays.

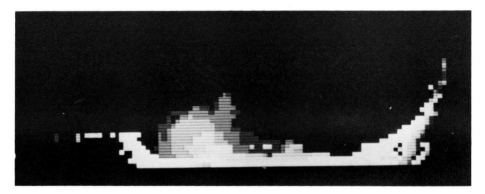

Fig. 5-19. Right parasellar chondrosarcoma (frontal view). This is an anteroposterior shaded pseudo-three-dimensional image in which gray scale no longer represents absorption value but distance from image plane. Objects shown had absorption values falling within a range low enough to encompass contrast-enhanced tumor and high enough to include bony structures. Lighter areas are closer to image plane; shaded areas are more posterior or further from image plane. Compare this single image with Fig. 5-11, which shows similar nonshaded coronal views of this right parasellar chondrosarcoma.

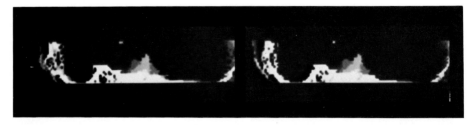

Fig. 5-20. Stereo images of right parasellar chondrosarcoma (lateral view). This pair of stereo images shows right petrous bone and mastoid air cells in foreground. Tumor mass is shown as a shaded gray area in background. Portions of the calvarium are seen at extreme left and right edges of these images.

CLINICAL EXAMPLES OF ALTERNATIVE DISPLAY FORMATS

The outline that follows, based on our initial 45 cases, summarizes the intracranial areas that may benefit from the multiplanar technique and the reasons why multiplanar capability has potential clinical benefit.[25] The example cases in this section illustrate many of these points:

1. Orbits
    a. Complementary views of intraorbital structures
    b. Increased definition from very thin CT planes that minimize partial volume artifacts, particularly adjacent to bone
    c. More complete evaluation of masses growing from frontal sinuses, posterior ethmoidal sinuses, or nasal cavity into the orbit (and vice versa)
    d. Better definition of cribriform plate and orbital apex lesions with extensions to or from medial sphenoid wing or anterior temporal lobe
2. Sellar and parasellar region
    a. Better demonstration of sellar floor, lateral walls of sphenoid sinus, and chiasmatic cistern
    b. Multiplanar studies replace or complement pneumoencephalography with polytomes and make possible postoperative or postirradiation assessment of sellar or parasellar tumors, aneurysms, etc.
3. Posterior fossa
    a. Improved definition of cerebellopontine angle or brain-stem lesions
    b. Further evaluation of interpeduncular cistern, pontine cistern, superior cerebellar cistern, and fourth ventricle
    c. Decreased need for pneumoencephalography (with tomography) for brain-stem evaluation
    d. Decreased need for pantopaque cisternography in some cases of cerebellopontine angle tumor
    e. Optimal midline visualization of cerebellar vermis abnormalities
4. Base of brain and other areas
    a. Minimized partial volume artifact adjacent to basal bone structures
    b. Good visualization of floor and anterior wall of middle fossa, orbital roof, and planum sphenoidale
    c. Increased accuracy in evaluation of the ventricular system and basal cisternal spaces
    d. Volume estimates of tumors, hemorrhages, aneurysms, etc.
    e. Aid in differentiating extra-axial versus intra-axial lesions
    f. More accurate detection of subdural hematomas using, for example, oblique CT coronal section similar to oblique angiographic films
    g. Better detection of multiple lesions using combined CT views for evaluation of patients with metastatic versus primary tumors
    h. Better definition of high-convexity lesions under tangential projections of bone

Fig. 5-21 demonstrates coronal and sagittal orbital views of a normal patient and of a patient with Graves' disease. Both an axial and a lateral view of the optic nerve are shown (Fig. 5-21, *B* and *C*). A comparison between normal and edematous superior muscles is provided (Fig. 5-21, *B* and *E*). Fig. 5-22 is an example of a right lacrimal gland tumor seen in coronal, sagittal, and transverse sections. The relationship of this tumor to the right globe and the extension of the tumor into the retrobulbar area is well documented in these sections. Other orbital cases (not shown) include an example of optic nerve meningioma extending from the right retrobulbar area into the orbital apex and and optic canal. Another case illustrated a metallic foreign body embedded in the wall of the globe.[25] Collectively, these cases suggest that multiplanar CT evalua-

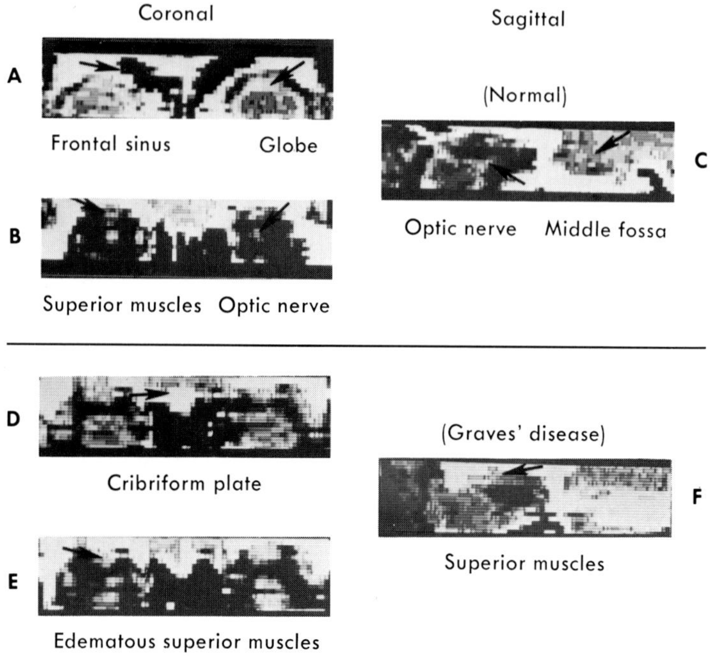

Coronal

Sagittal

A

Frontal sinus Globe

(Normal)

C

Optic nerve Middle fossa

B

Superior muscles Optic nerve

D

Cribriform plate

(Graves' disease)

F

Superior muscles

E

Edematous superior muscles

Fig. 5-21. Coronal and sagittal CT sections of orbits. *A* to *C* are from a normal patient and illustrate relationship of globes, frontal sinuses, superior muscles, and optic nerves. *D* to *F* illustrate abnormally large superior muscles in a patient with Graves' disease.

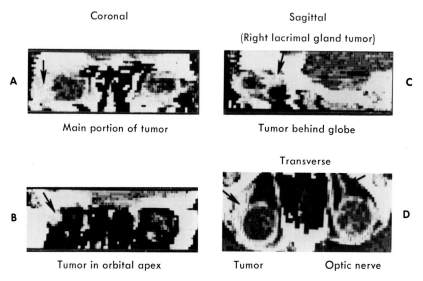

Coronal

Sagittal

(Right lacrimal gland tumor)

A

Main portion of tumor

C

Tumor behind globe

B

Tumor in orbital apex

Transverse

D

Tumor Optic nerve

Fig. 5-22. Multiplanar CT views of right lacrimal gland tumor. Selected coronal, sagittal, and transverse images show relationship of this tumor lateral to right globe and also tumor's extension behind right globe.

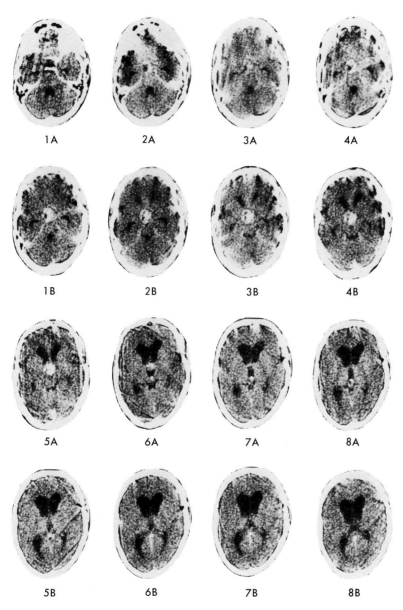

Fig. 5-23. Suprasellar tumor (transverse images). These horizontal CT sections are arranged in ascending order and represent eight pairs of scans obtained in an overlapped fashion at eight scan levels. (See Fig. 5-8.) Tumor demonstrates contrast enhancement (after 300 ml of 30% methylglucamine diatrizoate), which is not homogeneous, and on several images there appears to be a cystic or partially necrotic area of this lesion on the left. Its location as shown here is midline, near inferior portion of both frontal horns (*4B, 5A*) and just below third ventricle (*6A*). Histologically this proved to be a craniopharyngioma.

Coronal

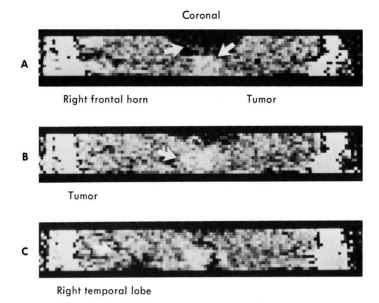

Right frontal horn   Tumor

Tumor

Right temporal lobe

Fig. 5-24. Suprasellar tumor (coronal sections). Relationship of this tumor to inferior portions of both frontal horns is easily seen in these coronal sections, which are reconstructed from transverse images in Fig. 5-23.

tion of the orbit is superior to ultrasound capabilities in the retrobulbar area and complementary to ultrasound for the more superficial and anterior structures in the orbit.[14, 15]

Figs. 5-23 to 5-25 are multiplanar views of a suprasellar tumor. The coronal views (Fig. 5-24) demonstrate the relationship of the tumor mass to the floor of both anterior horns. The sagittal views (Fig. 5-25) show the tumor's relationship to both the frontal horn of the lateral ventricle and the anterior inferior portion of the third ventricle. Other sellar and parasellar cases (not shown) include a case of partially empty sella (not confirmed at pneumo-encephalography), another case of suprasellar mass, a colloid cyst of the third ventricle, and a large lipomatous right parasellar lesion involving the right hypothalamic region.[25]

Figs. 5-26 and 5-27 represent our first case of posterior fossa abnormality, a left cerebellar hemangioblastoma.[28] The 2.0 mm horizontal sections at the bottom of Fig. 5-26 represent an improvement over the transverse visualization of this abnormality compared with the thicker 8.0 mm scans at the top of Fig. 5-26. Nonetheless, the low-absorption left cerebellar tumor was easily seen without contrast enhancement in both the coronal and sagittal sections (Fig. 5-27). Other cases of posterior fossa abnormalities (not shown) include several acoustic neurinomas and one tiny localized area of fatty tissue in the quadrigeminal cistern.[25] One of the acoustic neurinomas was quite small and therefore best demonstrated in an oblique plane parallel to the long axis of the petrous bone. The advantages of an oblique orientation in this case were twofold. First, the

Sagittal

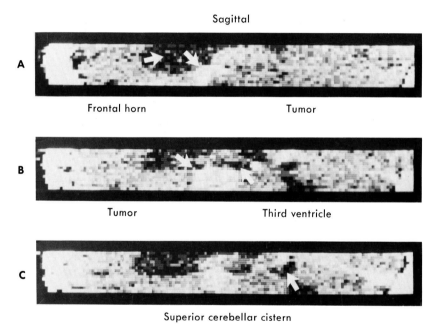

Fig. 5-25. Suprasellar tumor (sagittal images). Relationship of this tumor to anterior, inferior portion of third ventricle *(B)* is better characterized here than on either the transverse or coronal sections. These images also were reconstructed from transverse images of Fig. 5-23.

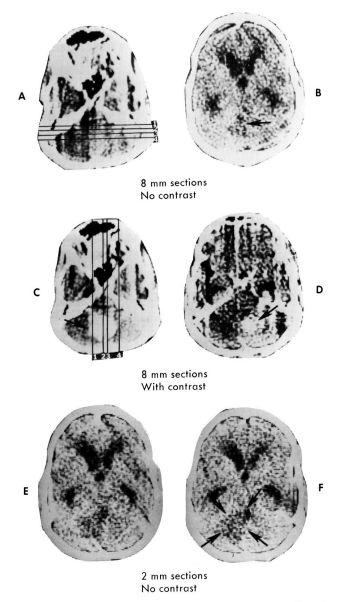

8 mm sections
No contrast

8 mm sections
With contrast

2 mm sections
No contrast

Fig. 5-26. Left cerebellar tumor (transverse images). *A* and *B* are selected views from this patient's initial CT study obtained without contrast material using "thick" 8.0 mm sections. At best, there is only the suspicion of an area of low absorption within left cerebellar hemisphere. *C* and *D* are similar 8.0 mm sections following contrast enhancement (with 300 ml of 30% methylglucamine diatrizoate). *C* shows an obvious area of increased vascularity in medial portion of left cerebellar hemisphere extending across midline. *E* and *F* represent 2.0 mm interpolated transverse planes. Partial volume artifact inherent in thicker sections has been removed in these images without contrast. The clearer delineation of an area of low absorption in these thin sections when compared with the thicker images of *A* and *B* is the same effect noted with the removal of partial volume artifact in the phantom experiment (Fig. 5-3). Numbered lines in *A* and *C* correspond to plane of reconstructed coronal and sagittal images in Fig. 5-27. Histologically this tumor proved to be a cerebellar hemangioblastoma. (From Glenn, et al.: Invest. Radiol. **10**:479, 1975.)

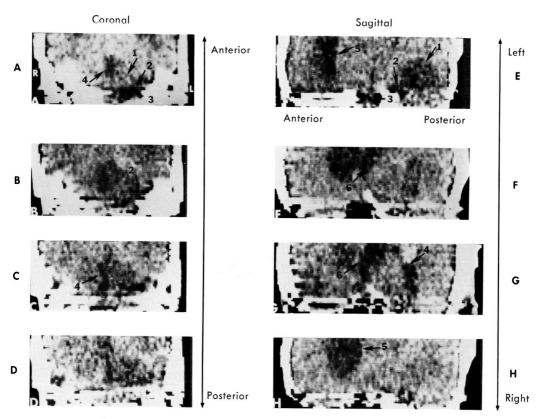

Fig. 5-27. Left cerebellar tumor (coronal and sagittal images). Locations of these anatomic sections are noted by numbered lines in Fig. 5-26, *A* and *C*. Coronal images show an area of slightly low absorption (*1*) corresponding to the tumor, low absorption changes (*2*) adjacent to posterior portion of left petrous pyramid (*3*), and the fourth ventricle (*4*). These structures are similarly numbered in the sagittal images *E* and *F*. In addition, anterior horns of lateral ventricles (*5*) as well as third ventricle (*6*) are shown in sagittal planes. These images without contrast left little doubt as to both the existence and the location of this patient's abnormality. (From Glenn, et al.: Invest. Radiol. **10**:479, 1975.)

tumor was visualized along its maximum diameter, and second, the oblique plane cut through the tumor but not the dense petrous bone immediately adjacent to the tumor. Another larger acoustic neurinoma was important in that the multiplanar technique provided the basis for stereotactically necrotizing the central core of this tumor with proton beam irradiation. This approach has been used several times to temporize in patients who are not immediate candidates for surgery but whose tumors are causing increasing symptoms.[25]

Fig. 5-28 is a series of coronal images showing various portions of the ventricular system as well as important basal cisternal spaces. Figs. 5-29 to 5-31 are multiplanar CT examples of the use of water-soluble metrizamide within the basal cisternal spaces. Comparison with Fig. 5-28 (no metrizamide) indicates equally good visualization of the ambient, quadrigeminal, and superior cerebellar cisterns. The metrizamide, however, offers an additional opportunity to visualize retropulvinar cisterns as well as the cistern velum interpositum in both the

Text continued on p. 119.

Coronal

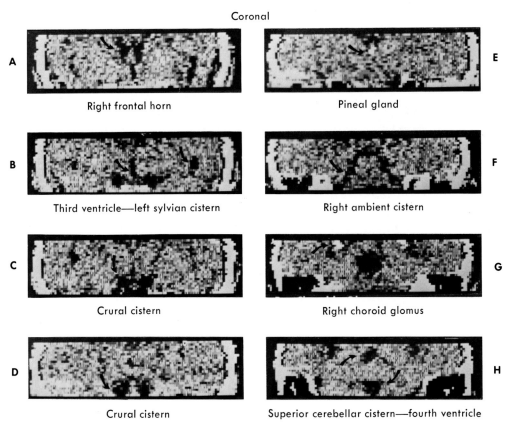

Right frontal horn   Pineal gland

Third ventricle—left sylvian cistern   Right ambient cistern

Crural cistern   Right choroid glomus

Crural cistern   Superior cerebellar cistern—fourth ventricle

Fig. 5-28. Normal basal cisternal spaces. This series of coronal images demonstrates right frontal horn *(A)*, third ventricle *(B)*, and fourth ventricle *(H)*. Important cisternal spaces include sylvian cistern *(B)*, crural cistern *(C* and *D)*, ambient cistern *(F)*, and superior cerebellar cistern *(H)*.

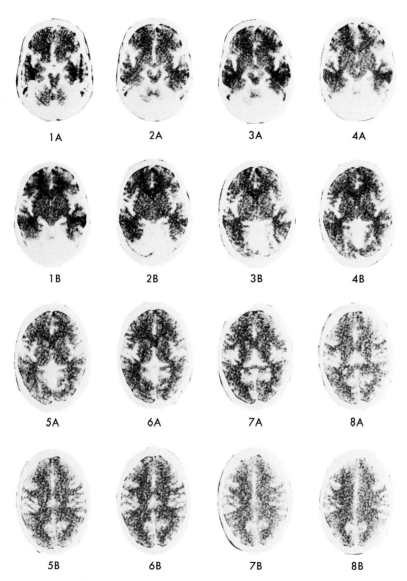

Fig. 5-29. Metrizamide enhancement of basal cisternal spaces. This series of transverse images arranged in ascending order represents eight pairs of CT scans obtained in an overlapped fashion at eight scan levels. (See Fig. 5-8.) These images provide the basis for the reconstruction of coronal and sagittal sections in Figs. 5-30 and 5-31. Positive contrast obtained with water-soluble metrizamide outlines sylvian cisterns (*1A* to *4B*), interhemispheric fissure (*1A* and *2A*), interpeduncular and ambient cisterns (*1A* to *3A*), retropulvinar cisterns (*4B* and *5A*), and superior cerebellar cistern (*4B* to *6A*). Contrast-enhanced area extending anterior from quadrigeminal cistern in *6A* is probably cistern velum interpositum.

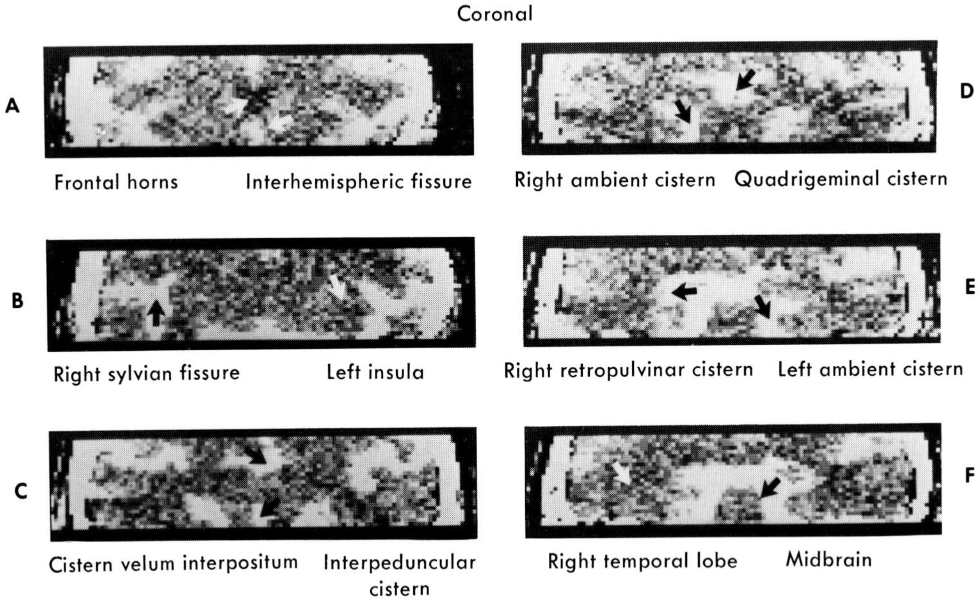

Coronal

Fig. 5-30. Metrizamide enhancement of basal cisternal spaces (coronal images). These reconstructed images from transverse sections in Fig. 5-29 should be compared with coronal sections (without metrizamide) in Fig. 5-28. Important CSF spaces demonstrated by metrizamide are interhemispheric fissure *(A)*, right sylvian fissure *(B)*, cistern velum interpositum *(C)*, interpeduncular cistern *(C)*, right ambient cistern *(D)*, quadrigeminal cistern *(D)*, and right retropulvinar cistern *(E)*. Midbrain *(F)* is outlined by positive contrast material in ambient and quadrigeminal cisterns.

Sagittal

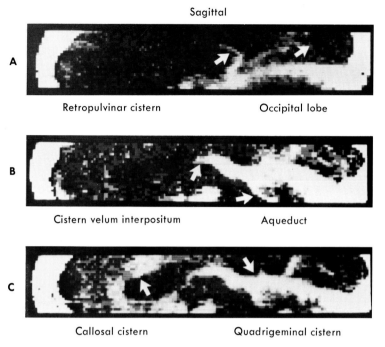

A

Retropulvinar cistern   Occipital lobe

B

Cistern velum interpositum   Aqueduct

C

Callosal cistern   Quadrigeminal cistern

Fig. 5-31. Metrizamide enhancement of basal cisternal spaces (sagittal images). These three sagittal sections from overlapped horizontal images of Fig. 5-29 demonstrate retropulvinar cistern *(A)*, cisternal velum interpositum *(B)*, aqueduct *(B)*, callosal cistern *(C)*, and quadrigeminal cistern *(C)*. Such views allow distinction of infratentorial from supratentorial abnormalities with relative ease. In midline section of *C*, cerebellar vermis is outlined superiorly by metrizamide within superior cerebellar cistern.

Coronal   Sagittal

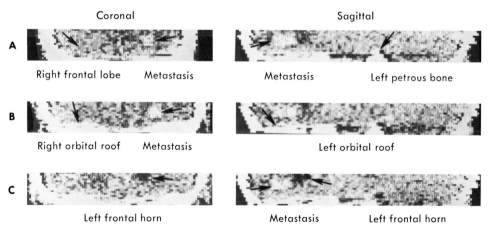

A

Right frontal lobe   Metastasis   Metastasis   Left petrous bone

B

Right orbital roof   Metastasis   Left orbital roof

C

Left frontal horn   Metastasis   Left frontal horn

Fig. 5-32. Solitary left frontal metastasis. These coronal and sagittal views demonstrate an elliptically shaped solitary metastatic lesion enhanced with contrast (300 ml of 30% methylglucamine diatrizoate). Lesion is located several millimeters above floor of anterior fossa. Posterior margin of this tumor is approximately 2.0 mm in front of anterior inferior portion of left frontal horn. Primary site of this tumor was the lung.

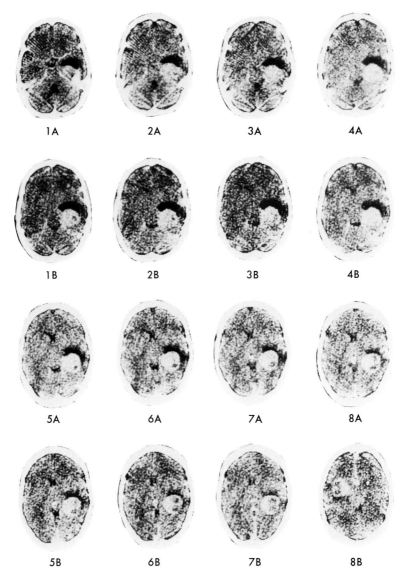

Fig. 5-33. Obstructed right temporal horn (transverse images). This series of transverse CT sections is arranged in ascending order and represents pairs of scans obtained in an overlapped fashion at eight scan levels. (See Fig. 5-8.) Right temporal tumor is enhanced with contrast (300 ml of 30% methylglucamine diatrizoate). Low absorption area directly anterior and lateral to this large tumor is an obstructed right temporal horn. Pathologic diagnosis of lesion was glioblastoma.

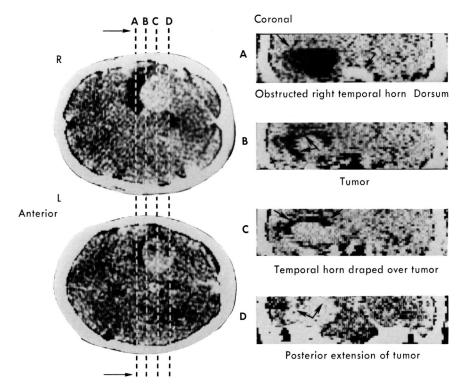

Fig. 5-34. Obstructed right temporal horn (coronal images). These coronal images show obstructed right temporal tip *(A)* and, further posteriorly, draping effect of temporal horn over tumor *(B* and *C)*. Some higher horizontal CT sections (Fig. 5-33, bottom transverse image) demonstrated what appeared to be a cystic portion of this tumor in area where temporal horn was draped over tumor. Coronal sections did not verify any cystic areas, and therefore cystic appearance on horizontal sections was attributed to partial volume averaging of contrast-enhanced tumor and a superiorly draped obstructed temporal horn.

coronal and sagittal views. The interpeduncular cistern (Fig. 5-30, *C*) and the callosal cistern (Fig. 5-31, *C*) are difficult to identify without metrizamide.

Fig. 5-32 shows reconstructed coronal and sagittal images of a single, small, contrast-enhanced metastatic lesion very closely related to both the left orbital roof and the anterior horn of the left lateral ventricle. This lesion was subjected to a single necrotizing dose of proton beam irradiation, with the combined multiplanar CT images again serving as the basis for this treatment.

Figs. 5-33 and 5-34 show the horizontal and coronal views of a temporal lobe tumor that has obstructed the tip of the right temporal horn. Note the displaced temporal horn draped over the tumor (contrast-enhanced). An interesting point was that in some of the higher horizontal sections this obstructing tumor appeared to be partially cystic in nature. Because a similar cystic appearance was not identified in the thin coronal and sagittal sections, it was concluded that the cystic appearance was artifactual and resulted from the horizontal thick slice partial volume averaging of tumor plus dilated temporal horn.

FUTURE DEVELOPMENTS

This project of exploring alternative CT display formats has progressed through the stages of plantom experiments, early anatomic correlations with cadaver data, and initial clinical use involving 45 patients.[25-28] The transition to routine clinical use, however, will depend on the availability of more rapid analysis facilities. For this next step, the Department of Radiology at Massachusetts General Hospital and the Image Analysis Laboratory at the University of Missouri-Columbia have been joined by a third medical center, the Department of Radiology at the Memorial Hospital Medical Center, Long Beach, California. At this third site, the following modifications have been implemented to provide the technical capability for routine clinical use of the proficiencies described in this chapter.

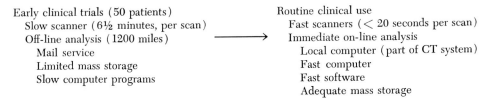

Early clinical trials (50 patients)
    Slow scanner (6½ minutes, per scan)
    Off-line analysis (1200 miles)   ⟶
      Mail service
      Limited mass storage
      Slow computer programs

Routine clinical use
    Fast scanners (< 20 seconds per scan)
    Immediate on-line analysis
      Local computer (part of CT system)
      Fast computer
      Fast software
      Adequate mass storage

Fig. 5-35 illustrates the computer-viewer configuration that will be used for reviewing CT images and carrying out any alternative image manipulation and display capabilities desired.

Recent success in transposing horizontal ultrasound data into alternative coronal and sagittal display formats provides an additional area for future investigation by the centers that have successfully participated in this CT work.

Reports on the feasibility of direct coronal CT scanning[30, 57] provide a different approach to alternative planes of view from the one presented here. The benefits of direct coronal scanning are the same as those presented in the coronal examples in this chapter. Both methods require a slightly higher irradiation dose, which is not considered a deterrent to either method, provided careful patient selection is made. The potential advantages of reprocessing horizontal data into the alternative display formats presented here compared to direct coronal CT scanning are as follows:

1. The CT sections are much thinner.
2. There are additional sagittal and oblique plane options.
3. The reformatted displays (sagittal, coronal, and oblique) represent a complete front-to-back or side-to-side series of parallel planes.
4. Our approach is equally valid for cranial scanning and body scanning; direct coronal scanning, on the other hand, is limited to cranial work only.
5. The multiplanar technique eliminates the need for patient positions (e.g., hyperextension of the neck) that may be difficult to attain or maintain.
6. The method is applicable to both early scanning systems and the newer, faster machines.

Although our overlap approach in gathering data is potentially susceptible to

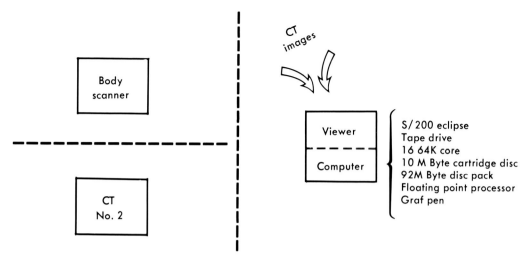

Fig. 5-35. CT viewing system separate from scanners. Schematic illustration of the separate CT viewing room equipped with a CT viewing console that has been directly interfaced to a dedicated computer. The radiology department at Memorial Hospital Medical Center of Long Beach, California, has augmented the viewing computer's peripheral equipment, as shown here, for the purpose of bringing into routine on-line clinical operation the advanced image manipulation and display capability discussed throughout this chapter. The facility is set up to process data originating from both in-house CT scanning systems as well as CT systems in other hospitals. The intent is to share with others the CT capabilities that have been developed until such time as those capabilities are routinely available from CT manufacturers.

patient motion, this caused difficulty in only 2 of the initial 45 cases. Faster scanners will further minimize this potential problem.

SUMMARY

The purpose of this chapter has been to summarize with clinical examples a number of image manipulation and display capabilities that have been developed to extend the well-documented usefulness of transverse computed tomography. For a significant number of patients undergoing CT examinations, present cross-sectional scanners can be used in a more specialized mode for diagnosis and as an adjunct in treatment. In cases in which a definite abnormality is established, the multiplanar technique provides a more careful assessment of the three-dimensional morphology, which not only assists in the differential diagnosis but also in the careful geometric considerations related to both the surgical approach and radiation therapy. When the case is less clear-cut and the presence of a lesion is not established with horizontal sections alone, the added CT perspectives may provide important additional information. By imparting a greater sense of confidence about the presence or absence of a lesion, these perspectives directly affect subsequent decisions about hospital admission and further diagnostic procedures. The trend toward increased cross-sectional resolution and faster scanning in the newer CT systems will significantly benefit the image manipulation and display capabilities described in this chapter.

Acknowledgment

We are indebted to Nadim Sawaya, Greg Larson, Ray Sprague, Stan Bennett, and Robert Crivello for their significant contributions to this project.

References

1. Abramowitz, K.: Economics of computerized scanning, Research paper, Harvard Business School, Cambridge, Mass., 1975.
2. Alfidi, R. J., et al.: Computed tomography of the thorax and abdomen; a preliminary report, Radiology **114**:257, 1975.
3. Ambrose, J.: Computerized transverse axial scanning (tomography); 2. Clinical application, Br. J. Radiol. **46**:1023, 1973.
4. Ambrose, J., and Hounsfield, G. N.: Computerized transverse axial tomography, Br. J. Radiol. **46**:148, 1973.
5. Ambrose, J., Lloyd, G.: and Wright, J.: A preliminary evaluation of fine matrix computerized axial tomography (emiscan) in the diagnosis of orbital space-occupying lesions, Br. J. Radiol. **47**:747, 1974.
6. Baker, H. L.: The impact of computed tomography on neuroradiologic practice, Radiology **116**:637, 1975.
7. Baker, H. L., Campbell, J. K., and Houser, D.: Computer-assisted tomography of the head; an early evaluation, Mayo Clin. Proc. **49**:17, 1974.
8. Baker, H. L., et al.: Computerized transaxial tomography in neuro-ophthalmology, Am. J. Ophthalmol. **78**:285, 1974.
9. Baker, H. L., et al.: Early experience with EMI scanning for study of the brain, Radiology **116**:327, 1975.
10. Baker, H. L., et al.: Computerized tomography of the head, J.A.M.A. **233**:1304, 1975.
11. Brownell, G. L., et al.: Transverse section imaging of radionuclide distributions in heart, lung and brain. In Ter-Pogossian, M. M., Phelps, M. E., and Brownell, G. L., editors: Workshop on Reconstruction Tomography in Diagnostic Radiology and Nuclear Medicine, P. R., April 17-19, 1975, Baltimore, 1977, University Park Press.
12. Budinger, T. F., and Gullberg, G.: Transverse section imaging with gamma ray emitting radionuclides. In Ter-Pogossian, M. M., Phelps, M. E., and Brownell, G. L., editors: Workshop on Reconstruction Tomography in Diagnostic Radiology and Nuclear Medicine, P. R., April 17-19, 1975, Baltimore, 1977, University Park Press.
13. Cho, Z. H., Ericksson, L., and Chan, J.: Preliminary results on circular ring transverse axial positron camera for dynamic function studies and static 3-D image reconstruction. In Ter-Pogossian, M. M., Phelps, M. E., and Brownell, G. L., editors: Workshop on Reconstruction Tomography in Diagnostic Radiology and Nuclear Medicine, P. R., April 17-19, 1975, Baltimore, 1977, University Park Press.
14. Coleman, D. J., et al.: High-resolution B-scan ultrasonography. V. Eye changes of Graves' disease; VI. Pseudotumors of orbit, Arch. Ophthalmol. **88**:465, 1972.
15. Coleman, D. J., Jack, R. L., and Franzen, L. A.: High resolution B-scan ultrasonography of the orbit; I. The normal orbit; II. Hemangioma of the orbit; III. Lymphoma of the orbit; IV. Neurogenic tumors of the orbit, Arch. Ophthalmol. **88**:355, 1972.
16. Conway, M. E., and Glenn, W. V., Jr.: Remote CT viewing system. In Computed Cranial Tomography: International Symposium and Course, Hamilton, Bermuda, March 10-15, 1975.
17. Crocker, E. F., Zimmerman, R. A., Phelps, M. E., and Kuhl, D. E.: The effect of steroids on the extravascular distribution of radiographic contrast material and technetium pertechnetate in brain tumors as determined by computed tomography, Radiology **119**:471, 1976.
18. Davis, D. O.: Anatomic-pathologic CT patterns and densities and their clinical utilization. In Ter-Pogossian, M. M., Phelps, M. E., and Brownell, G. L., editors: Workshop on Reconstruction

Tomography in Diagnostic Radiology and Nuclear Medicine, P. R., April 17-19, 1975, Baltimore, 1977, University Park Press.

19. Davis, D. O., and Pressman, B. D.: Computerized tomography of the brain, Radiol. Cl. North Am. **12**:297, 1974.

20. Davis, K. R., et al.: Diagnosis of epidermoid tumor by computed tomography, Radiology **119**:347, 1976.

21. Deck, M. D. F., Messina, A. V., and Sackett, J. F.: Computed tomography in metastatic disease of the brain, Radiology **119**:115, 1976.

22. DiChiro, G., et al.: Computerized axial tomography in syringomyelia, N. Engl. J. Med. **292**:13, 1975.

23. DiChiro, G., and Schellinger, D.: Computed tomography of spinal cord after lumbar intrathecal introduction of metrizamide (computer-assisted myelography), Radiology **120**:101, 1976.

24. Gawler, J., et al.: Computer-assisted tomography (EMI scanner). Its place in investigation of suspected intracranial tumors, Lancet **2**:419, 1974.

25. Glenn, W. V., Davis, K. R., and Dwyer, S. J.: Sagittal, coronal, and oblique computed cranial tomographic (CCT) images: clinical examples. (Submitted for publication.)

26. Glenn, W. V., et al.: Clinical feasibility of reconstructing coronal, sagittal, and thin transverse sections from overlapped 8.0 mm CT scans. In Ter-Pogossian, M. M., Phelps, M. E., and Brownell, G. L., editors: Workshop on Reconstruction Tomography in Diagnostic Radiology and Nuclear Medicine, P. R., April 17-19, 1975, Baltimore, 1977, University Park Press.

27. Glenn, W. V., Johnston, R. J., Morton, P. E., and Dwyer, S. J.: Image generation and display techniques for CT scan data: thin transverse and reconstructed coronal and sagittal planes, Invest. Radiol. **10**:403, 1975.

28. Glenn, W. V., Johnston, R. J., Morton, P. E., and Dwyer, S. J.: Further investigation and initial clinical use of advanced CT display capability, Invest. Radiol. **10**:479, 1975.

29. Greitz, T., and Hindmarsh, T.: Computer-assisted tomography of intracranial CSF circulation using a water-soluble contrast medium, Acta Radiol. [Diag.] **15**:497, 1974.

30. Hammerschlag, S. B., Wolpert, S. M., and Carter, B. L.: Computed coronal tomography, Radiology **120**:219, 1976.

31. Hounsfield, G. N.: Computerized transverse axial scanning (tomography). I. Description of system, Br. J. Radiol. **46**:1016, 1973.

32. Kramer, R. A., Janetos, G. P., and Perlstein, G.: An approach to contrast enhancement in computed tomography of the brain, Radiology **116**:641, 1975.

33. Kuhl, D. E., and Edwards, R. Q.: The Mark IV system for emission computerized tomography and quantitative reconstruction of brain radioactivity (abstr.), J. Nucl. Med. **16**:543, 1975.

34. Kuhl, D. E., and Edwards, R. Q.: Mark IV CT system for quantitative radionuclide imaging. In Ter-Pogossian, M. M., Phelps, M. E., and Brownell, G. L., editors: Workshop on Reconstruction Tomography in Diagnostic Radiology and Nuclear Medicine, P. R., April 17-19, 1975, Baltimore, 1977, University Park Press.

35. Lambert, V. L., Zelch, J. V., and Cohen, D. N.: Computed tomography of the orbits, Radiology **113**:351, 1974.

36. McCullough, E. C., et al.: An evaluation of the quantitative and radiation features of a scanning x-ray transverse axial tomograph: the EMI scanner, Radiology **111**:709, 1974.

37. McCullough, E. C., et al.: Performance evaluation and quality assurance of computed tomography scanners, with illustrations from the EMI, ACTA, and Delta scanners, Radiology **120**:173, 1976.

38. Metrizamide, a non-ionic water-soluble contrast medium, experimental and preliminary clinical investigations (series of papers), Acta Radiol. Supp. 335, pp. 1-390, 1975.

39. Naidich, T. P., et al.: Evaluation of pediatric hydrocephalus by computed tomography, Radiology **119**:337, 1976.

40. Naidich, T. P., et al.: Evaluation of sellar and parasellar masses by computed tomography, Radiology **120**:91, 1976.

41. New, P. F. J.: Present limitations of computed tomography of the head with the EMI scanner. In Ter-Pogossian, M. M., Phelps, M. E., and Brownell, G. L., editors: Workshop on Reconstruction Tomography in Diagnostic Radiology and Nuclear Medicine, P.R., April 17-19, 1975, Baltimore, 1977, University Park Press.

42. New, P. F. J., et al.: Computerized axial tomography with the EMI scanner, Radiology **110**:109, 1974.

43. New, P. F. J., et al.: Computed tomography (CT) with the EMI scanner in the diagnosis of primary and metastatic intracranial neoplasms, Radiology **114**:75, 1975.

44. Ommaya, A. K.: Computerized axial tomography of the head; the EMI scanner, a new device for direct examination of the brain, "in vivo," Surg. Neurol. **1**:217, 1973.

45. Paxton, R., and Ambrose, J.: The EMI scanner; a brief review of the first 650 patients, Br. J. Radiol. **47**:530, 1974.

46. Perry, B. J., and Bridges, C.: Computerized transverse axial scanning (tomography). 3. Radiation dose considerations, Br. J. Radiol. **46**:1048, 1973.

47. Pevsner, P. H., Garcia-Bunuel, R., Leeds, N., and Finkelstein, M.: Subependymal and intraventricular hemorrhage in neonates, Radiology **119**:111, 1976.

48. Phelps, M. E., et al.: II. Performance analysis of a positron transaxial tomograph (PETT). In Ter-Pogossian, M. M., Phelps, M. E., and Brownell, G. L., editors: Workshop on Reconstruction Tomography in Diagnostic Radiology and Nuclear Medicine, P. R., April 17-19, 1975, Baltimore, 1977, University Park Press.

49. Potchen, E. J.: Diagnostic radiology—planning for the future, (editorial), Radiology **120**:227, 1976.

50. Roberson, G. H., et al.: CSF enhancement for computerized tomography, Surg. Neurol. (In press.)

51. Sagel, S., Stanley, R. J., and Evens, R. G.: Early clinical experience with motionless whole-body computed tomography, Radiology **119**:321, 1976.

52. Schellinger, D., et al.: Early clinical experience with the ACTA scanner, Radiology **114**:257, 1975.

53. Scott, W. R., et al.: Computerized axial tomography of intracerebral and intraventricular hemorrhage, Radiology **112**:73, 1974.

54. Stephens, D. H., Hattery, R. R., and Sheedy, P. F.: Computed tomography of the abdomen, Radiology **119**:331, 1976.

55. Ter-Pogossian, M. M., Phelps, M. E., Hoffman, E. J., and Coleman, R. E.: I. Performance analysis of a positron transaxial tomograph (PETT). In Ter-Pogossian, M. M., Phelps, M. E., and Brownell, G. L., editors: Workshop on Reconstruction Tomography in Diagnostic Radiology and Nuclear Medicine, P. R., April 17-19, 1975, Baltimore, 1977, University Park Press.

56. Twigg, H. L., Axelbaum, S. P., and Schellinger, D.: Computerized body tomography with the ACTA scanner, J.A.M.A. **234**:314, 1975.

57. Wolf, B. S., Nakagawa, H., and Staulcup, P. H.: Feasibility of coronal views in computed scanning of the head, Radiology **120**:217, 1976.

6 Radiologic detection of breast cancer

John R. Milbrath, Katherine A. Shaffer, and James E. Youker

HISTORY OF MAMMOGRAPHY

Mammography was probably done soon after the discovery of x rays, but it was not until 1930 that Warren[52] first reported its usefulness in the diagnosis of breast disease. The initial enthusiasm subsided in the late 1930s, however, and mammography was all but abandoned. Interest was rekindled briefly some 20 years later when Leborgne[28] described his radiographic method and findings, but only Gershon-Cohen persisted in the use of mammography.[12] In 1960 Egan[11] reported on 1000 cases and described his mammographic technique, which still remains in use today. This report was a milestone in radiographic evaluation of the breast. Training programs were then conducted, demonstrating that other radiologists could also obtain consistently high-quality films. Mammography steadily increased in popularity as more physicians became skilled in interpretation.

Two recent developments, xeroradiography and film-screen mammography, are the most widely used alternatives to conventional film mammography. Other methods, including thermography, ultrasound, contrast mammography, and electron radiography, have been proposed to evaluate breast disease.

FILM MAMMOGRAPHY

The great impetus to mammography came when techniques were developed using double-emulsion, fine-grain industrial film.[11] This film is still considered by many to provide the ultimate in mammographic study. The film is placed in a cardboard holder and used without an intensifying screen. An exposure of 1800 mAs, a kVp of 26 to 32, and a tube-film distance of 30 to 40 inches are required. No filtration is used other than the inherent filtration of the tube. Although industrial film initially required hand processing, it may now be developed automatically.

The radiation exposure necessary for the fine-grain industrial film technique is generally acceptable for the symptomatic patient. However, the de-

Supported in part by American Cancer Society Grant DPBC No. 5 and National Cancer Institute Contracts NO1-CN-55308 and NO1-CN-55247.

125

sire to extend mammography to large groups of asymptomatic women has led
to a search for accurate techniques at lower radiation levels. A significant break-
through in film mammography occurred when a single-emulsion screen-film combination in vacuum cassette was developed.[21] This system provides excellent
images at greatly reduced radiation levels. The Regional Centers for Radiological
Physics recently measured radiation doses at the twenty-seven Breast Cancer
Demonstration Projects jointly sponsored by the American Cancer Society
(ACS) and National Cancer Institute (NCI). The median exposure for screen-
film combinations ranged from 0.8 to 1.9 R.[10]

A current development offering further reduction in radiation is the combination of film and rare-earth screens. These combinations use screens composed
of terbium-activated rare-earth oxysulfides (gadolinium and lanthanum oxysulfides).[2] These new rare-earth phosphors are of particular interest in mammography because in the 38 to 70 keV range, their x-ray absorption coefficients are
higher than calcium tungstate. The major disadvantage of these screens is that
they emit light primarily in the green spectral range, and thus green-sensitive
film is needed to replace the standard blue-sensitive film.[7] A rare-earth screen
that emits blue light and can be used with standard film has recently been developed.[38]

It is important to bear in mind that as the radiation dose to the patient
decreases, the degree of resolution of the image also decreases. However,
lower resolution does not necessarily lessen diagnostic accuracy.

XERORADIOGRAPHY

Although Carlson developed the process in 1939, xeroradiography was not
generally available to the medical community until Wolfe's[55] refinements in the
late 1960s. Since that time, this process has been widely used, particularly in
urban centers.

In xeroradiography the radiographic film used in conventional mammography
is replaced by a selenium-coated aluminum plate. Selenium, a photoconductor,
can retain an electrical charge. The charge can be dissipated by light or x rays
and is lost in proportion to the photon flux reaching the plate. Charged particles
of blue toner are used in developing the electrostatic image. Either a positive
or negative image can be produced. This image is then transferred to a piece
of plastic-coated paper creating a mirror image. The paper is heated, and the
toner particles become embedded in the plastic. The entire developing process
takes 90 seconds.

Routinely, mediolateral and craniocaudal images are taken of each breast. If
an abnormality is not well visualized on the mediolateral view, a contact
lateral or lateromedial view may be helpful. If areas are not seen on the routine
craniocaudal view, a second image should be taken with the patient rotated
either medially or laterally. Compression of the breast by balloon or other
means improves visualization and reduces radiation.

Quality control can be easily maintained by a well-motivated technologist who understands the most common causes of poor imaging (Fig. 6-1). Exposures are made at 300 mAs with a varying kVp. In a properly exposed image the halo around the breast is about 1 mm, the skin is partially imaged, and the subcutaneous structures are well visualized (Fig. 6-2, *A*). In an overexposed image the halo is less than 1 mm, the skin is well seen, and detail, particularly in the subcutaneous region, is lost (Fig. 6-2, *B*). In an underexposed image the halo is greater than 1 mm, the skin is barely visible, and the image is too blue (Fig. 6-2, *C*).

The radiation dose in xeroradiography is, in general, lower than in conventional film mammography but higher than with screen-film mammography. At the ACS-NCI Breast Cancer Demonstration Projects the median exposure for xeroradiography ranged from 1.9 to 4.1 R.[10] The dose for tubes equipped with molybdenum targets was consistently 0.5 to 1.0 R higher than similar tubes equipped with tungsten targets. In addition, contrast is higher with molybdenum targets; therefore most authorities[9, 55] recommend using tungsten targets for xeroradiography. By adding a 1.5 mm aluminum filter, we have reduced the radiation dose by as much as 55% without sacrificing image quality.

Generally, xeroradiography has lower contrast than film mammography; thus the entire breast is better visualized on the xeroradiographic image.

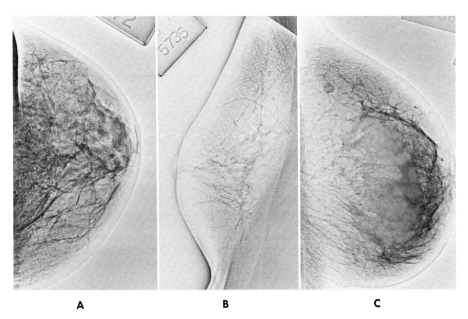

A   B   C

Fig. 6-1. Common causes of poor xeroradiographic imaging. **A,** Image smear is caused by loss of charge in the cassette and is seen as a complete loss of information in subcutaneous regions. Note same loss at edge of patient identification marker. **B,** With low back bias, image has greatly decreased contrast, and overall density is diminished. **C,** "Smudge" is caused when a second plate enters the processor before the first plate has been removed (piggybacking). Detail is lost mainly in central portion of image.

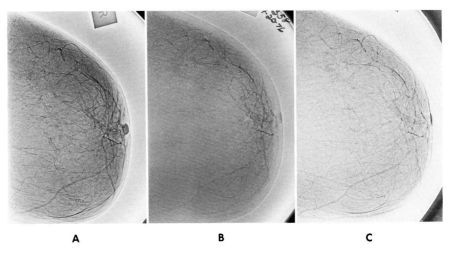

Fig. 6-2. Xeroradiographic images. **A,** Properly exposed. **B,** Overexposed. **C,** Underexposed.

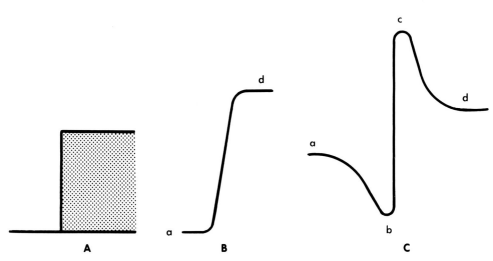

Fig. 6-3. Densitometry measurements from image of object (**A**) are represented for both film mammography (**B**) and xeroradiography (**C**). Overall contrast is represented as the difference between density *a* and density *d*. Note this difference is greater for film mammography. However, contrast at edge of object is enhanced on xeroradiographic image (*b* to *c*) and is greater than contrast on film.

A characteristic of xeroradiography is its edge enhancement due to fringing electrostatic fields.[55, 56] This increases contrast at abrupt changes in density (Fig. 6-3). Thus spicules and calcifications are clearly delineated.

Because xeroradiographs are viewed with reflected rather than transmitted light, large numbers of images can be read more easily. A darkroom is not required to process the images. Although there have been several reports advocating either xeroradiography[16, 60] or film mammography,[44] no controlled study has been done to demonstrate that the recording medium affects the accuracy of the mammographic examination.

RADIOGRAPHIC SIGNS OF MALIGNANCY

The classic radiographic signs of breast cancer are well documented and hold true for any imaging system. Most authors divide mammographic abnormalities into primary and secondary signs of malignancy.[12, 54, 55] A mass is the most frequent primary sign of breast cancer. Classically, the mass is spiculated, but on occasion it may be smooth and regular. The radiographic size of a malignant mass is characteristically smaller than the mass palpated on physical examination. Calcifications, another sign of malignancy, may be seen in the mass or in adjacent tissue. Secondary signs of breast cancer are less specific and can be produced by a variety of other causes. These signs include skin thickening, skin retraction, nipple retraction, increased vascularity, large axillary lymph nodes, and an asymmetric duct pattern.

Leborgne[28] emphasized the occurrence of calcifications in some breast carcinomas. His description of malignant calcifications is still used: ". . . innumerable punctate calcifications resembling fine grains of salt, generally clustered in a region of the breast."* Most current studies report that calcifications are seen in at least 50% of breast carcinomas.[40, 57] Two types of calcifications are virtually diagnostic of malignancy: multiple punctate calcifications seen in comedocarcinoma (Fig. 6-4) and rodlike calcifications, particularly when thin, branching, or curvilinear[31] (Fig. 6-5). The likelihood of malignancy increases with the number of calcifications in a cluster; however, a cluster with as few as three calcifications, particularly if they are irregular, may occur with carcinoma. Calcifications are commonly located within the malignancy in duct carcinoma, whereas in lobular carcinoma they are usually adjacent to the malignancy.[40, 45] Differentiating calcifications associated with malignancy from those of benign disease may be difficult (Figs. 6-6 and 6-7). A cluster of a few smooth, round, closely packed calcifications is usually benign.[58] Occasionally, the calcifications of carcinoma and sclerosing adenosis may be indistinguishable, particularly if the adenosis is not bilateral. Because calcifications may be associated with carcinoma, the radiologist must be particularly careful to look for them and to differentiate, if possible, benign calcifications from those requiring biopsy.

---

*Leborgne, R.: Diagnosis of tumors of the breast by simple roentgenography, Am. J. Roentgenol. Radium Ther. Nucl. Med. **65:**1, 1951.

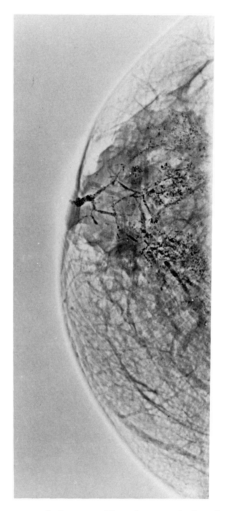

Fig. 6-4. Innumerable punctate calcifications. Note ducts packed with calcifications. Diagnosis: comedocarcinoma.

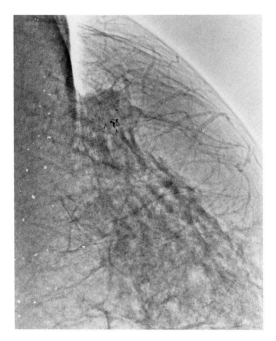

Fig. 6-5. Cluster of thin, linear calcifications within a mass. Pathognomonic of carcinoma.

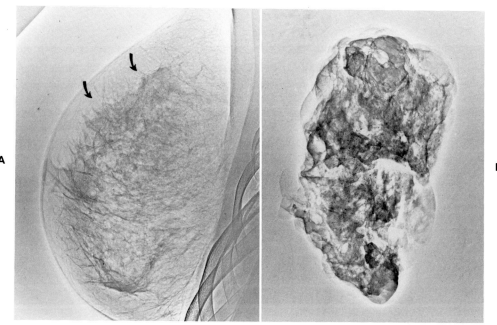

Fig. 6-6. A, Left mediolateral view demonstrating area of increased density with multiple, punctate, evenly distributed calcifications (arrows). Diagnosis: fibrocystic disease with atypical epithelial hyperplasia. **B,** Specimen xeroradiogram of **A.**

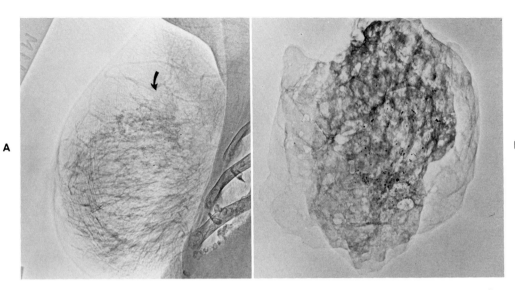

Fig. 6-7. A, Left mediolateral view with multiple irregular calcifications of varying size and some clustering (arrow). Diagnosis: intraductal carcinoma. **B,** Specimen xeroradiogram of **A.**

Interest is currently being generated by Wolfe's data, indicating that the parenchymal pattern on mammography is an important risk factor in determining subsequent development of breast cancer.[59] He evaluated the mammograms of 7214 women and classified them into four groups: N_1 (normal), P_1 (mild duct prominence—less than one fourth of the breast), P_2 (marked duct prominence), and DY (dysplasia). He estimates that the dysplasia group is twenty-two times more likely to develop breast cancer than is the normal group. Of 1000 women in the dysplasia group 448 are expected to develop carcinoma of the breast. Additional studies of large groups of women are needed to corroborate these data, which could have important implications in breast cancer screening.

IMAGE QUALITY

Some investigators have pointed out that the geometric factors of the total imaging system may be as important as the recording medium.[19] A short object-to-film distance is critically important in reducing geometric unsharpness. This is of particular importance in those mammography units in which the tube and film are close together.

Another factor that must be considered in improving image quality is the size of the focal spot. It should be as small as possible to minimize geometric unsharpness. A tube with a focal spot as small as 90 μ has been used successfully with rare-earth screen–film combinations.[30] In addition, compression of the breast improves image quality by decreasing the object-to-film distance as well as by minimizing motion.

The composition of the tube anode is important in determining not only the amount of radiation but also image quality. Molybdenum anodes are preferred with film mammography, and tungsten anodes are the choice for xero-radiography. The radiation dose to the patient is higher with molybdenum than with tungsten anodes.[13]

RADIATION EFFECTS

The carcinogenic effects of repeated mammography are not known. Mammography has never been shown to cause a breast cancer. However, Bailar[3] has recently theorized that repeated mammography in asymptomatic women may cause as many cancers as it finds. The only currently available data on carcinogenic effects of radiation to the breast are based on doses much greater than those used in mammography and of higher energy levels.[1] Also the women studied were younger than the average screening population. From these data, Bailar extrapolated the number of cancers that would be induced at the lower radiation levels used in mammography. In doing this, he assumed there is no threshold for inducing breast cancer and that a linear relationship exists between dose and effect. He also used the data from the Health Insurance Plan (HIP) study[49] to calculate the benefit of mammography in a screening program. However, the ACS-NCI Breast Cancer Demonstration Projects are detecting significantly more cancers by mammography alone (greater than 50%)[37] than were found during the HIP study. This is particularly true in the under-50 age-group. Also the cancers found on mammography alone are more likely to be minimal with a greater chance for cure.

Although we must recognize the need to reduce radiation without sacrificing diagnostic accuracy, we must not forget that mammography is the single best method for detecting breast cancer in a curable stage.

THERMOGRAPHY

In 1957 Lawson[27] first presented examples of thermographic imaging. Since that time, many investigators have advocated thermography,[8, 22, 46] and many others have demonstrated its ineffectiveness.[14, 15, 18, 24, 34] Thermography is a noninvasive, rapid technique. It is nonspecific and thus has a high false positive rate in the detection of cancer. Recent statistics from the ACS-NCI Breast Cancer Demonstration Projects show that thermography has an overall false negative rate of greater than 50%.[37] In our center the false negative rate is 61.2%. A recent study involving eleven expert thermographers indicates that in the detection of minimal or stage 1 cancer, thermography is no better than random selection.[34]

Opinion on the value of thermography has varied widely because (1) thermographic interpretation has often been biased because the thermographer knows the results of the physical examination, mammogram, or both, (2) conclusions correctly drawn from studies on symptomatic patients have been assumed to be true for asymptomatic screenees, (3) many conclusions have been drawn from statistically insignificant data, (4) many case reports are anecdotal and, perhaps most important, (5) uniform criteria for an abnormal thermogram have not been defined. However, a committee of thermographers has recently established standards for abnormal thermograms.[26] In addition, a program has been instituted to train thermography technologists.[*] Although thermography has not proved useful in the detection of breast cancer, it may be valuable in determining prognosis of breast cancer patients.[24]

SCREENING

The single most important factor in determining curability of breast cancer is the stage at which treatment is instituted. Strax[18] has shown that screening asymptomatic women can reduce the mortality rate by one third. His study was the impetus for establishing the ACS-NCI Breast Cancer Demonstration Projects. Each center screens 10,000 women between the ages of 35 and 75. Each screenee has mammography, thermography and a physical examination at least once a year for 5 years. There are plans for an additional 5 years' follow-up by letter. A comprehensive history form is completed during the initial visit and is updated on each subsequent visit. Each of the three examinations is interpreted independently, and results and recommendations are sent both to the screenee and to her personal physician.

A total of 10,250 screenees are enrolled in the program at The Medical College of Wisconsin. In the first year, 5000 women began the program, and the others entered the program during the second year. We are currently concluding our third year of screening. To date, a total of 86 cancers have been found in 80 women. Seventy-one of these cancers were diagnosed as a result of 255 biopsies recommended for suspicious findings on mammography, physical examination, or both. The remaining 184 biopsies showed benign disease, although many revealed atypical epithelial changes. Eight cancers were found in 152 biopsies done for masses that appeared benign on either mammography or physical examination. The remaining 7 cancers were found when 59 biopsies (interval biopsies) were done for abnormalities noted within 12 months of a normal screening examination. Thus 79 cancers were diagnosed as a result of biopsies recommended by our center for abnormalities noted during the patient's routine screening examination (57 on the initial visit, 1 during the first year follow-up visit, 14 during the second year, and 7 during the third year), and 7 cancers were diagnosed in the interval between routine screenings. No cancers have been found in 67 breasts that had aspirations recommended for suspected cysts. Of 71 patients who had axillary lymph nodes removed, 80% showed no evidence of metastases. Twenty-three (29%) of the patients had minimal cancer (either noninvasive or, if invasive, 5 mm or less in size). Patients with minimal cancer have a 95% chance of surviving 10 years or more.[51]

Our experience has shown that to be most effective, screening must include a combination of mammography and physical examination.[29] Because thermogra-

---

[*]University of Oklahoma Health Sciences Center, Oklahoma City, Okla.

phy has both low sensitivity and low specificity, it has little value in screening for breast cancer.[29, 34]

A comprehensive course for radiologists and radiologic technologists is offered at seven centers throughout the United States. These centers have been established by the National Cancer Institute in cooperation with the American College of Radiology to teach methods of breast cancer detection, including mammography, thermography, and physical examination.

LOCALIZATION OF BREAST ABNORMALITIES

With improved mammographic techniques and the availability of xeroradiography, more asymptomatic women are undergoing mammography and a greater percentage of malignancies are being discovered before they metastasize to the lymph nodes. Although nonpalpable breast abnormalities can be readily detected on mammography, locating them for biopsy remains a significant problem for both radiologists and surgeons.

Numerous techniques have been tried for directing the surgeon to the abnormality shown on the mammogram. By themselves, measurements based on the image[6, 47] are frequently inaccurate. Although some investigators have used markers placed on the breast[17] or needles positioned in the breast[39, 50] to locate nonpalpable lesions, we prefer a variation of the "spot" method.[43] With this method the mammogram is usually repeated without compression to reduce distortion of the breast (Fig. 6-8, *A*). The distance between the abnormality and the nipple is measured on the image, and coordinate measurements are made on the breast. The location of the abnormality is then estimated by triangulation. The skin overlying the suspicious area is prepared with antiseptic solution. A mixture of equal amounts of iodinated radiographic contrast and vital dye* totaling 0.1 to 0.3 ml is injected through a 25-gauge needle. More than one injection is rarely necessary. No local anesthetic is required. Mammograms are obtained again without compression (Fig. 6-8, *C*). The iodinated contrast serves as a radiographic marker for the blue dye, and the distance between the contrast "spot" and the abnormality is measured. The injection does not have to be at the exact location of the abnormality, only near it, to provide a reference point for the surgeon. To minimize diffusion of the blue dye, the mixture should be injected no more than 2 or 3 hours before surgery. Since the radiographic contrast is rapidly absorbed by the lymphatics, it does not interfere with the specimen radiograph.

SPECIMEN RADIOGRAPHY

Many breast biopsies are now being done for nonpalpable abnormalities. A radiograph of the biopsy specimen may verify that the nonpalpable lesion has been removed.[5] If the abnormality contains calcifications, specimen radi-

---

*Evans Blue, Warner-Chilcott Co., Morris Plains, N.J.

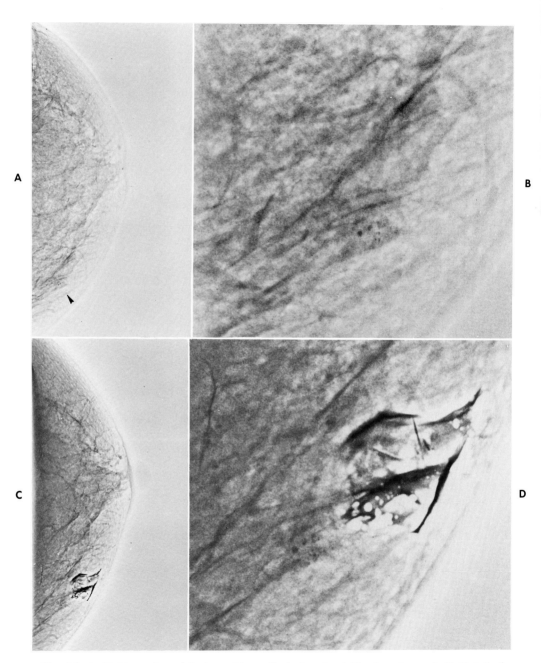

Fig. 6-8. A, Right craniocaudal view with small cluster of calcifications (arrow). B, Detail of A. C, Right craniocaudal view following injection of contrast mixture to localize calcifications. D, Detail of C. E, Clustered calcifications in xeroradiogram of biopsy specimen. F, Calcifications (arrow) demonstrated in radiograph of sliced specimen.

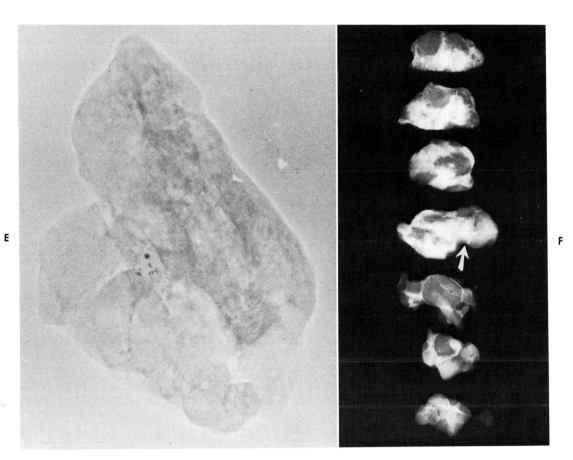

E   F

Fig. 6-8, cont'd. For legend see opposite page.

ography is invaluable; if it does not, specimen radiography is of less value.[41]

In our institution, specimens suspected of containing calcifications are immediately taken to the radiology department. An image of the specimen is taken (Fig. 6-8, *E*) and compared to the original mammogram. This comparison is particularly important in cases in which there are numerous calcifications on the mammogram, but only one area is suspicious. The radiologist notifies the surgeon whether or not the suspicious calcifications are contained in the tissue specimen. The specimen is then sent to the pathology department where it is sliced "bread-loaf" style into sections 2 to 3 mm thick. The slices are arranged in sequence on a sheet of clear film for support and are radiographed again (Fig. 6-8, *F*)—this time in a self-contained x-ray unit* located in the surgical pathology laboratory. The radiologist marks the areas of suspicion on the films to guide the pathologist in selecting areas to examine histologically.[35]

Specimen radiography is most useful when a biopsy is done for suspicious calcifications discovered on mammography or when the entire specimen is so large it cannot be conveniently examined histologically. It is also helpful when blind biopsies have been done on the contralateral breast.[45]

ULTRASOUND

Diagnostic ultrasound, which does not expose the patient to ionizing radiation, has been used to study the breast. Kossoff, Jellins, Reeve, and Barraclough[23] have demonstrated small cancers on a highly sophisticated water bath B scanner. The criteria for diagnosing malignant and benign lesions by ultrasound have been thoroughly described.[25] However, to date, its main value is in differentiating between solid and cystic lesions of the breast.

CONTRAST MAMMOGRAPHY

Routine mammograms may be supplemented with either positive or negative contrast studies. In negative contrast mammography, cyst fluid is replaced with air. Solitary or even multiple masses can be aspirated by sterile technique. If no aspirate is obtained, or if the aspirate is bloody, an excisional biopsy should be done. The aspirate may be sent for cytologic examination.[32, 33] Cyst wall irregularities, papillary excrescences, or papillary intracystic tumors may be delineated by filling the cyst with air.[53] The addition of a small amount of positive contrast medium may enhance visualization of the inner cyst margins.

Positive contrast mammography was first used in 1939 when Hicken[20] injected thorium dioxide (Thorotrast) into the mammary ducts. Since the advent of water-soluble contrast, interest in this method has been renewed. Most women have five to seven ducts and, correspondingly, five to seven lobes in the breast.[42] The ducts may be cannulated with either a blunt 25-gauge needle or a breast duct catheter.† Cannulation is easier when there is a nipple discharge.

---

*Faxitron, Field Emission Corp., McMinnville, Ore.
†Travenol Laboratories, Inc., Morton Grove, Ill.: (available in 0.15 and 0.2 mm OD).

With the aid of a dissecting microscope, the ducts may be cannulated even in the absence of discharge. Radiographic contrast medium is injected into the duct system before mammograms are taken. Moderate pain may occasionally follow injection. Inflammation occurs infrequently and may require antibiotics.[4]

Sartorius[36] uses mammary duct injection in all cases where the cytologic examination of the breast fluid is abnormal. In a series of thirty-two cancers, cytology combined with galactography was more accurate than mammography alone in detecting lesions smaller than 8 mm in size.[42] A normal galactogram will show the gradually narrowing branches of the ductal system. Carcinoma of the breast may cause extravasation of contrast material, filling defects, and obstruction or irregular narrowing of the ducts (Fig. 6-9). Papillomas and epithelial hyperplasia are usually seen as filling defects (Fig. 6-10). Fibroadenomas and cysts communicating with the duct system have characteristic appearances.[42] Although mammary duct injection offers promise in the detection of breast cancer, further evaluation is necessary.

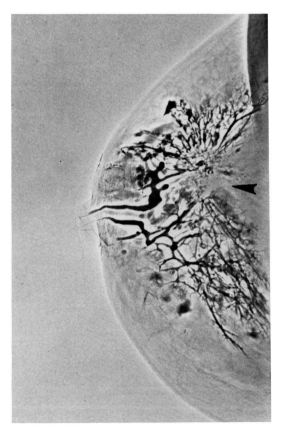

Fig. 6-9. Galactogram of woman with carcinoma. Xeroradiogram of medial and lateral central ducts reveals malignancy (arrow) involving the lateral system. Some ducts are obstructed, while others are irregularly narrowed. Note distortion without obstruction of medial ducts.

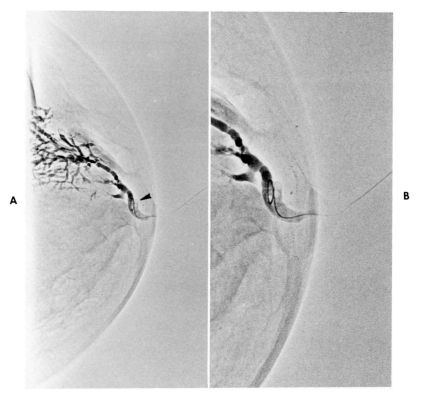

Fig. 6-10. A, Galactogram of patient with bloody discharge. Note lobulated filling defect (arrow) where catheter is coiled. Diagnosis: focal intraductal papillomatosis. **B,** Detail of **A.**

Acknowledgment

We are indebted to Dianna Stearman Lawrence, technical editor, for her assistance in the preparation of this manuscript.

References

1. Advisory Committee on the Biological Effects of Ionizing Radiation: The effects on populations of exposure to low levels of ionizing radiation (BEIR Report), Washington, D.C., 1972, National Academy of Sciences, National Research Council.
2. Ardran, G. M., Langmead, W. A., and Crooks, H. E.: Exposure reduction using new screen/film combination, Br. J. Radiol. **48:**233, 1975.
3. Bailar, J. C.: Mammography: a contrary view, Ann. Intern. Med. **84:**77, 1976.
4. Barth, V., Muller, R., and Mayle, M.: Galactography of female breast, Dtsch. Med. Wochenschr. **100:**1213, 1975.
5. Bauermeister, D. E., and Hall, M. H.: Specimen radiography—a mandatory adjunct to mammography, Am. J. Clin. Pathol. **59:**782, 1973.
6. Berger, S. M., Curcio, B. M., Gershon-Cohen, J., and Isard, H. J.: Mammographic localization of unsuspected breast cancer, Am. J. Roentgenol. Radium Ther. Nucl. Med. **96:**1046, 1966.
7. Buchanan, R. A., Finkelstein, S. I., and Wickersheim, K. A.: X-ray exposure reduction using rare-earth oxysulfide intensifying screens, Radiology **105:**185, 1972.
8. Byrne, R. R., and Yerex, J. A.: The three roles of breast thermography, Appl. Radiol. **4:**53, 1975.

9. Carlile, T.: Mammography—an assessment of its present capabilities. In Gallager, H. S., editor: Early breast cancer detection and treatment, New York, 1975, John Wiley & Sons, Inc.

10. Centers for Radiological Physics: Second report on Breast Cancer Demonstration Project Dosimetry, New York, Aug. 4, 1975 (unpublished).

11. Egan, R. L.: Experience with mammography in a tumor institution, Radiology **75**:894, 1960.

12. Egan, R. L.: Mammography, ed. 2, Springfield, 1972, Charles C Thomas, Publisher.

13. Evans, A. L., James, W. B., McLellan, J., and Davison, M.: Film and xeroradiographic images in mammography. A comparison of tungsten and molybdenum anode materials, Br. J. Radiol. **48**:968, 1975.

14. Feasey, C. M., Evans, A. L., and James, W. B.: Thermography in breast carcinoma: results of a blind reading trial, Br. J. Radiol. **48**:791, 1975.

15. Feig, S. A.: How good is thermography in breast cancer screening? Am. Fam. Physician **12**:78, 1975.

16. Frankl, G., and Rosenfeld, D. D.: Breast xeroradiography: an analysis of our first 17 months, Ann. Surg. **178**:676, 1973.

17. Frankl, G., and Rosenfeld, D. D.: Xeroradiographic detection of occult breast cancer, Cancer **35**:542, 1975.

18. Furnival, I. G., et al.: Accuracy of screening methods for the diagnosis of breast disease, Br. Med. J. **4**:461, 1970.

19. Haus, A. G., et al.: The effect of geometric and recording system unsharpness in mammography, Invest. Radiol. **10**:43, 1975.

20. Hicken, N. F.: Mammography: the roentgenographic diagnosis of breast tumors by means of contrast media, Surg. Gynecol. Obstet. **64**:593, 1937.

21. Isard, H. J., and Baker, A. S.: Low-dose mammography. In Gallager, H. S., editor: Early breast cancer detection and treatment, New York, 1975, John Wiley & Sons, Inc.

22. Isard, H. J., Becker, W., Shilo, R., and Ostrum, B. J.: Breast thermography after 4 years and 10,000 studies, Am. J. Roentgenol. Radium Ther. Nucl. Med. **115**:811, 1972.

23. Jellins, J., Kossoff, G., Reeve, T. S., and Barraclough, B. H.: Ultrasonic grey scale visualization of breast disease, Ultrasound Med. Biol. **1**:393, 1975.

24. Jones, C. H., et al.: Thermography of the female breast: a five-year study in relation to the detection and prognosis of cancer, Br. J. Radiol. **48**:532, 1975.

25. Kobayashi, T., Takatani, O., Hattori, N., and Kimura, K.: Differential diagnosis of breast tumors: the sensitivity-graded method of ultrasonotomography and clinical evaluation of its diagnostic accuracy, Cancer **33**:940, 1974.

26. Lapayowker, M., et al.: Criteria for obtaining and interpreting breast thermograms, Cancer **38**:1931, 1976.

27. Lawson, R. N.: Thermography: new tool in investigation of breast lesions, Can. Serv. Med. J. **13**:517, 1957.

28. Leborgne, R.: Diagnosis of tumors of the breast by simple roentgenography, Am. J. Roentgenol. Radium Ther. Nucl. Med. **65**:1, 1951.

29. Lewis, J. D., Milbrath, J. R., Shaffer, K. A., and DeCosse, J. J.: Implications of suspicious findings in breast cancer screening, Arch. Surg. **110**:903, 1975.

30. Logan, W.: Film—rare earth screen mammography in conjunction with microfocal spot, presented at 24th Annual Meeting of the Association of University Radiologists, Boston, May, 1976.

31. Martin, J.: Calcifications, presented at 15th Annual Conference on Detection and Treatment of Early Breast Cancer, Las Vegas, Nev., March, 1976.

32. Masukawa, T.: Breast cytology, Am. J. Med. Technol. **39**:397, 1973.

33. Masukawa, T.: Breast cytology. In Wied, G. L., Koss, L. G., and Reagan, J. W., editors: Compendium on diagnostic cytology, vol. 3, no. 1, Chicago, 1974, Tutorials of Cytology.

34. Moskowitz, M., et al.: Lack of efficacy of thermography as a screening tool for minimal and stage 1 breast cancer, N. Engl. J. Med. **295**:249, 1976.

35. National Cancer Institute: Standardized management of breast specimens, Am. J. Clin. Pathol. **60**:789, 1973.

36. Petrakis, N. L., and Sartorius, O. W.: Application of breast pump to obtain breast secretions, presented at Annual Program Review Conference, Breast

Cancer Task Force, National Cancer Institute, San Antonio, Texas, Feb., 1975.

37. Pomerance, W.: Report of project officer, presented at Project Directors Meeting, Breast Cancer Demonstration Projects, Bethesda, Md., Feb., 1976.

38. Price, J. L., and Butler, P. D.: A new screen/film combination applicable to mammography, Br. J. Radiol. **48:**872, 1975.

39. Rosato, F. E., Thomas, J., and Rosato, E. F.: Operative management of non-palpable lesions detected by mammography, Surg. Gynecol. Obstet. **137:**491, 1973.

40. Rosen, P., Snyder, R. E., Foote, F. W., and Wallace, T.: Detection of occult carcinoma in the apparently benign breast biopsy through specimen radiography, Cancer **26:**944, 1970.

41. Rosen, P., Snyder, R. E., Urban, J., and Robbins, G.: Correlation of suspicious mammograms and x-rays of breast biopsies during surgery, Cancer **31:**656, 1973.

42. Sartorius, O.: Personal communication, 1975.

43. Simon, N., Lesnick, G. J., Lerer, W. N., and Bachman, A. L.: Roentgenographic localization of small lesions of the breast by the spot method, Surg. Gynecol. Obstet. **134:**572, 1972.

44. Snyder, R.: Comparison study of xero-mammography and low-dose mammography. In Gallager, H. S., editor: Early breast cancer detection and treatment, New York, 1975, John Wiley & Sons, Inc.

45. Snyder, R. E., and Rosen, P.: Radiography of breast specimens, Cancer **28:**1608, 1971.

46. Stark, A. M., and Way, S.: Screening for breast cancer, Lancet **2:**407, 1970.

47. Stevens, G. M., and Jamplis, R. W.: Mammographically directed biopsy of nonpalpable breast lesions, Arch. Surg. **102:**292, 1971.

48. Strax, P.: Results of mass screening for breast cancer in 50,000 examinations, Cancer **37:**30, 1976.

49. Strax, P., Venet, L., and Shapiro, S.: Value of mammography in reduction of mortality from breast cancer in mass screening, Am. J. Roentgenol. Radium Ther. Nucl. Med. **117:**686, 1973.

50. Threatt, B., Appelman, H., Dow, R., and O'Rourke, T.: Percutaneous needle localization of clustered mammary micro-calcifications prior to biopsy, Am. J. Roentgenol. Radium Ther. Nucl. Med. **121:**839, 1974.

51. Urban, J. A.: Changing patterns of breast cancer, Cancer **37:**111, 1976.

52. Warren, S. L.: A roentgenologic study of the breast, Am. J. Roentgenol. Radium Ther. Nucl. Med. **24:**113, 1930.

53. Willemin, A.: Mammographic appearances, New York, 1972, S. Karger.

54. Witten, D. M.: The breast. In Hodes, P. J., editor: An atlas of tumor radiology, Chicago, 1969, Year Book Medical Publishers, Inc.

55. Wolfe, J. N.: Xeroradiography of the breast, Springfield, 1972, Charles C Thomas, Publisher.

56. Wolfe, J. N.: Xeroradiography: image content and comparison with film roentgenograms, Am. J. Roentgenol. Radium Ther. Nucl. Med. **117:**690, 1973.

57. Wolfe, J. N.: Analysis of 462 breast carcinomas, Am. J. Roentgenol. Radium Ther. Nucl. Med. **121:**846, 1974.

58. Wolfe, J. N.: Unpublished data, 1974.

59. Wolfe, J. N.: Breast patterns as an index of risk for developing breast cancer, Am. J. Roentgenol. Radium Ther. Nucl. Med. **126:**1130, 1976.

60. Wolfe, J. N., Dooley, R. P., and Harkins, L. E.: Xeroradiography of the breast: a comparative study with conventional film mammography, Cancer **28:**1569, 1971.

7 Some metabolic considerations in bone disease

Joseph P. Whalen, Lennart Krook, and Eladio A. Nunez

Much has been learned recently concerning the cellular mechanisms of bone function and their endocrine control. The discovery of the importance of the osteocyte in the resorption of bone has required reexamination of all physiologic and pathologic processes of bone that require or result in resorption. The discovery in 1962 of calcitonin (thyrocalcitonin) by Copp et al.[9] has led to much work in attempting to determine its role in calcium and phosphorus metabolism and, more recently, in modeling.[22, 46, 48]

The discovery of calcitonin was closely followed by the discovery of more active forms of vitamin D, which require an intact liver and kidney for their production.[2, 10] A tremendous insight was then gained in understanding the various mechanisms causing osteomalacia in both experimental and clinical situations. There has also been much research on the interactions of vitamin D, calcitonin, calcium, and phosphorus with parathyroid hormone and their effects on bone. This chapter will attempt to bring the radiologist up to date on the most recent information on these interactions and to interrelate the mechanisms involved in the pathogenesis of osteomalacia, "osteoporosis," and hyperparathyroid disease. We will also endeavor to more clearly elucidate the definition of these conditions and the terms used in discussing metabolic bone disease. Parts of this chapter will reflect our own original experimentation carried out specifically for the writing of this chapter to demonstrate the interrelations of a number of these factors. For example, an understanding of the bone changes in renal osteodystrophy requires a knowledge of many of these interrelations. We believe a correlation of the radiographic appearance of the bones in renal osteodystrophy with blood calcium and phosphorus levels offers an explanation for the lucent and sclerotic bone changes in this entity. We shall show experimental data on nutritional secondary hyperparathyroid disease (NSH) in growing pigs that simulate both the decreased and increased bone density in renal secondary hyperparathyroid disease (RSH).

The mechanisms of action of parathyroid hormone, calcitonin, and vitamin D and their activation will be reviewed. Furthermore, their interreaction in secondary hyperparathyroid disease, both renal and nutritional, will be demonstrated. We will discuss, for instance, why in vitamin D deficiency the growing skeleton develops rickets or osteomalacia, whereas pure dietary calcium deficiency with adequate phosphorus in the growing skeleton results primarily in hyperparathyroid disease. Histologically, why does phosphorus deficiency in experimental animals closely resemble the appearance of human rickets? Why does clinical rickets develop either in the hypertrophic or atrophic form? The possibilities of calcitonin deficiency or excess syndromes will also be briefly discussed.

The cellular mechanisms by which bone is formed, shaped, and renewed will be illustrated along with the acceptance of the major role of the osteocyte in resorbing both bone and calcified tissue in both calcium homeostasis[47] and bone modeling.[42, 44, 49] This histologic review is necessary to make the picture of their pathologic alteration more meaningful both radiologically and histologically. It must, however, be clearly understood that all the answers are not known. In areas of conflict we will attempt to present all sides objectively, but with our views prevailing.

Metabolic bone diseases are most commonly characterized by either "too little" or "too much" bone. A partial classification of the characteristics of some of these diseases follows[1]:

I. Osteopenia
   A. Too little formation of bone matrix (osteoblastic insufficiency)
      1. Osteoporosis
         a. Osteogenesis imperfecta
         b. Dietary deficiency of protein or vitamin C
   B. Too little mineralization of bone matrix
      1. Rickets in young people
      2. Osteomalacia in adults
   C. Too much resorption of bone tissue
      1. Generalized osteodystrophia fibrosa (hyperparathyroidism)
         a. Primary hyperparathyroidism
         b. Renal secondary hyperparathyroidism (RSH)
         c. Nutritional secondary hyperparathyroidism (NSH)
      2. ?Calcitonin deficiency
         a. Hereditary bone dysplasia with hyperphosphatasemia
         b. Lytic phase of Paget's disease
II. Osteomegaly
   A. Too little resorption of bone
      1. Osteopetrosis in children (cause unknown, ?calcitonin excess)
      2. Nutritional hypercalcitoninism (dietary calcium excess)
      3. Vitamin D toxicosis
      4. Heavy metal toxicity (lead, phosphorus)
   B. Too much production of bone
      1. Acromegaly (growth hormone)
      2. Sclerotic renal dystrophy (phosphate effect)

BONE STRUCTURE AND DEVELOPMENT

Human bone is either woven or lamellar in structure. Woven bone shows disorganization, reflecting rapid turnover.[45, 46] In developing bone there is a gradual transition from woven to lamellar type, and by the age of 11 years all woven bone is replaced by lamellar bone. Jaffe[23] states that this substitution takes place without notable involvement of the osteoclast and refers to this as creeping replacement. The term woven bone is used interchangeably with the terms immature, fetal, or coarse-fiber bone. Some researchers believe that this is the type of bone initially laid down. We believe, however, that this bone results primarily from the rapid turnover during growth or from certain pathologic situations that result in accelerated resorption. During growth, early in life, modeling requires accelerated production and resorption. Resorption carried out by the osteocyte in this gowth process, we believe, results in the characteristic appearance of this type of bone, and therefore reflects enhanced osteocytic osteolysis and chondrolysis.[42] This concept is most important in appreciating the histologic appearance of various disease states, such as Paget's disease[5] and hereditary bone dysplasia with hyperphosphatasemia,[22, 45] in which pathologic acceleration of bone resorption occurs with a secondary increase in bone production. To understand this concept, the role of the osteocyte in bone resorption must be appreciated. A brief review of the processes of bone production and resorption follows.

Bone production

Bone is formed only by osteoblasts. If formed on preexisting cartilage, it is termed endochondral; if not, it is termed intramembranous. Endochondral bone formation involves the simultaneous removal of cartilage and formation of bone to replace the cartilage tissue. In the past the cellular mechanism has been explained by a clastic cell, either a chondroclast or an osteoclast.[11] The cartilage is the template, or core, on which bone is formed by osteoblasts. It is then "deep" to bone, and if removed by a cellular mechanism, the cell also must be deep and adjacent to the core. This, then, must be the function of the osteocyte. We have termed this process osteocytic chondrolysis,[49] which will be discussed later.

Bone resorption

Resorption of bone involves the simultaneous removal of both bone matrix and mineral. It occurs by two different mechanisms—osteoclasia and osteolysis.

Osteoclasia. Osteoclasia is a surface resorption of bone tissue brought about by the action of osteoclasts. These cells are multinucleated giant cells typically located in Howship's lacunae during their active phase of resorption. Osteoclasia may occur on the surfaces of trabeculae (Figs. 7-4 and 7-31), subperiosteally (Fig. 7-35), on the medullary cavity, and on the surfaces of haversian and Volkmann's canals.

Osteolysis. Osteolysis is a deep-seated resorption centered around the activity of older osteocytes. This concept was first proposed in 1910 by von Recklinghausen but was discarded and not fully elucidated until the 1960s by the many contributions of Belanger.[3]

Osteocytic osteolysis is characterized histologically by enlargement of the osteocyte and the adjacent lacunar space. The lacunar rim stains metachromatically with toluidine blue and basophilically with hematoxylin and eosin stain, re-

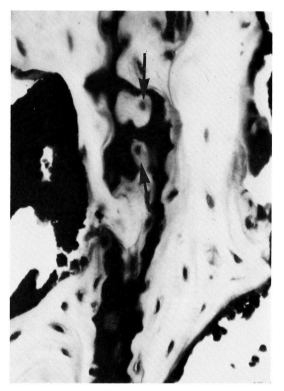

Fig. 7-1. Normal rat, 60 days of age. Section in metaphysis at junction of primary and secondary spongiosa. Cartilaginous core is partially removed and replaced by lamellar bone. Note enlarged osteocytes (arrows) adjacent to receding cartilaginous core. No spaces are present, since they are replaced by lamellar bone. (Toluidine blue; ×350.)

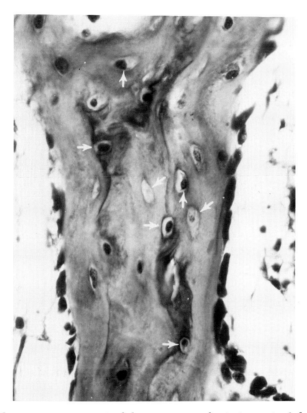

Fig. 7-2. Secondary spongiosa, proximal humerus metaphysis in a pig fed normal amounts of vitamin D, calcium, and phosphorus for 8 weeks from weaning at 6 weeks of age. Surfaces are lined by large osteoblasts; apposition is active, but there are no osteiod seams. Osteocytic osteolysis (vertical arrows) and osteocytic chondrolysis (horizontal arrows) are evidenced by large osteocytes and a basophilic lacunar rim. Osteocytes (oblique arrows) have completed the osteocytic cycle and are fading away. (H & E; ×450.)

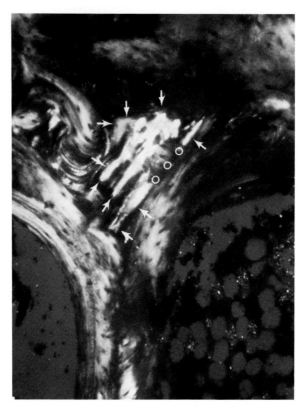

Fig. 7-3. Secondary spongiosa, proximal humerus metaphysis in a normal 3-year-old horse. Area within arrows is a chondroid core surrounded by bone tissue on all sides. Removal of this core within the trabecula is by osteocytic chondrolysis. Enlarged osteocytes have caused dissolution of the core; note excavation to left of circles. (Toluidine blue; ×140, polarized light.)

flecting the degradation of the polysaccharides (Figs. 7-1 to 7-3). Osteocytic osteolysis appears to be the initial resorbing mechanism in either physiologic conditions or pathologically enhanced resorption states.[5, 42, 45, 47] Osteoclasia appears to be concerned with the removal of bone already altered as in fracture healing or in bone that has been partially resorbed or modified by osteocytic osteolysis (Fig. 7-4).

Fig. 7-6 is a diagram illustrating the concept of osteocytic osteolysis and chondrolysis. This concept is required to understand the correlative histologic and radiographic pictures of the pathologic entities and their pathogenesis discussed in this chapter.

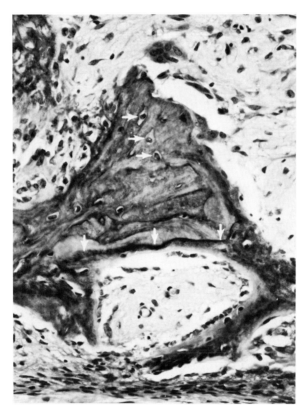

Fig. 7-4. Nutritional secondary hyperparathyroidism. Trabecular bone from a turbinate in a 6-month-old pig fed a low-calcium (0.35%) and high-phosphorus (1.40%) diet from weaning at 6 weeks of age. There is intense osteocytic osteolysis at top of bone tissue (horizontal arrows) and osteoclastic resorption at surface on top right. Vertical arrows point to a cementing line. Trabecular surface beneath this line is lined by a wide osteoid seam. (H & E; ×250.)

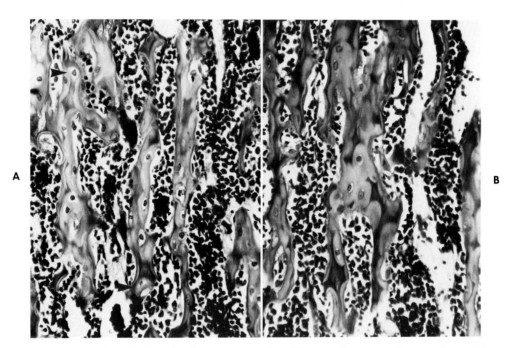

Fig. 7-5. Metaphyseal trabecular bone in area of visible secondary spongiosa. **A,** Osteocytic removal of cartilaginous core (arrowheads) in trabeculae is occurring with normal thinning in modeling of growth. **B,** After calcitonin injections, there is inactivity of osteocytes, persistence of cartilaginous core, and thickened trabeculae. (H & E; ×300.)

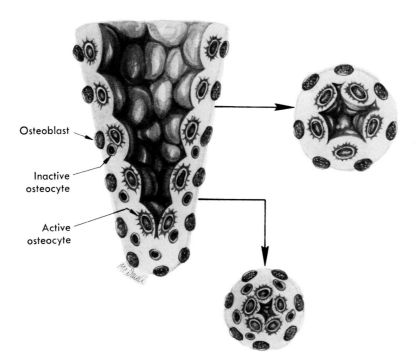

Fig. 7-6. Diagrammatic representation of primary spongiosa. The cartilaginous core (dark shading) is enveloped by bony tissue. Osteoblasts are on surface actively laying down bone. Inactive osteocytes are deep to the surface "entrapped" by bony tissue. Deeper, adjacent to cartilaginous core, osteocytes are actively removing cartilage to be replaced by trabecular bone. Schematic cross sections to the right at different levels illustrate central position of core, its relationship to deep-seated osteocytes, and its eventual disappearance without cavity formation in the progression to secondary spongiosa.

HORMONAL CONTROL OF BONE PRODUCTION AND RESORPTION
Parathyroid hormone

Parathyroid hormone is a polypeptide hormone secreted by the cells of the parathyroid glands (Figs. 7-8 and 7-10). Its secretion and synthesis are controlled by the blood calcium level. An elevated blood calcium level inhibits its elaboration; a low blood calcium level stimulates its production. These physiologic actions are aimed at raising a hypocalcemic level toward normal, and in doing this, parathyroid hormone acts on three organ systems and on vitamin D.

Low Ca^{++} ──────→ Parathyroid hormone

- Enhances bone resorption
- Inhibits calcification of osteoid
- Phosphorus diuresis (decreases tubular reabsorption)
- Increases renal calcium reabsorption
- Enhances absorption of calcium and phosphorus from gut
- Promotes active form of vitamin D (1,25-DHCC)

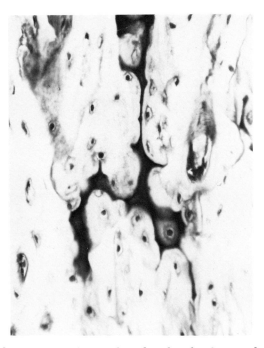

Fig. 7-7. Accelerated resorption of metaphyseal trabecular bone induced by parathyroid hormone in a 60-day-old growing rat. Note increased activity of osteocytes adjacent to cartilaginous core. Core is decreased when compared to normal growing rat depicted in Fig. 7-1. (Toluidine blue; ×350.)

Action on bone. Parathyroid hormone has a *direct* action on bone tissue by stimulating osteocytes and osteoclasts (Figs. 7-4 and 7-7). There is some evidence to suggest that osteoclastic activity is "triggered" by osteocytic activity which first modifies the bone.[12, 48]

The effect of parathyroid hormone on bone production is controversial. Some investigators believe it causes increased bone production[24, 38]; others think it diminishes bone production[26]; still others believe it may stimulate osteoblastic formation of osteoid, but osteoid that is not calcifiable.[31] In the latter case osteoid seams would then be a part of the histologic picture of the parathyroid hormone effect on bone. This osteoid seam is not pathogenically related to osteomalacia. (We will discuss osteoid seams further in the section on renal osteodystrophy.) If parathyroid hormone in physiologic doses did act to enhance bone production, it would be counterproductive to its primary action of elevating a low blood calcium to a normal one. It may well be that the divergent findings of the various investigators are a function of the dose of parathyroid hormone used in experimentation.

In summary, the effect of parathyroid hormone on bone is to enhance resorption by both osteolysis and osteoclasia. In addition, it "creates" an osteoid seam by the prevention of calcification of osteoid, though excessive osteoid may be

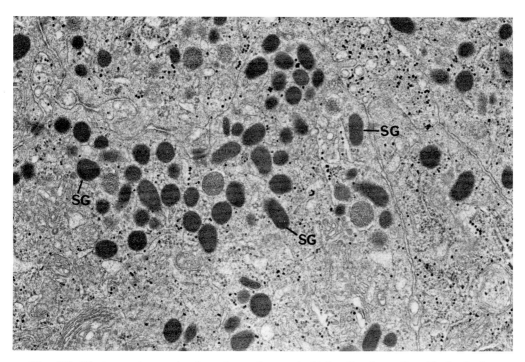

Fig. 7-8. Electron micrograph of portions of several chief cells of parathyroid gland of a normal young pig. Cells are characterized by many small dense secretory granules *(SG)*. These granules are the intracellular storage sites of parathyroid hormone. (×20,000.)

present. Both these actions on bone attempt to elevate a low blood calcium level toward normal.

Action on kidney. Parathyroid hormone also has a direct action on the kidney. It acts to inhibit tubular resorption of phosphorus, resulting in hyperphosphaturia and therefore hypophosphatemia.[1] This results in a compensatory rise in the blood calcium level to maintain an appropriate $Ca^{++}/HPO_4^=$ product. Furthermore, it inhibits the filtration and resorption of calcium. Again, all these actions are directed at raising the blood calcium level.

Action on gastrointestinal tract. The hormone acts directly on the gastrointestinal tract to promote the absorption of both calcium and phosphorus.[37]

Effect on vitamin D. Parathyroid hormone acts to enhance the most active form of this compound, 1,25-dihydroxycholecalciferol (1,25-DHCC).[10] See the discussion on vitamin D for more detail.

Calcitonin

Calcitonin was first discovered by Copp et al. in 1962.[9] He clearly described the action of this hormone but falsely attributed its origin to the parathyroid gland. Shortly after this exciting discovery Hirsch, Gautier, and Munson[20] clearly established its source as the thyroid gland.

Calcitonin, like parathyroid hormone, is a polypeptide. Its primary action, opposite to that of parathyroid hormone, is that of lowering an elevated blood calcium level, and it acts directly on bone, causing inhibition of bone resorption.[43] Calcitonin appears to have no influence on bone production but acts directly on the osteocyte[47] and osteoclast.[36]

Calcitonin appears to promote the inactive form of vitamin D (24,25-DHCC).[2, 10] (See the discussion on vitamin D.)

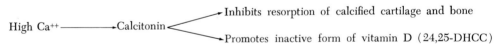

High Ca⁺⁺ ⟶ Calcitonin ⟨ Inhibits resorption of calcified cartilage and bone / Promotes inactive form of vitamin D (24,25-DHCC)

Calcitonin is produced in the thyroid gland and is synthesized and secreted by the parafollicular cell of the gland (Figs. 7-9 and 7-11). The parafollicular cell was first described in 1932 by Nonidez,[32] but no function could be attributed to it until the discovery of calcitonin in 1962 by Copp et al.[9]

The stimulus for calcitonin release is hypercalcemia. Its physiologic role initially appeared to be strictly that of calcium homeostasis, with its stimulus for secretion and its action on bone reciprocal to that of parathyroid hormone. Supporting this hypothesis was the demonstration of increased activity of the parafollicular cell and increased amounts of calcitonin in the active phase of hibernating animals and a decreased activity during the inactive phase of hibernating mammals at a time when the dietary intake of calcium was zero.[47]

It became apparent that control of bone resorption was also required in modeling and remodeling of bone. Only recently calcitonin was found to be important in controlling resorption in these processes. Calcitonin may thus be a hormone controlling the normal remodeling of bone by regulating the rate of

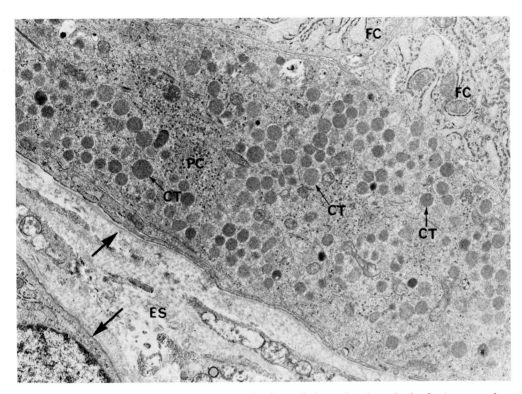

Fig. 7-9. Electron micrograph of a parafollicular cell from the thyroid gland of a normal young pig. Parafollicular cell *(PC)* is wedged between the lining follicular cells *(FC)* and the basement membrane (large arrows) of the follicle. Basement membranes border extracellular space *(ES)* between adjacent follicles. The parafollicular cell is distinguished by a large number of calcitonin-containing granules *(CT)* that fill the cytoplasmic matrix. (×20,000.)

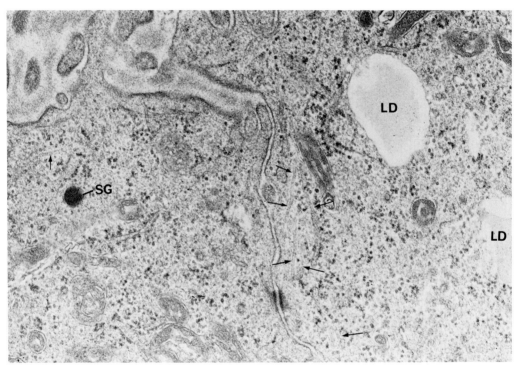

Fig. 7-10. Electron micrograph of portions of several chief cells from parathyroid gland of a young pig on a low-calcium diet for a 12-week period. Cells now contain only a few dense secretory granules *(SG)*. However, many microtubules (arrows) and large lipid droplets *(LD)* are found in cytoplasm of these stimulated chief cells. (×20,000.)

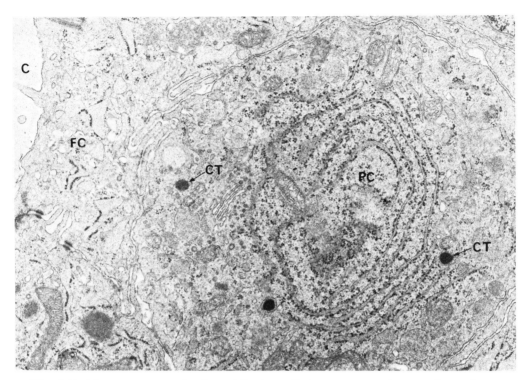

Fig. 7-11. Electron micrograph of parafollicular cells from a young dog on a high-calcium diet for 12 weeks. Stimulated parafollicular cell contains only a few calcitonin storage granules *(CT)*. Also seen are follicular cells *(FC)* and a portion of the colloid *(C)*. (×20,000.)

resorption. It is interesting to note that parafollicular cells are very rare in the human adult thyroid gland.[6] However, human prenatal and neonatal thyroid glands contain large numbers of parafollicular cells that are fully granulated (loaded with calcitonin storage granules).[8] One could speculate that the large numbers of parafollicular cells in the neonate represent secretion of calcitonin during the growth period. Calcitonin may therefore act as a regulatory mechanism of the osteocyte's removal of the cartilaginous core. In adult bone this is no longer required.

It also has been shown that introducing relative excess amounts of calcitonin in growing mammals, either by excessive dietary calcium intake[19] or by injection of calcitonin, results in modeling errors[46] produced by the inhibition of osteocytic resorption (Figs. 7-5, *B*, and 7-24, *B*). There has been some suggestion that calcitonin stimulates bone production,[13] but the evidence is inconclusive. There is no good evidence of gastrointestinal or renal response to calcitonin.

Vitamin D

Vitamin D is converted in the liver to 25-hydroxycholecalciferol (25-HCC). It is further hydroxylated in the kidney to its most active form, 1,25-dihydroxycholecalciferol (1,25-DHCC) (Figs. 7-14 and 7-25).[10] The fact that there is endogenous production of vitamin D_3 and a negative feedback regulating its metabolism suggests that it has a hormonal activity, and its name "vitamin D" may be inappropriate.[2]

In the past some controversy existed about which elements promote the active form of vitamin D. Parathyroid hormone was thought by some to deactivate the active form to the more inactive form, 24,25-DHCC.[51] This theory of the action of parathyroid hormone was an attempt to explain osteoid seams in cases of primary hyperparathyroid disease, but it is apparent that this mechanism would not be consistent with the role of the hormone to elevate blood calcium levels. It has been more recently shown that parathyroid hormone action is the reverse—to promote 1,25-DHCC,[2] thereby elevating the blood calcium level. It also would appear that the action of calcitonin affects the metabolism of vitamin D by promoting the formation of the inactive form over the active form, the reverse action of parathyroid hormone.[2] Again, the purpose of this action is to lower the blood calcium level.

Vitamin D action on bone is probably dose related. Its direct action is controversial, but by enhancing calcium intestinal absorption, it stimulates hypercalcemia followed by calcitonin release, thereby inhibiting bone resorption (Fig. 7-26). The actions of vitamin D are summarized:

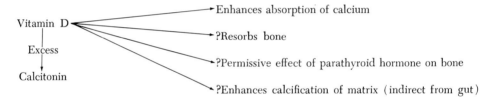

Vitamin D
|
Excess
|
Calcitonin

→ Enhances absorption of calcium

→ ?Resorbs bone

→ ?Permissive effect of parathyroid hormone on bone

→ ?Enhances calcification of matrix (indirect from gut)

OSTEOPOROSIS

Osteoporosis is defined as a generalized metabolic bone disease characterized by osteopenia caused by too little formation of bone matrix. This is a morphologic-pathologic definition. Clinicians and radiologists often use this term synonymously with osteopenia. We will adhere to this morphologic-pathologic definition. The classic disease causing osteoporosis is osteogenesis imperfecta. The dietary deficiency of protein and vitamin C that can occur through failure of intake or failure of absorption can cause inhibition of osteoblastic function and is another major cause of osteoporosis.

The pathologic anatomy of osteoporosis is, by definition, too little bone. It has been described as too little normal bone with the osteoblasts decreased in number and therefore more widely separated along the appositional surface. The osteoblasts are somewhat atrophic and the bone trabeculae more slender (Fig. 7-12). The cortical bone is thinner.

We shall discuss only briefly those states which in the past have been classified as osteoporosis after skeletal maturity such as senile or postmenopausal osteoporosis. It is our belief that these entities are a result of enhanced resorption of bone rather than defect in formation. Furthermore, we believe a common

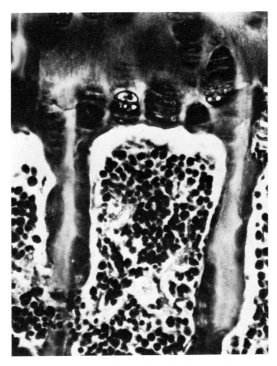

Fig. 7-12. Osteoporosis. Transition zone of epiphyseal plate and metaphysis of proximal tibia in a 14-week-old pig fed 2.8% protein from weaning at 6 weeks of age. (Normal dietary protein is 18%.) There are a few cartilage cells, all small in narrow columns; vesicular cartilage is completely missing. A thin bar of transverse bone—the distal terminal plate—is sealing off the plate distally. Only two secondary spongiosa trabeculae are present. There is no osteoblastic lining of these trabeculae. There is no primary spongiosa. (H & E; ×400.)

cause of this excess resorption is a long-term relative calcium deficiency.[30] These entities are then best classified as secondary nutritional hyperparathyroid diseases.

OSTEOMALACIA

Osteomalacia is defined as a generalized metabolic bone disease characterized by osteopenia caused by too little mineralization of the bone matrix because of a depressed $Ca^{++}/HPO_4^=$ product (Fig. 7-13). Osteomalacia is termed rickets when it occurs in the growing skeleton before epiphyseal closure.

Etiology. Osteomalacia develops when the product of the levels of blood calcium and phosphate decreases below a critical level, impeding the normal mineralization of osteoid. If the product is lowered because of a depressed blood calcium level, the condition is called low calcium rickets or osteomalacia. If the product is reduced because of a lowered blood phosphate level, the condition is termed low phosphate rickets or osteomalacia. Any mechanism whereby the total product is reduced becomes of etiologic importance. Vitamin D deficiency, from

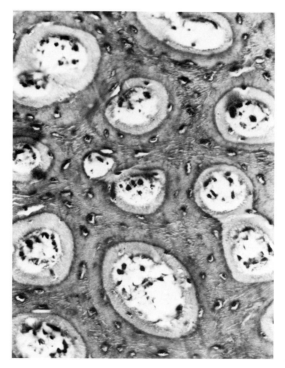

Fig. 7-13. Rickets. Transverse section of middiaphysis of tibia of a 21-day-old chicken raised on vitamin D–free feed. There are very wide osteoid seams lining all haversian canals; the canals are wider than normal for the age. Pronounced osteocytic osteolysis of peripheral osteonic lamellae and of interstitial lamellae is present. (H & E; ×400.)

whatever cause, will result in a lowering of this product and ultimately in osteo-malacia. If, however, the $Ca^{++}/HPO_4^=$ product is not significantly reduced but the blood serum calcium is, regardless of the cause, the parathyroid gland is stimulated and hyperparathyroid disease supervenes. Fig. 7-14 illustrates most of the factors involved in altering this important $Ca^{++}/HPO_4^=$ product. The numbers throughout the diagram illustrate the sites of potential lesions whereby a diminished product may result in osteomalacia and/or hyperparathyroidism or hyper-calcitoninism. Figs. 7-15 to 7-23 show some examples of the radiographic appearance of these lesions.

Pathologic anatomy. In rickets, the diagnostic features occur in the metaphysis and the epiphysis—the areas of most actively growing bones. Mineralization does not occur in the zone of provisional calcification. The distal row of vesicular cartilage cells is not penetrated by the vessels from the metaphysis. The vessels continue to grow into the cartilaginous matrix. The large cartilage cells grow down into the metaphysis, either in single rows or in large conglomerates. The epiphyseal plate is therefore irregular. There is tremendous osteoblastic activity, resulting in trabeculae with wide osteoid seams.

In osteomalacia of the adult, the diagnosis rests on the demonstration of osteoid seams alone, since the epiphyseal plates are closed.

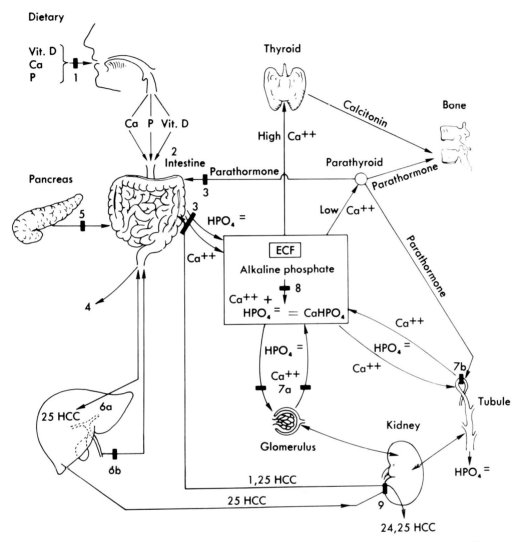

Fig. 7-14. Interrelationships of dietary calcium, phosphorus, vitamin D, and the controlling mechanism in maintaining calcium and phosphorus blood levels. Numbers refer to lesions that may result in altering the Ca^{++} and $HPO_4^{=}$ blood levels and their product and therefore osteomalacia, hyperparathyroidism or hypercalcitoninism. Any alteration resulting in a decrease of this product results in osteomalacia. If blood calcium level is decreased, regardless of the product, hyperparathyroidism results. If serum calcium level is increased, hypercalcitoninism results. *1,* Dietary deficiency of calcium, phosphorus, or vitamin D (NSH, osteomalacia). *2,* Gastrectomy (osteomalacia). *3,* Hypoparathyroid disease, Hypovitamin D (osteomalacia). *4,* Absorption defect (calcium, phosphorus, vitamin D) (NSH, osteomalacia). *5,* Pancreatic abnormality (vitamin D absorption failure) (osteomalacia). *6a,* Liver disease (failure of formation of 25-HCC) (osteomalacia); anticonvulsant drugs (osteomalacia); prematurity (osteomalacia). *6b,* Biliary obstruction (osteomalacia). *7a,* glomerular renal disease (loss of calcium and phosphorus) (RSH). *7b,* Tubular renal disease (hyperphosphaturia) (RSH); vitamin D resistant. *8,* Familial hypophosphatasia (osteomalacia). *9,* Renal disease (failure of 1,25-DHCC formation) (osteomalacia).

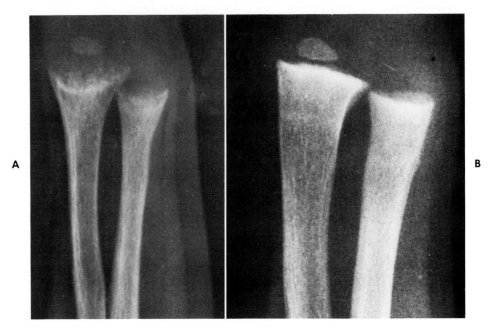

Fig. 7-15. A, Vitamin D deficiency with an adequate dietary calcium resulting in classical rickets. The major change is at the physis, showing minimally calcified cartilage and osteoid at growth plate. There is some osteopenia of the shaft but not in proportion to the metaphyseal change (hypertrophic-type rickets). **B,** Three months after vitamin D therapy there is calcification of previously noncalcified cartilage and osteoid. This area is actually sclerotic and has ill-defined margins typical of calcified osteoid, rather than discrete trabeculae.

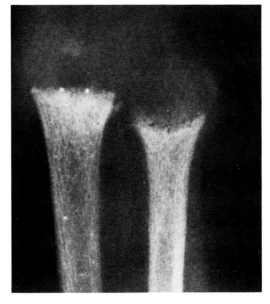

Fig. 7-16. Vitamin D and calcium deficiency resulting in rickets and also marked osteopenia of cortex of shaft. There is more resorption in cortical and diaphyseal trabecular areas than in Fig. 7-22, *A.* Patient's serum calcium level was depressed to well below normal (atrophic-type rickets).

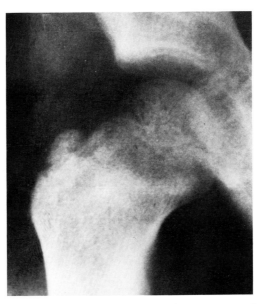

Fig. 7-17. Active rickets after a month of treatment. Features of rickets are still showing, but there are areas of sclerotic change representing calcification of osteoid. This is somewhat reminiscent of sclerotic bone changes seen in renal disease.

Radiographic findings

Rickets. The radiographic findings in rickets reflect its histologic appearance. The epiphyses appear rarefied and irregular. The metaphyses are widened (cupped). Rarefaction of the cortex and spongiosa of the diaphysis also occurs (Figs. 7-15 to 7-23).

It must be pointed out that pathologically and radiographically rickets may be classified as either hypertrophic or atrophic. The atrophic form shows minimal metaphyseal change radiographically, although histologically wide ricketic zones may be found. A more striking change is a thin and porous diaphyseal cortex and thin, spongy trabeculae (Fig. 7-16). The hypertrophic form shows more cupping of the metaphysis and thickening of the perichondrial ring.[50] The thinning of the cortex is much less evident than in the atrophic form (Fig. 7-15).

Several explanations have been given for the form in which this disease presents. Caffey[7] believes that the activity of muscle pull promotes the cupping in the hypertrophic form. The atrophic form occurs in more severe cases with limited mobility. Jaffe[23] believes the atrophic form occurs in undernourished infants and the hypertrophic form in better-nourished infants. Our opinion is that the atrophic form of rickets is due to osteomalacia and secondary hyperparathyroid disease, which is due to a vitamin D deficiency associated with low calcium intake. This deficiency results in a more severe hypocalcemia and therefore hyperparathyroid disease in addition to the osteomalacia. It is to be remembered that the calcium-phosphorus ratio influences parathyroid hormone

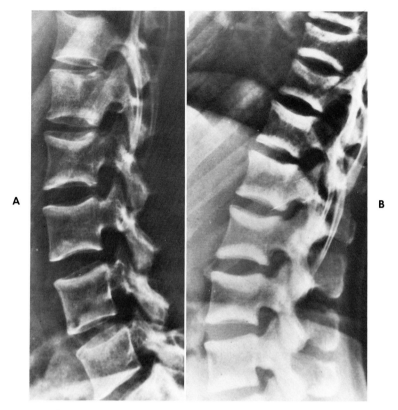

Fig. 7-18. Osteomalacia of a growing spine. **A,** Osteopenia but with some sclerosis of sub-chondral surfaces of all vertebral bodies. **B,** After a month of therapy with vitamin D and calcium, there is marked sclerosis of subchondral surfaces of vertebral bodies. These areas merely represent metaphyses of vertebral bodies and are reminiscent of the "rugger jersey spine" seen in renal disease.

activity. This will be discussed further in the section on nutritional secondary hyperparathyroid disease. Suffice it to say that a diet with a reversed calcium-phosphorus ratio will result in a state resembling hyperparathyroid disease. A diet with a distortion of the calcium-phosphorus ratio in favor of calcium, in the absence of vitamin D, will produce rickets. An absolute low phosphorus diet usually results in rickets, radiographically and histologically, since the product is reduced, although the blood calcium level may be normal. Thus it may well be that atrophic rickets has a prominent hyperparathyroid component stimulated by a low calcium level. Hypertrophic rickets may well be primarily an osteo-malacia without a significant hyperparathyroid effect.

Osteomalacia. The radiographic appearance of adult osteomalacia is entirely due to the presence of noncalcified osteoid in place of normally calcified lamellar bone. The bones are osteopenic. It has been stated that the trabeculae in spongy areas appear indistinct because of the "covering" osteoid. In practice this may be difficult to ascertain, and fine detail radiography may be required.

Text continued on p. 169.

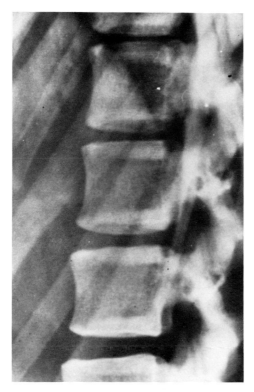

Fig. 7-19. Patient with osteomalacia on phenytoin (Dilantin) therapy for seizures. He was treated for a month prior to this radiograph. Calcification of "metaphysis" of vertebral body, where "osteoid seams" were present is seen, again reminiscent of sclerotic renal osteodystrophy. (Corresponds to *6a* of Fig. 7-14.)

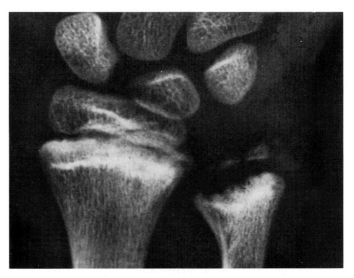

Fig. 7-20. Wilson's disease showing ricketic change. There are some areas of increased density corresponding to calcified osteoid with other areas of lucency closer to growth plate corresponding to osteoid seams. (Corresponds to *6a* of Fig. 7-14.)

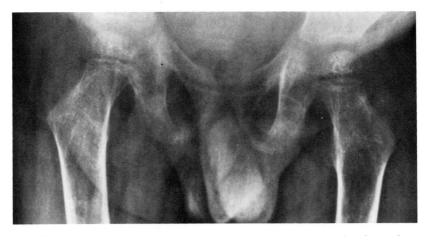

Fig. 7-21. Child with intrahepatic biliary atresia showing osteopenia and ricketic changes of metaphysis. Presence of ascites at top of radiograph is a clue to the diagnosis. (Corresponds to *6b* in Fig. 7-14.)

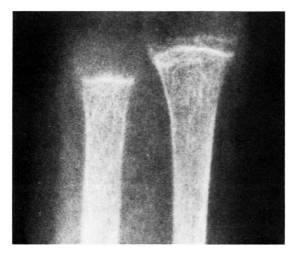

Fig. 7-22. Six-month-old infant with biliary atresia with atrophic ricketic pattern. (Corresponds to *6b* in Fig. 7-14.)

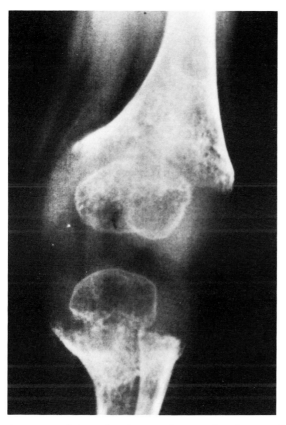

Fig. 7-23. Child with congenital hypophosphatasia showing the changes of hypertrophic-type rickets. (Corresponds to 8 in Fig. 7-14.)

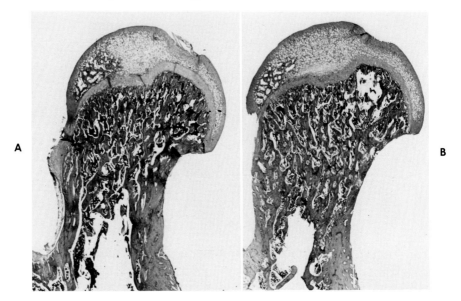

Fig. 7-24. A, Section through neck of femur of a 55-day-old rat showing normal modeling. **B,** Calcitonin-treated rat of similar age with a broader, poorly modeled femoral neck and failure of resorption during growth.

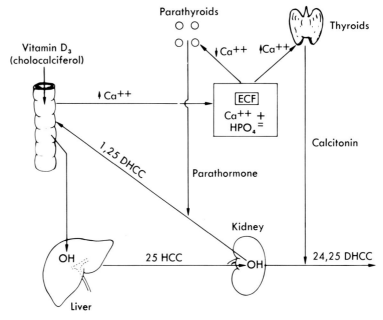

Fig. 7-25. Diagrammatic representation of effect of parathyroid hormone and calcitonin on formation of 1,25-DHCC and 24,25-DHCC. Vitamin D is first hydroxylated in the liver to become 25-HCC. Further hydroxylation in the kidney occurs to form either 1,25-DHCC (which is enhanced by parathyroid hormone) or 24,25-DHCC (which is enhanced by calcitonin). A depressed serum calcium level stimulates parathyroid hormone formation, and an elevated serum calcium level stimulates calcitonin formation. 1,25-DHCC enhances intestinal absorption of calcium.

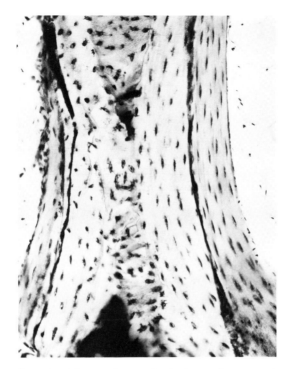

Fig. 7-26. Section of proximal humeral metaphysis (secondary spongiosa) in a 3-year-old horse "poisoned" with *Cestrum diurnum*, a plant containing 1,25-DHCC. There are no signs of osteocytic osteolysis; osteocytes are small and elongated and lack metachromasia of lacunar rim. There are two cementing lines, both merging from areas of diffuse metachromasia. The horse was hypercalcemic, and there was evidence of calcitonin release. Vitamin D action in this case resulted in dense bones mediated by hypercalcemia, triggering calcitonin release.

Looser's zones are, however, highly suggestive of osteomalacia. They represent fractures that do not completely involve the entire cortical surface from the endosteal to the periosteal surface. They are true fractures and, though incomplete, should not be called pseudofractures. The incomplete calcification of the osteoid form at the fracture site results in the characteristic lucency. Characteristically, the areas of involvement are those where stress occurs. The sites most frequently involved are the medial borders of the femoral necks, the ischial and pubic rami, the axillary portion of the scapula, and the ribs. Looser's zones are not seen exclusively in this disease but can occur in any disease process where abnormal bone is subject to stress fractures and delayed healing.

HYPERPARATHYROIDISM

Hyperparathyroidism is a condition of excess secretion of parathyroid hormone. The disease results in "too little" bone because of "too much" resorption. Two types of hyperparathyroid disease will be discussed: primary and secondary.

Primary hyperparathyroidism

Etiology. Primary hyperparathyroidism is caused by primary hyperparathyroid hyperplasia, parathyroid adenoma, or parathyroid carcinoma. Primary hyperparathyroidism, from whatever cause, serves no useful function. The skeletal disease results from the uncontrolled excessive production of parathyroid hormone.

Pathogenesis. The clinical and morphologic appearance of primary hyperparathyroid disease is the result of excess parathyroid hormone. There is bone resorption with consequent hypercalcemia, which results in a compensatory hypophosphatemia. Because of the action of parathyroid hormone on the kidney, there is further hyperphosphaturia resulting in increasing hypophosphatemia. The alkaline phosphatase blood level is elevated.

Pathologic anatomy. Following are pathologic changes in bone in generalized osteodystrophia fibrosis:

1. Excessive bone resorption
2. Fibrosis, replacing the resorbed bone
3. Hemorrhages into fibrotic tissue with hemosiderosis
4. Cyst formation
5. Brown nodes
6. Osteoid seams

Excessive resorption is the first and most important pathologic feature; all other findings are consequential. In experimental studies in which animals were given excess parathyroid hormone and necropsies were carried out at different time intervals, the earliest mode of resorption was found to be osteocytic. Osteoclastic resorption occurred later and appeared to be concerned with the removal of bone already altered by osteolysis[4] (Fig. 7-4).

The resorbed bone is replaced by fibrous tissue. The degree of proliferation of fibrous tissue varies greatly, and the tissue is often subject to trauma. Hemorrhages occur and hemosiderin-laden macrophages appear within the fibrous tissue. Extravasated blood undergoes hemolysis, and with further hemorrhage into the area the fibrous tissue is pushed peripherally, causing the formation of a cyst. The cyst is lined by the compressed fibrous tissue. A brown node consists of loose connective tissue with hemorrhage and hemosiderosis, a large accumulation of osteoclasts, and perhaps a few remaining bone spicules.

Increased osteoblastic activity also occurs as an attempt to replace lost bone. The newly formed bone matrix is poorly mineralized and osteoid seams reflect one of the functions of parathyroid hormone—to retard mineralization of osteoid (Fig. 7-27). As stated previously, if the calcium gained by bone resorption were immediately deposited on the abundant newly formed osteoid, there would be no net increase in blood calcium.

Radiographic findings. The radiographic changes closely reflect the pathologic findings. The cystic lesions and brown nodes appear as well-marginated areas of bone replacement, which often expand bone (hyperostatic osteodystrophy fibrosa). The most frequent sites for this occurrence are the pelvis, long bones, hands, and ribs.

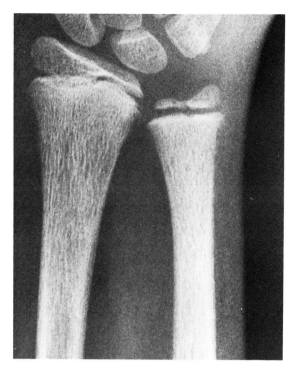

Fig. 7-27. Primary hyperparathyroidism in a growing child showing osteopenia. Ulnar cortex appears laminated. We believe this represents periosteal new bone incompletely calcified, rather than stimulated excess new bone formation. This radiographic picture may be confused with so-called tunneling.

Excessive resorption is the most commonly seen abnormal radiographic appearance. It may appear as generalized osteopenia, but there are common sites of confluent bone destruction. Following are some of the most common sites that are diagnostic of parathyroid hormone excess:

1. Subperiosteal bone of phalanges of the hand (particularly the medial side of the middle phalanges)
2. Lateral portions of the clavicle
3. Sacroiliac joints
4. Medial surface of proximal tibia
5. Medial surface of the symphysis pubis
6. Ischial tuberosities
7. Posterior-inferior calcaneus
8. Proximal medial humerus

Secondary hyperparathyroidism

Secondary hyperparathyroidism is induced by hypocalcemia, and its actions are compensatory to the depressed blood calcium level. There are two types of secondary hyperparathyroid disease: renal (RSH) and nutritional (NSH).

RSH. Hyperplasia of the parathyroid glands associated with renal insufficiency is well known.

Pathogenesis. Chronic renal insufficiency causes hypophosphaturia and therefore hyperphosphatemia. According to the mass law equation

$$\frac{Ca^{++} \times HPO_{\bar{i}}}{Ca\ HPO_i} = Kph$$

hyperphosphatemia induces hypocalcemia. The parathyroids are then stimulated and excessive bone resorption occurs. A partial, but usually incomplete, compensation of the hypocalcemia results. The insufficient kidneys do not respond, and hyperphosphatemia is progressive.

Furthermore, since 25-HCC is converted to its most active form, 1,25-DHCC, in the kidney, renal insufficiency blocks the activation of vitamin D (Figs. 7-14 and 7-25). This metabolite is involved in the formation of a calcium-binding protein in the intestine.[41] Decreased formation of this metabolite results in diminished intestinal absorption of calcium, hypocalcemia, and parathyroid gland stimulation. Renal osteodystrophy will be discussed later in the chapter.

Radiographic findings. The radiographic appearance of renal secondary hyperparathyroid disease is changing with the advent of dialysis and renal transplant. For the most part, however, generalized and subperiosteal resorption may occur (Figs. 7-28 and 7-29) as in primary hyperparathyroid disease, the common sites being the clavicle, hands, sacroiliac joints, and pelvic symphy-

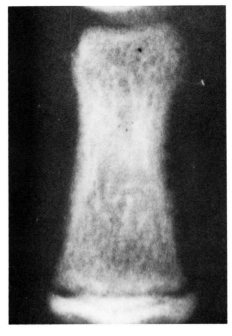

Fig. 7-28. Renal secondary hyperparathyroid disease in a growing child showing subperiosteal resorption of a phalanx.

sis. Brown nodes may occur, but cysts are not common.[16] Soft tissue and vascular calcifications commonly occur, especially in the later stages. This is more common and extensive than in primary hyperparathyroid disease. The greatly elevated phosphate level in RSH, compared to the low phosphate level in primary hyperparathyroid disease, accounts for this difference.

NSH. Nutritional secondary hyperparathyroid disease is a well-known entity in animals.[25, 27] It is less well known in humans but is believed by some to be a significant cause of "osteoporosis"—the clinical postmenopausal and senile entities. We believe "osteoporosis" is most commonly caused by increased resorption of bone, and a common cause of this resorption is dietary calcium deficiency with or without a relative phosphorus excess.[30] For this reason we include this entity under secondary hyperparathyroid disease (NSH).

Calcium-deficient diets result in bone loss and in striking bony alterations such as general osteitis fibrosa and bone atrophy.[35] It has been proposed that the parathyroid glands play an important role in the development of bone changes occurring as a result of prolonged calcium deficiency.[27] Others, however, have suggested that the bone changes are due to the calcium deficiency per se.

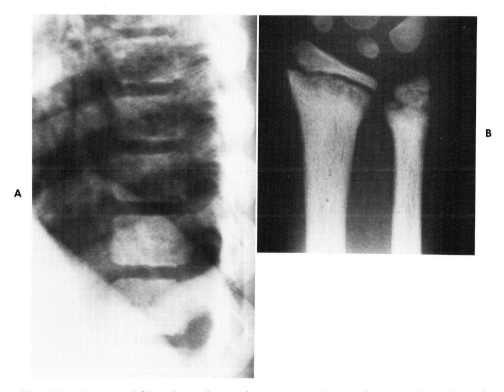

Fig. 7-29. Growing child with renal secondary hyperparathyroid disease with an elevated phosphate level. **A,** Dense vertebral bodies. **B,** Both osteopenia and sclerosis of bones of the wrist.

In an attempt to better define the possible role and endocrine mechanism of bone loss in dietary calcium restriction and subsequent repletion, we performed an experiment.

Experiment materials and methods. Six weanling (6-week-old) Yorkshire pigs of both sexes were fed a control diet containing 1.2% calcium and 1.0% phosphorus. The control pigs were designated C animals. Six other pigs, matched by litter and sex, were fed a diet containing 0.8% calcium and 1.6% phosphorus. These animals were designated T (test) animals. After 10 weeks, at age 16 weeks, two control pigs (C-1 and C-2) and two test pigs (T-1 and T-2) were sacrificed. The remaining test pigs (T-3 through T-6) were then switched to the control diet. One pair of control and test pigs were sacrificed after 1, 2, 3, and 4 weeks, respectively, on the control diet—at ages 17, 18, 19, and 20 weeks (pigs C-3 through C-6 and T-3 through T-6).

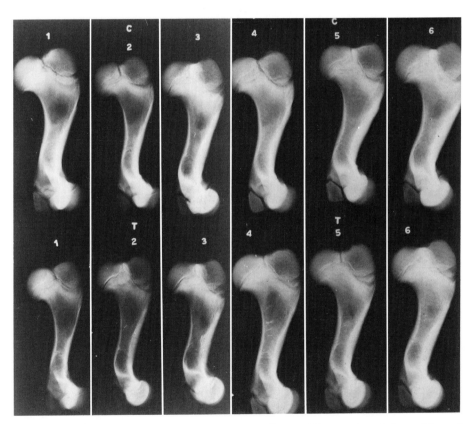

Fig. 7-30. Top row, radiographs of femurs of control pigs *(C)*. Pigs *1* and *2* are 16 weeks of age. Pigs *3, 4, 5,* and *6* are 17, 18, 19, and 20 weeks of age, respectively. Bottom row, test pigs *(T)*. Pigs *1* and *2* are 16 weeks of age and maximally experimentally depleted. Pigs *3, 4, 5,* and *6* are those repleted for 1, 2, 3, and 4 weeks, respectively. Note decreased density and cortical thickness of pigs *T-1* and *T-2* compared to their controls *(C-1* and *C-2)*. There is progressive increase in cortical thickness and metaphyseal density with progressive repletion.

The animals were sacrificed by intraperitoneal injection of pentobarbital sodium (Nembutal). Humeri were removed and specific gravity analysis and radiographic and histologic examinations were made. The parathyroid and thyroid glands were removed and processed for electron microscopy.

For radiographic examination the femurs of the pigs were stripped of all soft tissue and carefully positioned to ensure constant alignment. Technical factors were as follows: 55 kVp, 300 ma, 0.5 second; GAF 400/800 film was used and developed by hand, employing Kodak liquid developer at 68° F for 5 minutes. Measurements of the radiographs were taken with calipers at the area of maximal cortical thickness of the diaphysis. The total cortical thickness and the total diameter at that level were recorded. The cortex was then expressed as a percentage of the total diameter (the percent cortical thickness).

The stripped bones were weighed in air and water, and the specific gravities were determined by the following formula: the ratio of the mass of a body to the mass of an equal volume of water at 4° C.

Experiment results. The radiographs of the humeri are shown in Fig. 7-30. Radiographs of the humeri at 16 weeks demonstrated marked osteopenia of the T group characterized by decreased density of the trabecula and diminished percent cortical thickness (T-1 and T-2 animals) when compared to the C group at that time (C-1 and C-2). Progressively, after a repletion diet the trabecular density of the T animals (T-3 to T-6) increased, as did the percent

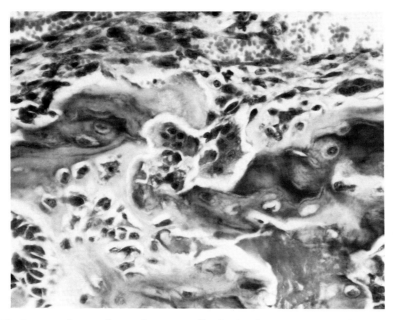

Fig. 7-31. Section of metaphysis of a maximally depleted pig showing evidence of marked resorption by active osteocytes. In addition, there is marked osteoclasia in areas where lysis has occurred. Little of the calcified cartilaginous core remains. There is also fibrous ingrowth. (H & E; ×350.)

cortical thickness. The cortical thickness of the maximally repleted animal (T-6) was similar to the 20-week control (C-6). The trabecular pattern was actually more dense than in the control. This could be best observed in the metaphysis or active enchondral growth area (Figs. 7-32 and 7-33).

At 16 weeks the specific gravity of bone of the depleted pigs was less than the controls of that age. With repletion there was progressive increase in the specific gravity. At 20 weeks (4 weeks' repletion diet) the specific gravity of T-6 was similar to that of C-6 (Fig. 7-34).

The histologic appearance of the bone and the results of electron microscopy of the parathyroid chief cells and parafollicular cells are the subjects of a separate report.[33] However, to explain briefly, during the depletion stage, the chief cells of the parathyroid gland were characterized by hyperactivity, reflecting the elaboration of parathyroid hormone. Repletion, however, resulted in prompt return of the parathyroid chief cell activity to normal. The parafollicular cells of the test group appeared indistinguishable from the control group, indicating that calcitonin may have no involvement in the appearance of bone associated with a diet that is calcium depleted and then repleted.

Histologically, during the depletion diet there was marked resorption of both

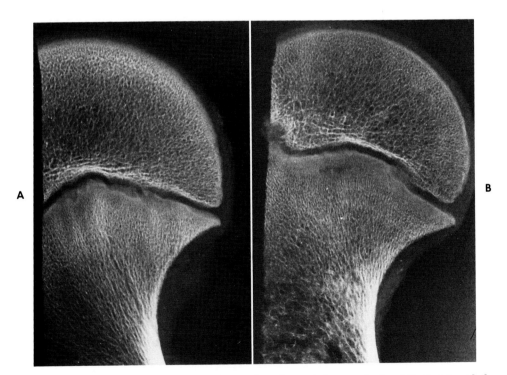

Fig. 7-32. A, Magnified radiograph of metaphyseal area of control pig *C-2*. **B,** Magnified radiograph of metaphyseal area of maximally depleted pig *(T-2).* Note marked osteopenia, compared to control. This is most apparent in the subchondral epiphyseal bone. In addition, just beneath the epiphyseal line there is evidence of lack of distinct trabeculae. Diaphyseal trabeculae are likewise sparser and thinner.

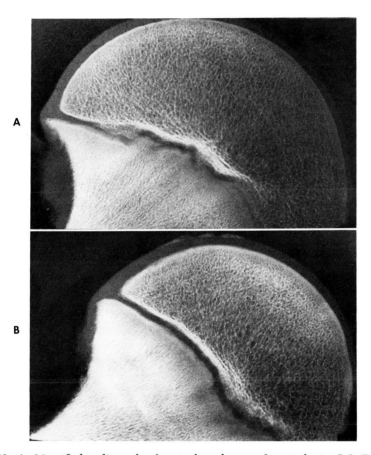

Fig. 7-33. A, Magnified radiograph of metaphyseal area of control pig *C-6.* **B,** Magnified radiograph of metaphyseal area of a maximally repleated pig *(T-6).* There is increased density of the primary and secondary trabeculae compared to control in **A** and a convex medial border of the metaphysis. Increased density is somewhat chalky in appearance and reminiscent of healing rickets or sclerotic renal osteodystrophy.

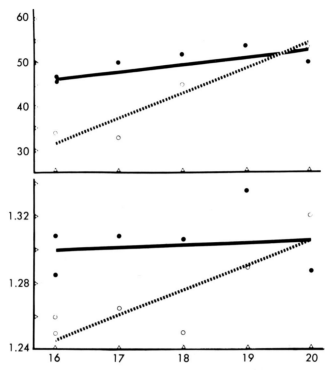

Fig. 7-34. Percent cortical thickness of middiaphysis of femur as measured on the radiography (ordinate) above and the specific gravity (ordinate) below as a function of age in weeks (abscissa). Controls are the solid lines and the test groups are the broken lines. Regression line equations for percent cortical thickness:

$$C: Y = 1.325 \ X + 26.425; \ r = + \ 0.723, \ P > 0.05$$
$$T: Y = 5.300 \ X - 50.300; \ r = + \ 0.897, \ P < 0.01$$

bone and calcified cartilage by active osteocytes and osteoclasis (Fig. 7-31). After the repletion diet, osteolysis was diminished with a gradual return of the cartilaginous core to normal. The histologic appearance then correlated well with the radiographic appearance and the specific gravity of bone. In addition, prominent osteoid seams were found in the depleted phase.

The administration of a low calcium diet to growing pigs (test animals) resulted in osteopenia, as seen radiographically and as determined by specific gravity. Histologically, the bones of the growing pigs on the calcium-poor diet were characterized by increased osteocytic osteolysis, osteoclasia, and accelerated removal of the cartilaginous core. These observations agree with the "osteoporotic" changes noted in other young animals fed a low calcium diet. In the rat, for example, loss of bone tissue, osteocytic activation, appearance of resorption cavities, and thinness of the compacta have been observed.[18, 35]

Accelerated osteocytic resorption seen in the long bones of the test pigs was found in the proximity of the cartilaginous core; thus, when the core was within

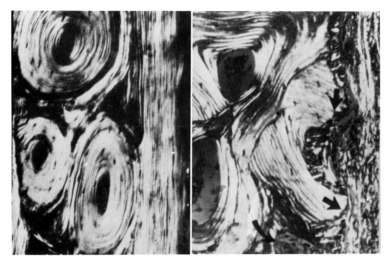

Fig. 7-35. Transverse section of middiaphysis of humerus of a 14-month-old horse with nutritional secondary hyperparathyroid disease (right) and age match control (left). In the normal horse, haversian canals are narrow and outer circumferential lamellae, which support the periosteum, are well defined. Bone of the hyperparathyroid horse is characterized by extensive subperiosteal resorption with complete loss of circumferential lamellae. Haversian canals are wider, and osteonic lamellae are severed by osteoclasts (straight arrows). There is a large resorption cavity within intersititial lamellae (curved arrow). (H & E; ×120, polarized light.) (From Krook, L., and Lowe, J. E.: Supplementum ad Pathologia Veterinaria, vol. 1, Basel, 1964, S. Karger.)

range of this osteocytic activity, it could be removed. Such resorption would be similar to that proposed by Belanger[3] in bone resorption by deep-seated osteocytes. In the present case, however, the target of the resorbing osteocyte is cartilage, not bone. This has been called osteocytic chondrolysis.[46] Repletion of the test pigs by instituting a normal calcium-phosphorus ratio in the diet inhibited the osteocytic chondrolysis, returning it to normal levels. This also resulted in a normal amount of retention of the cartilaginous core and returned the bone density to control levels.

The present study strongly indicates that the parathyroid gland plays an important role in the development of the "osteoporosis" (osteopenia) associated with the low calcium diet and in the reversal of these changes.

The average American diet is relatively low in calcium (milk and cheese) and relatively high in phosphorus (meat). We believe that this may be an important etiologic cause of the clinical entity osteoporosis. This concept has been extensively reviewed by Krook et al.[30] In Fig. 7-36 the plasma calcium and phosphorus levels are contrasted in the three forms of hyperparathyroid disease discussed.

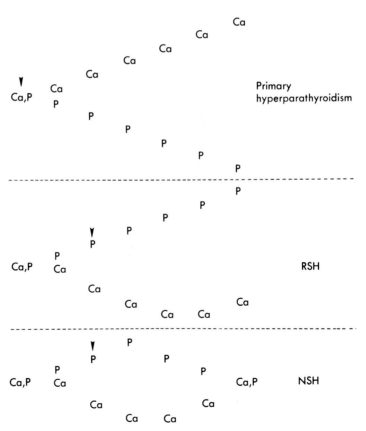

Fig. 7-36. Summary of plasma calcium and phosphorus in hyperparathyroidism.

RENAL OSTEODYSTROPHY

A separate, brief discussion of renal osteodystrophy is included, since almost all the previously discussed factors influencing bone are involved, and it is a bone lesion frequently presented to the radiologist.

The pathogenesis of the changes causing osteopenia in renal disease have been well established. They are caused by osteomalacia and hyperparathyroidism. The mechanism of the production of sclerotic bone changes in renal disease, however, is not well established. Many theories of its pathogenesis have been advanced. Garner and Ball[5] attributed the increased bone density to the formation of large amounts of unmineralized bone. If one defines osteomalacia by the presence of osteoid seam, the sclerotic change, according to their explanation, would then be due to osteomalacia. Shapiro[40] postulated that the sclerotic changes seen in the so-called rugger-jersey spine resulted from calcified osteoid, newly laid down, which was resistant to resorption. Selye[38] demonstrated increased bone density in mice with parathyroid gland extract and Doyle et al.[24] further demonstrated increased bone density in thyroparathyroidectomized rats given large doses of parathyroid hormone, excluding a secondary calcitonin effect as the cause of osteosclerosis. In our laboratory we were unable to detect increased bone density with doses of 5 to 40 IU given daily to growing rats over a 3-week period, although a dose-related elevation of blood calcium and alkaline phosphatase and a decrease in blood phosphorus were found[34] (Fig. 7-37).

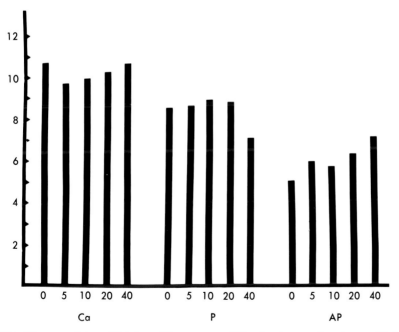

Fig. 7-37. Plasma calcium *(Ca)* in milligrams per 100 ml, plasma phosphorus *(P)* in milligrams per 100 ml, and alkaline phosphatase *(AP)* in sigma units per 100 ml (ordinate) as a function of parathyroid hormone injected intravenously (abscissa).

Selye[39] noted that moderate doses of parathyroid gland extract stimulated new bone formation, whereas larger doses promoted bone resorption. It may be that bone density secondary to parathyroid hormone is a function of dose or perhaps, in addition, the local concentration of calcium and phosphorus.

Bony sclerosis is most commonly seen in the metaphysis of growing bone with long-standing renal disease. It occurs rarely in primary hyperparathyroidism, but when it does it is most commonly seen in the growing metaphysis.[12] In primary hyperparathyroidism there are always areas of osteopenia in other portions of bone when sclerosis occurs. When it occurs in renal osteodystrophy, it is always preceded by and coexists with osteopenia from both secondary hyperparathyroidism and osteomalacia. Further correlation of bone density, as determined by photon absorption with various biochemical parameters, yields interesting results. In patients on dialysis there is a significant correlation of increasing bone density with elevated serum creatinine levels and serum phosphorus levels.[17] Thus it appears the most likely circumstances for sclerotic renal osteodystrophy are the following:

1. A growing child
2. Metaphyseal location
3. Preexisting osteomalacia and hyperparathyroid disease
4. Elevated serum creatinine levels
5. Elevated serum phosphorus levels

The radiographic appearance of sclerotic renal osteodystrophy has been graphically described by British authors, who note the rugger-jersey spine and the rotting stump of the femoral neck. These have characteristic radiographic appearances.[21] If it is remembered that the vertebral bodies have two growth areas and therefore two metaphyseal areas, each of these corresponding to the sclerotic area of the rugger-jersey spine, it is easy to correlate these two radiographic observations and descriptions. The chalky sclerotic densities in both cases are metaphyseal. The "rotted" portion of the femoral neck corresponds to the noncalcified osteoid with the inferior sclerotic border corresponding to newly calcified osteoid (nonlamellar bone). Most of these changes are seen in growing children with renal disease, secondary hyperparathyroidism, and osteomalacia. In addition, most of these patients have elevated phosphate levels.

We believe all these factors are important in the pathogenesis of sclerotic changes. The mere presence of excess osteoid does not seem a plausible explanation, since osteoid is of soft tissue density. The rarity of sclerosis in primary hyperparathyroid disease makes it extremely unlikely that the pathogenesis is that of parathyroid effect. The unusual case of sclerosis in primary hyperparathyroid disease may, however, be a function of the parathyroid hormone level coupled with the local level of calcium and phosphorus. In renal disease that produces sclerosis there is always preexisting and concurrent hyperparathyroid effect and osteomalacia. The areas involved are those where either cartilage core or osteoid are being most actively laid down. We believe that the osteopenic phase, characterized by osteoid seams and noncalcified cartilage produced by both parathyroid hormone effect and inactive vitamin D, is fertile ground for avid calcification to occur, once the calcium and phosphorus product rises and is supersaturated. This is particularly true when the product is a result of a tremendously elevated phosphorus level, which generally occurs at a time when calcification also occurs in the soft tissues and blood vessels. This concept is diagrammatically explained in Fig. 7-38. Figs. 7-39 and 7-40 show osteopenic and osteosclerotic bone changes in 2 patients with renal insufficiency correlated with their blood calcium and phosphorus levels.

The sclerotic changes seen in the test pigs described in the experiment on NSH resulted from the production of osteoid seams by parathyroid hormone elaboration and the subsequent calcification of these abundant seams in the growing areas of bone, brought about by repleting the animals. These changes are reminiscent of those seen in sclerotic renal osteodystrophy and in healing rickets. The common denominator of all these is preexisting osteoid seams and the consequent availability of calcium or phosphorus to avidly calcify them.

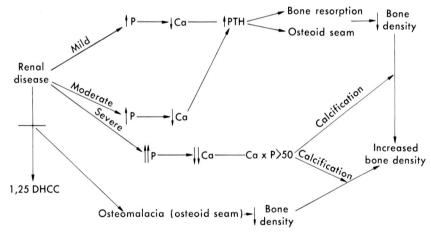

Fig. 7-38. Diagrammatic representation of pathogenesis of bone changes in renal disease. Initially, in mild renal disease, there is slight elevation of serum phosphate level, requiring a decrease in blood calcium level, resulting in parathyroid hormone release. This causes bone resorption and formation of osteoid seams, giving a radiographic appearance of decreased bone density. In moderate renal disease, there is accentuation of these changes with further decrease in bone density. There is diminished formation of 1,25-DHCC, causing increasing superimposed osteomalacia (osteoid seams), which causes more diminished bone density. As severe renal disease ensues, further phosphate retention occurs causing higher serum phosphate levels, which leads to marked increase in the product of calcium and phosphorus. The decrease in serum calcium level cannot compensate completely for this increased product. Calcification then occurs in soft tissues, blood vessels, and most actively in the available osteoid in bone, resulting in increased bone density, particularly in areas of metaphyseal growth, where most new osteoid is laid down.

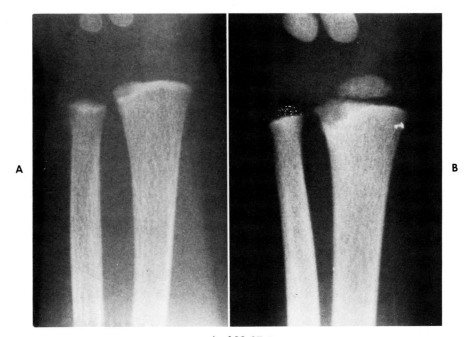

A. 122 87 71

Date	Ca	P	Ca x P
1/5/71	7.4	4.4	33
2/5/71	9.0	4.6	41
*3/4/71	9.8	2.4	24
1/6/72	7.0	6.1	43
*3/7/73	8.6	5.2	45

Fig. 7-39. Radiographs of a growing child taken 2 years apart. **A,** The major change is osteopenia at a time when the calcium and phosphorus product is relatively low. **B,** Taken at a time when the calcium and phosphorus product is increased primarily because of the increased phosphate level. Sclerosis is due to increased product. There are still areas of osteopenia, presumably because of the low serum calcium level, which stimulates parathyroid hormone production. **C,** Blood chemistries over the approximate 2-year span. Asterisks correspond to times of radiographs in **A** and **B.**

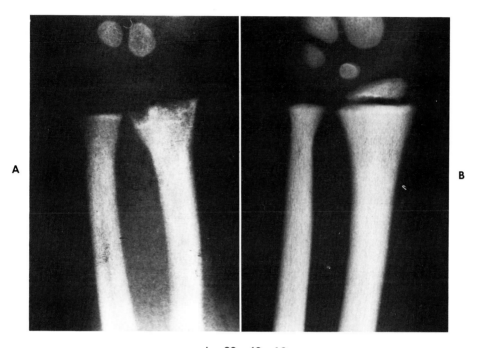

J. 99 69 12

	Date	Ca	P	Ca x P
	6/65	8.1	5.9	48
C	*6/66	10.0	4.3	43
	5/67	10.2	4.7	48
	*9/69	10.2	6.2	63

Fig. 7-40. Radiographs of a growing child taken 39 months apart. **A,** Combined osteopenic and osteosclerotic change. **B,** Overwhelming change is that of osteosclerosis, corresponding to a greatly increased calcium and phosphorus product caused mainly by an elevated phosphate blood level. **C,** Blood chemistries over a 4¼-year period. Asterisks correspond to times of radiographs in **A** and **B.**

HYPERCALCITONINISM

As stated earlier, the role of calcitonin in bone metabolism and modeling is still difficult to determine. There are, however, several areas where pathologic excess is demonstrable in bone disease.

Dietary calcium excess

Krook et al.[28] described a syndrome they termed nutritional hypercalcitoninism in bulls that had been fed a diet containing excess calcium equivalent to that fed milking cows. This diet resulted in marked parafollicular cell activity and calcitonin release with tremendously overgrown bones causing marked hypertrophic bone changes (Fig. 7-41). The histologic hallmark of this disease state was a marked decrease in osteocytic osteolysis (Fig. 7-42). Furthermore, when growing dogs were fed a diet containing excess calcium, the results were parafollicular hyperactivity, calcitonin excess, and pathologically dense bones, which were at times debilitating.[19] There is no evidence that dietary excess of calcium in humans results in bone disease, but there is evidence of calcitonin release after the ingestion of excess calcium protecting the body from hypercalcemia.[15]

?Osteopetrosis

Osteopetrosis has been properly called the disease of universal failure of modeling. All bones fail to model whether classified as endochondral or membranous, although the most striking changes occur in those preformed in cartilage. Jaffe[23] states that the histologic hallmarks of this disease are the accumulation and persistence of calcified cartilage normally resorbed in the course of

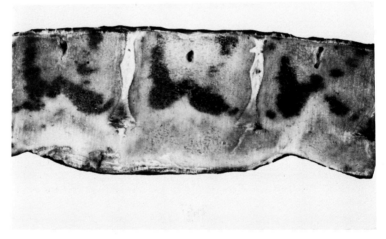

Fig. 7-41. Lumbar region of an 11½-year-old bull fed five times the recommended levels of calcium for his entire life. Nutritional hypercalcitoninism is characterized by osteopetrosis, with dense bone "squeezing" out red marrow in vertebral bodies. (From Krook, et al.: Cornell Vet. **61**:625, 1971.)

modeling and a reduced number of osteoclasts. According to Jaffe, the osteogenesis is not due to osteoblastic activity but to metaplasia of cartilage. Furthermore, he states that cartilage is laid down as a primitive, nonlamellar-type bone with very little of it being transformed into more mature lamellar type. He thus attributes the pathologic picture to two factors—decreased osteoclastic activity and cartilage metaplasia causing abnormal bone formation.

Our opinion is in agreement with the histologic description, but we disagree on the pathogenesis in that we believe the histologic appearance is caused by inhibited osteocytic osteolysis and chondrolysis.[29] Since osteocytic chondrolysis accounts for the removal of calcified cartilage, inhibition of osteocytic chondrolysis explains its retention.[46, 49] Also since osteocytic activity is largely responsible for normal bone modeling,[42, 44] its absence accounts for failure of modeling. The histologic picture of osteopetrosis also shows cementing lines, which we believe reflect arrested osteocytic osteolysis. The histologic hallmarks of osteopetrosis are then indistinguishable from the effects of excess calcitonin on growing bones listed here:

1. Persistence of calcified cartilaginous core
2. Inactive osteocytes
3. Decreased number of osteoclasts, only in proportion to diminished osteocytic resorption
4. Cementing lines
5. Nonlamellar-type bone in areas where lamellar-type bone should be present

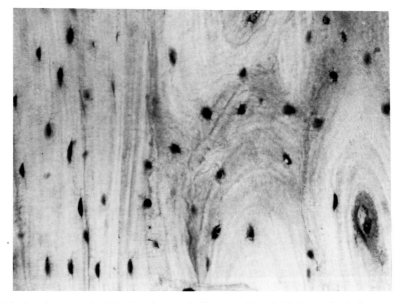

Fig. 7-42. Lumbar vertebral body of same bull as in Fig. 7-41. Instead of the normal cancellous with anastomosing trabeculae, there is severe osteopetrosis. Osteocytic osteolysis is minimal or absent. (Toluidine blue; ×300.)

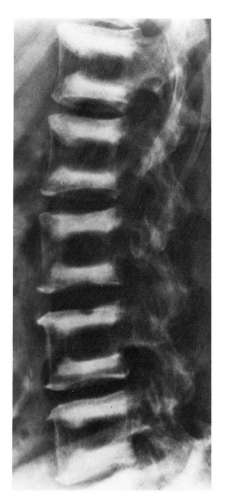

Fig. 7-43. Radiograph of lumbar spine in a patient with human osteopetrosis. Note increased density in subchondral area of vertebral bodies (the metaphysis). This corresponds to nonresorbed calcified cartilage. Appearance is reminiscent of healing rickets and sclerotic renal osteodystrophy.

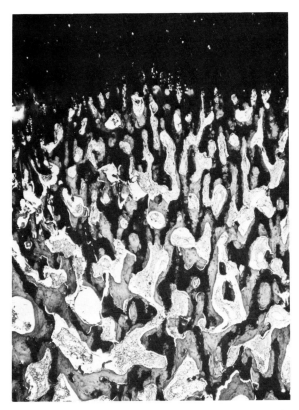

Fig. 7-44. Histologic section of iliac crest of a child with osteopetrosis. Apophyseal cartilage at top is inactive. Thick trabeculae contain large amounts of chondroid core. (H & E; ×25.)

Radiographically, the modeling error is apparent. The marked increased density results from a combination of the persistent calcified cartilaginous core and the failure of resorption of bone in the modeling process (Figs. 7-43 and 7-44), all secondary to inhibited resorption. The role of excess calcitonin in this disease is yet to be determined.

?HYPOCALCITONINISM
?Hereditary bone dysplasia with hyperphosphatasemia

Although there is no established syndrome of calcitonin deficiency, hereditary bone dysplasia with hyperphosphatasemia may be related to such a deficiency. This disease is characterized by tremendously accelerated bone resorption with compensatory bone production, resulting in completely disorganized, or woven, bone structure. The disease responds to calcitonin therapy,[22, 45] which slows bone turnover and appears to convert the immature, woven bone to more mature, lamellar-type bone. Studies are in progress to establish calcitonin deficiency in this disease.

?Paget's disease

The hallmarks of Paget's disease, all reflecting excessive bone turnover, are well known both histologically and biochemically.[23] The histologic picture is similar to that of hereditary bone dysplasia with hyperphosphatasemia. Belanger et al.[5] pointed out excessive osteocytic osteolysis in this disease process. The promising results with calcitonin treatment[52] further suggest the pathogenesis of this disease to be that of primary bone resorption with compensatory bone production. The possibility of calcitonin deficiency, however, is less likely than in hereditary bone dysplasia with hyperphosphatasemia, since Paget's disease tends to be a localized rather than a systemic disease.

References

1. Albright, F., and Ellsworth, R.: Studies on the physiology of the parathyroid glands. I. Calcium and phosphorus studies on a case of idiopathic hypoparathyroidism, J. Clin. Invest. 7:183, 1929.
2. Alvioli, L. V., and Haddad, J. G.: Vitamin D: current concepts, Metabolism 22:507, 1973.
3. Belanger, L. F.: Osteocytic osteolysis, Calcif. Tissue Res. 4:1, 1969.
4. Belanger, L. F., et al.: The two faces of resorption. In Fleisch, H., Blackwood, H. J. J., and Owen, M., editors: Proceedings of the Third European Symposium on Calcified Tissues, New York, 1966, Springer Publishing Co., Inc.
5. Belanger, L. F., Jarry, L., and Uhthoff, H. K.: Osteocytic osteolysis in Paget's disease, Rev. Can. Biol. 27:37, 1968.
6. Braunstein, H., and Stephens, C. L.: Parafollicular cells of human thyroid, Arch. Pathol. 86:659, 1968.
7. Caffey, J. P.: Pediatric x-ray diagnosis, ed. 6, Chicago, 1972, Year Book Medical Publishers, Inc.
8. Chan, A. S., and Conen, P. E.: Ultrastructural observations on cytodifferentiation of parafollicular cells in the human fetal thyroid, Lab. Invest. 25: 3:249, 1971.
9. Copp, D. H., et al.: Evidence for calcitonin. A new hormone from the parathyroid that lowers blood calcium, Endocrinology 70:638, 1962.
10. DeLuca, H. F.: Recent advances in our understanding of the metabolism of Vitamin D and its regulation, Clin. Endocrinol. 5:975, 1976.
11. Dodds, G. S.: Osteoclasts and cartilage removal in enchondral ossification of certain mammals, Am. J. Anat. 50:97, 1932.
12. Doyle, F. H.: Radiologic assessment of endocrine effects on bone, Radiol. Clin. North Am. 5:289, 1967.
13. Foster, C. V.: Effect of thyrocalcitonin on bone, Lancet 2:1426, 1966.
14. Garner, A., and Ball, J.: Quantitative observation on mineralized and unmineralized bone in chronic renal azotemia, J. Pathol. 91:545, 1968.
15. Gray, T. K., and Munson, P. L.: Thyrocalcitonin: evidence for physiological function, Science 166:512, 1969.
16. Griffiths, H. J., Ennis, J. T., and Bailey, G.: Skeletal changes following renal transplantation, Radiology 113:621, 1974.
17. Griffiths, H. J., Zimmerman, R. E., Bailey, G., and Snider, R.: Use of photon absorptiometry in the diagnosis of renal osteodystrophy, Radiology 109: 277, 1973.
18. Harrison, M., and Fraser, R. J.: Bone structure and metabolism in calcium-deficient rats, J. Endocrinol. 21:197, 1960.
19. Hedhammar, A., et al.: Overnutrition and skeletal disease. An experimental study in growing Great Dane dogs, Cornell Vet. 64(suppl. 5):128, April, 1974.
20. Hirsch, P. F., Gauthier, G. F., and Munson, P. L.: Thyroid hypocalcemic principle and recurrent laryngeal nerve injury as factors affecting the response to parathyroidectomy in rats, Endocrinology 73:244, 1963.
21. Hodson, C. J.: Endocrine and metabolic bone disease. In Sutton, D., and Grainger, R. G., editors: Textbook of radiology, Baltimore, 1969, The Williams & Wilkins Co.
22. Horwith, M., et al.: Hereditary bone dysplasia with hyperphosphatasemia: re-

sponse to synthetic human calcitonin, Clin. Endocrinol. **5**(suppl.):341s, Feb., 1976.

23. Jaffe, H. L.: Metabolic, degenerative and inflammatory diseases of bones and joints, Philadelphia, 1972, Lea & Febiger, Publishers.

24. Kalu, D. N., Doyle, F. H., Pennock, J., and Foster, G. V.: Parathyroid hormone and experimental osteosclerosis, Lancet **1**:1363, 1970.

25. Krook, L.: Dietary calcium and phosphorus and lameness in the horse, Cornell Vet. **58**(suppl. 1):59, 1968.

26. Krook, L.: Metabolic bone disease of endocrine origin. In Pallaske, G., Dobberstein, J., and Stünzi, H., editors: Ernst Joests Handbuch der Speziellen pathologischen Anatomie der Haustiere, vol. I, Berlin, 1969, Parex.

27. Krook, L., Barrett, R. B., Usui, K., and Wolke, R. E.: Nutritional secondary hyperparathyroidism in the cat, Cornell Vet. **53**:224, 1963.

28. Krook, L., et al.: Nutritional hypercalcitoninism in bulls, Cornell Vet. **61**: 625, 1971.

29. Krook, L., et al.: Osteopetrosis: the role of osteocytic chondrolysis in its pathogenesis. (In preparation.)

30. Krook, L., Whalen, J. P., Lesser, G. V., and Berens, D. L.: Experimental studies on osteoporosis. In Jasmin, G., and Cantin, M., editors: Methods and achievements in experimental pathology, vol. VII, Basel, 1975, S. Karger.

31. McLean, F. C.: The parathyroid glands and bone. In Bourne, G. H., editor: The biochemistry and physiology of bone, New York, 1956, Academic Press, Inc.

32. Nonidez, J. F.: The origin of the parafollicular cell. A second epithelial component of the thyroid of the dog, Am. J. Anat. **49**:479, 1932.

33. Nunez, E. A., Krook, L., and Whalen, J. P.: Effect of calcium depletion and subsequent repletion on parathyroids, parafollicular (C) cells and bone in the growing pig, Cell Tissue Res. **168**:373, 1976.

34. O'Donohue, N., Krook, L., Whalen, J. P., and Nunez, E. A.: Effect of parathormone on the growing skeleton, Invest. Radiol. **9**:311, 1974.

35. Ornoy, A., Wolinsky, I., and Guggenheim, K.: Structure of long bones of rats and mice fed a low calcium diet, Calcif. Tissue Res. **15**:71, 1974.

36. Raisz, L. G.: Stimulation of bone resorption by parathyroid hormone in tissue culture, Nature **197**:1015, 1963.

37. Rasmussen, H., and DeLuca, H. F.: Calcium homeostasis, Ergeb. Physiol. **63**: 108, 1963.

38. Selye, H.: On the stimulation of new bone formation with parathyroid extract and irradiated ergosterol, Endocrinology **16**:547, 1932.

39. Selye, H.: Mechanism of parathyroid hormone action, Arch. Pathol. **34**:625, 1942.

40. Shapiro, R.: Radiologic aspects of renal osteodystrophy, Radiol. Clin. North Am. **10**:557, 1972.

41. Wasserman, R. H., and Taylor, A. N.: Vitamin D_3-induced calcium-binding protein in chick intestinal mucosa, Science **152**:791, 1966.

42. Whalen, J. P., et al.: Mechanisms of bone resorption in human metaphyseal remodelling: a roentgenographic and histologic study, Am. J. Roentgenol. Radium Ther. Nucl. Med. **112**:526, 1971.

43. Whalen, J. P., et al.: Growing bone: the role of internal resorption and its control. In Kaufman, H. J., editor: Progress in pediatric radiology, vol. 4, Basel, 1973, S. Karger.

44. Whalen, J. P., et al.: Neonatal transplacental rubella syndrome: its effect on normal maturation of the diaphysis, Am. J. Roentgenol. Radium Ther. Nucl. Med. **121**:166, 1974.

45. Whalen, J. P., et al.: Calcitonin treatment in hereditary bone dysplasia with hyperphosphatasemia. A radiographic and histologic study of bone, Am. J. Roentgenol. Radium Ther. Nucl. Med. (In press.)

46. Whalen, J. P., Krook, L., MacIntyre, I., and Nunez, E. A.: Calcitonin, parathyroidectomy and modelling of bones in the growing rat, J. Endocrinol. **66**: 207, 1975.

47. Whalen, J. P., Krook, L., and Nunez, E. A.: A radiographic and histologic study of bone in the active and hibernating bat (Myotis lucifugus), Anat. Rec. **172**:97, 1972.

48. Whalen, J. P., Krook, L., Nunez, E. A., and MacIntyre, I.: Bone, bones and calcitonin. Endocrinology 1973. In Taylor,

S., editor: Proceedings of the Fourth International Symposium, London, 1973, William Heinemann Medical Books, Ltd., London, pp. 143-152.

49. Whalen, J. P., O'Donohue, N., Krook, L., and Nunez, E. A.: Pathogenesis of abnormal bone remodelling: effects of yellow phosphorus in the growing rat, Anat. Rec. 177:15, 1973.

50. Winchester, P., et al.: The growing metaphysis. The roentgen significance of the perichondral ring. (In preparation.)

51. Woodhouse, N. J. Y., Doyle, F. H., and Joplin, G. F.: Vitamin D deficiency and primary hyperparathyroidism, Lancet 2: 283, 1971.

52. Woodhouse, N. J. Y., et al.: Human calcitonin in the treatment of Paget's bone disease, Lancet 1:1139, 1971.

8 Bone imaging

Alfred Eric Jones and Gerald S. Johnston

Bone scanning (scintigraphy) is a valuable diagnostic tool that is gaining acceptance for the detection of malignant metastases. In addition, this imagery can be useful in the detection of primary bone tumors, osteomyelitis, fractures, and certain traumatic and metabolic diseases involving bone that may not be clearly delineated by conventional radiographs. Since these latter cases are relatively few in number, the great majority of bone studies are performed to show the presence or absence of primary or metastatic osseous tumors. Considering the frequency with which bony metastases accompany cancer in other organs,[1, 37] the potential benefit from this technique through the early detection of metastases is enormous.

The information provided by bone scans can be crucial in the management of malignant disease. The images provide clear-cut data that answer important, frequently asked questions about the extent of disease, sites involved, likelihood of spread or recurrence, and response to treatment. The various scanning agents concentrate in areas of reactive bone formation with high specificity. Scanning agents have been developed that meet high nuclear medical criteria for localization and for rapid clearance from the blood and other tissues.[46]

After the diagnosis of malignancy is made, bone scintigraphy can help those concerned with the patient's care to decide on the kind of treatment to be used. Radical mastectomy could well be a useless and unnecessary ordeal for a patient with breast cancer if it could be shown that metastasis to the skeleton was already established.

Whether the first bone scan is normal (Fig. 8-1) or abnormal, it can be used as a baseline marker for study of a tumor's behavior under therapy, thus providing the oncologist with additional means by which to monitor the advance or regression of disease.

Although conventional radiographs may detect many metastatic lesions, in many instances bone scintigraphy has shown metastatic disease when radiographs were negative or equivocal*—sometimes as long as 18 months before they become abnormal[24] (Fig. 8-2). At times, however, the bone scan has remained normal despite widespread metastatic disease evidenced by radiography (Fig.

---

*References 8, 28, 31, 38, 47, 63.

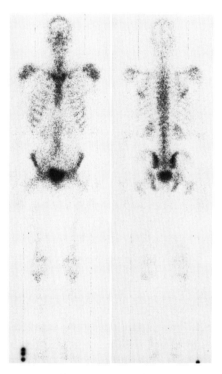

Fig. 8-1. Normal bone scan performed with 5 to 1 reduction on a whole-body scanner 3 hours following an intravenous, 10 mCi dose of technetium 99m diphosphonate. Anterior view with bladder activity is on left, and posterior view with kidney visualization is on right. Patient was a 20-year-old man with stage II-B Hodgkin's disease.

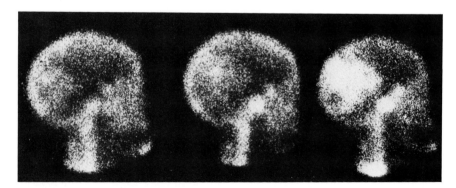

Fig. 8-2. This series of bone scans shows a lesion in right occiput of skull, which progressed from March 24 (left) through June 18 (center) to large lesion on right on October 20. Patient was a 59-year-old woman with breast carcinoma. Skull x-ray films remained normal, despite striking bone scan appearance.

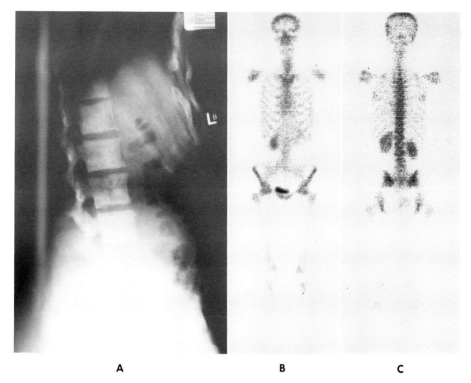

Fig. 8-3. A, This 45-year-old woman has breast cancer with widespread bony metastases shown on x-ray examination. **B** and **C,** Her bone scans were normal on four occasions from 1973 to 1975.

8-3). Since each method provides information of a different kind, the bone scan and radiograph complement one another and should be used in conjunction. The bone scan reflects aspects of the metabolic status of skeletal tissue, whereas radiographs record the net result of bone destruction and new bone formation.

From all this, one would expect bone scintigraphy to have a very prominent place in the diagnosis and staging of tumors and other diseases involving the skeletal structure. Unfortunately, this has not been the case. Although bone scintigraphy is being used with increasing frequency in specialized cancer centers and in some general hospitals as a routine preoperative surgical procedure for cancer patients, its full potential has not been realized. This is explained in part by the relative newness of the procedure and the rapid succession of newly developed imaging agents and techniques, which has caused some confusion.

HISTORY

Radioisotopes of calcium and strontium have lent themselves nicely to the study of calcium turnover throughout the body and in bones specifically. In 1941 the concentrations of calcium 45 and strontium 89 were demonstrated in bone tumors, and attempts were made to use these radionuclides as therapeutic agents.[44, 45] Since then, radioisotopic tagging methods have been used to study bone metabolism in normal and many disease states.[*] The specific in vivo detection of tumor sites was first done by hand-probe scanning in 1959.[3]

Radioisotopes of gallium were studied for their tendency to localize in primary and metastatic bone tumors. These radionuclides were also employed as possible therapeutic agents[13, 40] in the late 1940s and in the 1950s. Although the intravenous use of radionuclides of calcium, strontium, and gallium was established as an inadequate approach to the treatment of tumor in bone, the differential concentration of radioactivity in the lesions was recognized as a powerful diagnostic tool.

Strontium 85, with its relatively good imaging characteristics but high radiation dosage, was used for obtaining bone scans in patients with known malignancy and became the standard bone-imaging agent of the 1960s.[9, 10, 12, 16, 49] As with gallium 68,[67] the strontium 85 bone scans detected bone metastases before the lesions were delineated radiographically. Although bone scintigraphy with strontium 85 was cumbersome, it was used to advantage in helping delineate portals for irradiation therapy,[55] in determining the extent of primary bone tumor involvement prior to amputation, and in searching for metastatic bone involvement.[54]

Fluorine 18 was introduced as a superior imaging agent in 1962.[4, 23, 66] At that time high cost and general unavailability prevented its wide use. By the early 1970s radiopharmaceutical manufacturers had made this short-lived, positron-emitting, bone-localizing nuclide more generally available at a lower price.[52] However, it could not be used with the widely popular conventional scintillation camera because of its energetic photon emission. A short-lived, low radiation dose material that could be used with the gamma scintillation camera was needed.

In 1971 the technetium 99m-tagged polyphosphates[58] were received as an answer to the shortcomings of earlier bone-imaging agents. High doses of these bone-seeking compounds soon became available and provided the capability of rapid bone visualization with low radiation dose and improved resolution using either gamma cameras or scanning devices (Fig. 8-4).[35] The only drawback was the variable stability of the early preparations. At present, technetium 99m diphosphonate (disodium ethane-1-hydroxy-1, 1-diphosphonate), the first reliable stable form of these agents, appears to be the most widely used.[6] However, good preparations of technetium 99m-tagged polyphosphate, pyrophosphate, or diphosphonate give comparable imaging results.[64, 33]

Comparative studies of the use of fluorine 18, technetium 99m diphosphonate, and radiographic skeletal survey have demonstrated the superiority of technetium 99m diphosphonate in the detection of metastases.[35, 46, 65] In one study fluorine 18 detected 56% of all lesions seen by technetium 99m diphosphonate, whereas approximately one third of the lesions were detected by skeletal radiography.[53]

---

[*]References 2, 11, 36, 42, 43, 50, 57, 61, 63.

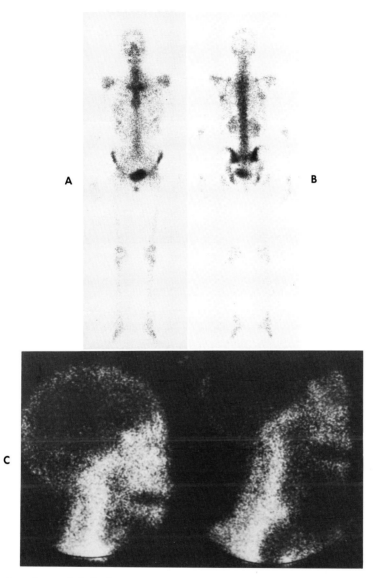

Fig. 8-4. **A** and **B**, Whole-body scan of a 40-year-old patient with breast carcinoma without metastatic disease to bone. **C**, Lateral head view was obtained using gamma scintillation camera. Lateral neck view reveals increased activity in neck to be thyroid cartilage.

BONE PHYSIOLOGY AND MECHANISM OF LOCALIZATION OF BONE-IMAGING AGENTS

The apatite crystal is generally presented as the basic mineral component of bone. Atoms in the crystals form a lattice arrangement in which each ion is surrounded by ions of the opposite charge. At the surface, however, unbalanced charges exert a force that attracts oppositely charged ions.[40] This surface activity has been termed chemisorption. Ions that are incorporated into bone are initially attracted by this method to enter a hydration shell around bone in a rather uniform fashion. Ionic exchange in or about the hydroxyapatite crystal is fundamental to the process of localization of a bone tracer for scintigraphic purposes. The process of heterionic exchange whereby an ion that is characteristic of bone is exchanged for a dissimilar one ("bone seeker" ion or molecule) is a basic concept in bone tracer localization.[48]

Heterionic exchange is extremely dynamic, especially in regions of high blood flow[25, 39] such as growing bone or tumor. Solid neoplasms are always accompanied by neovascularization. The tumor cells apparently possess the ability to promote neovascularization by release of a diffusible messenger capable of stimulating endothelial cells and termed tumor angiogenesis factor (TAF).[17] It may be postulated that the increased blood flow in the region of a proliferating bone tumor will bring more tracer to the affected region of bone and encourage a more important role for heterionic exchange and localized deposition of the bone-seeking agent.

Although available bone-imaging agents vary markedly, the end result is essentially the same. All these substances are attracted to bone generally and localize more in the regions where bone remodeling is in progress. Radioisotopes of calcium mix with stable calcium and are included in the general metabolism of this mineral. Strontium isotopes do this by being analogous enough to calcium to partially follow the metabolic routes of calcium. Fluorine is substituted for hydroxyl ions in the shell of hydration around the apatite crystal. The polyphosphates, disphosphonate,[19] and pyrophosphate are probably adsorbed by osteoid and by the apatite crystal.[32] All are more concentrated in areas of new or reactive bone formation. Variations in hormone levels and the availability of calcium, phosphate, and other ions as well as physical stress and growth can introduce nonuniformity of chemisorption and stimulate bone remodeling. This remodeling may be extensive or limited, depending on the stimulus. Reactive bone formation is associated with remodeling. A site of bone formation attracts greater amounts of involved ionic constituent than surrounding bone. If such constituent is radioactive, it can be used to locate sites of reactive bone formation, which in turn reflect sites of bone stress.

Three hormones[48] are primarily important in mineral homeostasis of bone metabolism: parathyroid hormone (PTH), calcitonin, and 1,25-dihydroxycholecalciferol ($1,25(OH)_2D_3$). Other hormones that influence skeletal remodeling are thyroxine, adrenal glucocorticoids, gonadal hormone, and growth hormone. Abnormally high or low levels of one or more of the hormones can influence the appearance of the bone scan, generally as well as locally.

PTH appears to regulate the rate of activation of bone metabolic units and to maintain plasma calcium concentration at an optimal level. It also regulates the renal synthesis of $1,25(OH)_2D_3$ from 25-hydroxycholecalciferol $(25(OH)D_3)$. The main functions of PTH are to (1) increase calcium and decrease phosphate in plasma, (2) increase urinary concentration of phosphate and hydroxyproline peptides but decrease excretion of calcium in urine, (3) increase the rate of bone resorption and skeletal remodeling, (4) increase osteocytic osteolysis and the number of osteoclasts and osteoblasts in bone, (5) increase the rate of conversion of $25(OH)D_3$ to $1,25(OH)_2D_3$ in renal tissue, and (6) increase gut absorption of calcium. Increased levels of PTH in patients may increase the concentration of bone-imaging agents (Fig. 8-5).

Calcitonin modulates the effects of PTH by (1) decreasing the bone resorption activity of osteoblasts and osteocytes, (2) decreasing the rate of formation of preosteoblasts and osteoblasts, and (3) increasing the production of osteo-

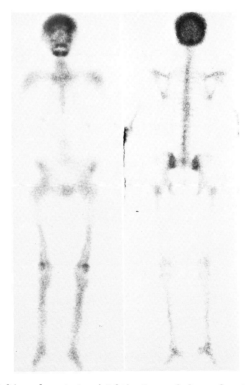

Fig. 8-5. Anterior (left) and posterior (right) views of the technetium 99m diphosphonate bone scan of a woman with hyperparathyroidism. Increased concentration in skull, lower femurs, and tibias is extraordinary and is commonly seen in this condition. Skeleton seems subdued when compared to very high skull concentration.

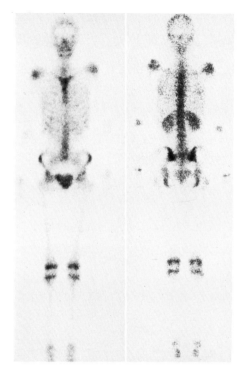

Fig. 8-6. Whole-body scan of 18-year-old woman with medullary carcinoma and hyper-calcitonin levels shows excellent concentration of technetium 99m diphosphonate. Scan has a better-than-normal appearance. Long bone epiphyses are distinct.

blasts. As a result of increased osteoblastic activity, the concentration of bone-imaging agents could also be augmented (Fig. 8-6).

The effects of $1,25(OH)_2D_3$ are to increase calcium and phosphate retention and control bone matrix mineralization. This hormone also causes sufficient retention of mineral ions to ensure proper bone calcification and causes PTH to maintain the proper ratio of calcium to phosphate in extracellular fluid (ECF). The presence of renal disease or other disruption of vitamin D metabolism should be considered in the interpretation of the activity of bone-scanning agents.

CONTROL OF SKELETAL REMODELING

Six cell pools[48] have been identified and arranged in the cellular scheme of bone formation. The cell progression, with appropriate stimulation, appears to be that mesenchymal (osteoprogenitor) cells have the capacity to differentiate into preosteoclasts, which give rise to osteoclasts. Osteoclasts can then differentiate into preosteoblasts, which form osteoblasts,[30] and, finally, osteoblasts can be incorporated in bone and become osteocytes. Although this seems to be the usual route of cell progression, there is evidence that a direct path from mesenchymal cell to preosteoblast formation can occur. On the other hand, in some pathologic states, osteoblastic activity may be spotty or not occur at all (Fig. 8-3).

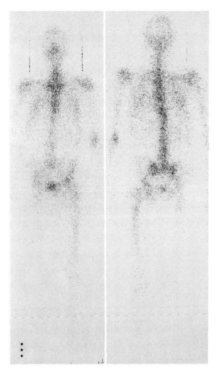

Fig. 8-7. Fluorine 18 bone scans of a 50-year-old man with melanoma of right calf. No metastatic disease in bone nor primary tumor concentration of fluorine 18 was noted. However, leg asymmetry is apparent and is due to decreased innervation of right leg secondary to poliomyelitis in childhood. Pelvic and sacroiliac asymmetry and spinal scoliosis are also present.

The major determinants of skeletal remodeling are the rate at which new bone metabolic units are activated and the balance between resorption and formation within the units. These events are determined by (1) the rate of bone mesenchymal cell differentiation into osteoclasts, (2) osteoclast activity, (3) rate of osteoclast transformation into osteoblasts, and (4) activity of osteoblasts.

Mechanical stresses placed on the skeleton and the concentration of inorganic phosphate in plasma and ECF can also result in osteoblast formation and increased bone formation (Fig. 8-7). With all bone remodeling, the body's effort seems directed to preserving the strongest bone structure under the prevailing circumstances.

TECHNIQUE OF BONE SCINTIGRAPHY

The imaging agent is administered intravenously to the patient, and sufficient time is allotted to achieve a good target-to-background ratio. Since the skeleton rapidly concentrates the bone-seeking agent, this time is required for excretion of other-than-bone activity. With strontium 85, several days are required for background activity to decrease enough for imaging to produce the best results. With other agents, imaging can be performed in 2 to 6 hours.

The patient who is referred for whole skeletal radionuclide imaging is usually known to have a malignancy and will often have had other radionuclide studies such as a liver and/or brain scan and possibly a whole-body gallium 67 scan. When these studies have preceded bone scintigraphy, adequate time must be allowed for the patient to clear the preceding tracer activity. It is best to allow 48 hours to elapse following pertechnetate brain and/or liver or thyroid gland scintigraphy (Fig. 8-8). When gallium 67 scans have been obtained, approximately 1 week should elapse before whole skeletal scintigraphy is performed.

At present there are two major forms of imaging devices with which bone scans may be produced—the rectilinear scanner and the gamma scintillation camera. The most useful rectilinear scanner has employed two opposed detectors with focusing collimators, which are paired and move in concert, facing one another. The patient is usually placed supine with an upper scanning probe tracing out an anterior skeletal image and a lower probe surveying the posterior skele-

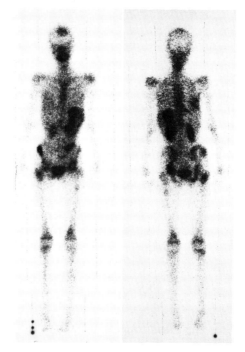

Fig. 8-8. These anterior and posterior technetium 99m diphosphonate views of a 15-year-old girl with Ewing's sarcoma show activity in mouth and stomach, as seen when a brain scan is obtained just before the bone scan. A similar appearance results when there is partial dissociation of the technetium 99m from the phosphate, which actually occurred in this instance. In addition, abnormal concentrations are seen in left parietal skull, midcervical spine, right paraspinal region, left ribs laterally, right iliac crest, both ischia, both femoral heads, and left proximal and distal femur. An area of decreased uptake is seen in left proximal tibia following radiation therapy.

ton. The rectilinear scanner is capable of producing a 1:1 image of a limited portion of the skeleton, but more commonly it is used to produce a whole skeletal image reduced five times or more in size to fit on a 14 by 17 to 8 by 10-inch sheet of x-ray film. Skeletal structures located within the focal plane of either the anterior or posterior probe will be efficiently imaged, but portions of the skeleton not located in either focal plane may harbor undetected pathology because of less optimal resolution. This difficulty is most evident when a whole skeletal scan is required of an obese patient or of a patient with ascites (Fig. 8-9).

Head-to-toe radionuclide skeletal scans require approximately 90 minutes, utilizing a dual probe, 5-inch crystal rectilinear scanning device. Newer devices such as the whole-body scanning cameras require approximately an hour for combined anterior and posterior whole skeletal scans. It is possible that significant data will not be lost if a posterior whole skeletal scan only is acquired with the scanning camera and accompanied by spot camera views of questionable areas. The scanning camera is not limited by fixed depth of field collimation, since it utilizes a parallel hole collimator. Multicrystal rectilinear scanners can perform a whole-body bone scan with both anterior and posterior views in about 25 to 40 minutes.

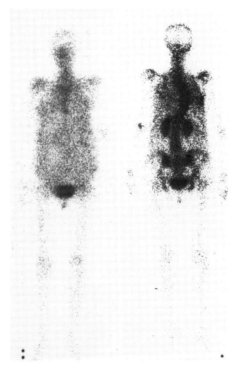

Fig. 8-9. Technetium 99m diphosphonate whole-body scan of 51-year-old woman with ovarian carcinoma, bilateral pleural effusion, and ascites. Anterior view (left) shows marked diffusion of radioactivity and poor skeletal delineation. Posterior view (right) clearly outlines spine, pelvis, and posterior ribs.

The whole-body image has been routinely collected on double-emulsion x-ray film. The clarity of the skeletal image produced on double-emulsion film appears to be less satisfactory than on single-emulsion film, which is gaining in popularity.

It is especially important that the physician be familiar with the normal scan pattern before attempting to evaluate bone abnormalities. Techniques of scanning and film processing vary from clinic to clinic, and these variations influence the interpretation.[26] Some physicians recommend hydration of the patient before dosing with bone-seeking compounds that are cleared by the kidney.[59] Bone-seeking tracers or compounds accumulate unevenly throughout the skeleton in the normal patient, with more activity localizing at the ends rather than in the shafts of the bones (Fig. 8-6). Normality is largely judged by the bilaterally symmetrical localization of activity. This symmetry may be altered by improper positioning of the patient as well as by disease. If, for example, the knees are at different distances from the focused detector of a rectilinear scanner, there will be artifactual variation in their appearance. This can usually be accounted for by considering the activity seen in both knees on the anterior as well as the posterior scan.

Although a whole-body scan has many advantages, the more limited gamma scintillation camera views can be quite helpful and are often indispensable. The whole-body scan provides perspective for easier identification of asymmetry. Spot camera views should be obtained in addition to allow for high resolution re-examination of radioactively suspicious areas and of symptomatic regions not well delineated on the whole-body scan. For example, the anterior and posterior rectilinear head views obtained on the whole skeletal rectilinear scan should be accompanied by lateral views of the skull (Fig. 8-4). Lateral views alone or anterior and posterior rectilinear views alone do not provide a thorough approach to the detection of skull lesions—supplemental views are recommended.

Gamma scintillation camera views can be helpful in delineating extravasation at the injection site, radioactive contamination of clothing from the injection site, the alcohol sponge used to cover the injection site and located in a pocket of the patient's clothing, urine leakage from ileostomy collection devices or incontinence, prevoiding and postvoiding views of the bladder, and the shielding effects of breast prostheses, pocket contents, belt buckles, jewelry, hearing aids, and pacemakers.

Normal anatomic variations may occur in scintiphotos and can cause confusion. Apparent areas of increased radioactivity may be seen in the skull, usually because of tangential positioning. These are best resolved by multple gamma camera views. The region of the temporomandibular joints may be prominent in the absence of demonstrable disease other than changes in dentition. Sites of dental disease or surgery (Fig. 8-10) are so frequently seen on bone images that they represent a normal variation of sorts.

The thyroid cartilage tends to concentrate the phosphate agents and is best delineated on a lateral view of the neck with the gamma camera (Fig. 8-4).

This camera view can also reveal abnormal involvement of cervical vertebrae not suspected from the anterior or posterior views obtained with the rectilinear scanner.

In the chest many variations may be seen. Normal (Fig. 8-11) or diseased breasts may be prominent (Fig. 8-4), as may the sternal joints such as the sternoclavicular manubriosternal and sternosternal ossification centers. One shoulder is often slightly more prominent, indicating handedness.[59] The scapulae may be clearly outlined, or only the tips may be seen.

Extremity asymmetries are very common and usually reflect differences in use. The injection site should always be noted on the patient's study requisition, since it may frequently be seen on the scan and be a source of error or confusion.

In addition to the sites already mentioned, extraskeletal uptake occurs in recent surgical sites (Fig. 8-10), hematomas, myocardial infarction, and a number of tumors such as osteosarcoma metastases (Fig. 8-12), melanoma, those of Hodgkin's disease, bronchogenic carcinoma, sarcoma, and brain tumor.[27]

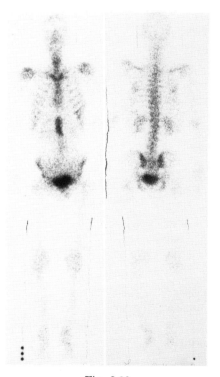
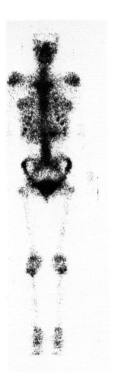

Fig. 8-10   **Fig. 8-11**

Fig. 8-10. Whole-body bone scan using technetium 99m diphosphonate shows concentration of the agent in a midabdominal laparotomy-splenectomy scar. Surgery was performed a month prior to scan as a lymphoma staging procedure. Bone scan is normal otherwise.

Fig. 8-11. Normal breasts are prominent on this normal bone scan of a 20-year-old woman with sarcoma of the vulva. Manubrium and sternoclavicular joints are also prominent.

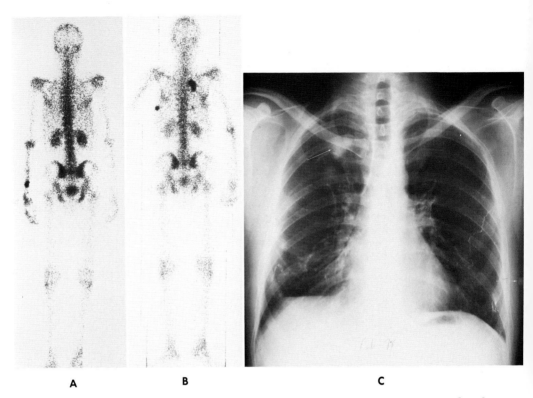

A   **B**   **C**

Fig. 8-12. A 30-year-old man had an osteosarcoma of the left distal radius resected in late 1972. **A,** Scan shows recurrence. Arm was amputated in 1973. **B,** Follow-up scan in early 1975 shows marked uptake of technetium 99m diphosphonate in soft tissue metastases in right lung and left chest wall, which were also apparent (arrows) in radiograph, **C.**

Concentration of activity in epiphyseal centers is a normal appearance and must be expected in radionuclide skeletal images of children (Fig. 8-6).

In occasional cases localization of activity may be diminished at the site of bony abnormality, as observed with radiation therapy (Fig. 8-8). The defective localization may be due to decreased vascularity following irradiation as well as depressed osteoblastic activity. "Cold" bone lesions have been reported to correspond to osteolytic metastases observed on bone radiographs, and if not carefully looked for, they may result in false negative interpretations.[62] The localization of tracer may extend beyond the apparent limits of a variety of skeletal lesions, be they benign or malignant or due to trauma or infection. It has been postulated that these "extended patterns" are due to increased blood flow around lesions.[60]

Although the usual interpretation of the bone scan would hold that the concentration of the radioactive imaging agent increases in proportion to the progression of disease, this is not always true. Successful treatment of malignant metastatic bone lesions removes, at least partially, the osteoclastic effect of the disease.

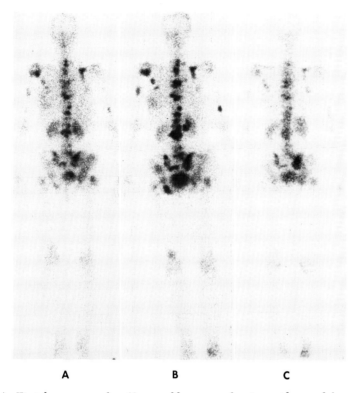

A   B   C

Fig. 8-13. A, First bone scan of a 48-year-old woman showing widespread bony metastases from breast carcinoma in April, 1974. Chemotherapy was begun, and patient improved clinically. **B,** Second bone scan in July, 1974, showed increased prominence to the metastatic lesions in spine, pelvis, ribs, shoulders, humeri, femurs, and right ankle. Scan was repeated in January, 1975, with no further therapy other than radiation of left acetabulum. **C,** All metastatic lesions had decreased in prominence.

Usually, a rapid increase in new bone formation at these sites can be seen to incorporate greater amounts of radioactive bone-scanning agents. Then the usual sign of disease progression—increased activity at disease sites on bone scan—becomes a sign of efficacy of therapy (Fig. 8-13). This situation underlines a tenet of nuclear medicine that scans can best be interpreted in light of the individual patient's presentation. Individual studies may be read as normal or abnormal. However, interpretation of the reading becomes hazardous unless the complete clinical picture is considered.

Bone scans can be helpful in diagnosing many skeletal disorders, including those caused by metabolic disease and trauma. However, except for patients whose symptoms are difficult to evaluate with radiography, the technique is, and should be, used mainly to aid in cancer diagnosis and treatment. The method can detect bone tumors and cysts and find and follow the progress of bony metastases, provided that osteoblastic activity and resulting reactive bone formation are stimulated.

The nonspecificity of bone imaging has been disappointing in some respects and may have discouraged some clinicians from its use. This aspect has received the attention of several investigators.[18, 59] The pertechnetate-labeled phosphates and fluorine 18 are largely cleared by the kidneys. It is expected on the normal whole skeletal scan that both kidneys will be visualized, and the urinary bladder is always visible even though it is routinely requested that the patient void just prior to beginning the scan. On completion of the skeletal scan, the urinary bladder is seen as a central retropubic accumulation of activity. A distortion in the location or outline of the bladder may be an indication of intrapelvic pathology or recent pelvic surgery. Uterine fibroids, sigmoid colon contents, and tumors adjacent to the bladder have been observed to alter the configuration of the scan.[21]

A unilateral discrepancy in the intensity of radioactivity or a major variation in the size or position of the kidney may indicate renal disease. Depending on the cause, one kidney may accumulate more radionuclide than the other, suggesting obstruction; less radionuclide in the kidney may indicate secretory disease. It is difficult to determine the laterality of renal disease by the intensity of radionuclide localization. Approximately 35% of patients with unequal radionuclide concentration in the kidneys have unilateral renal abnormalities, whereas those with equal renal concentrations are unlikely to have renal disease.[51] Urograms are most helpful in assessing patients whose skeletal images show unilateral alteration in the appearance of a ureter or a distortion of the urinary bladder.

While providing clues to renal, retroperitoneal, or pelvic abnormalities, the genitourinary system may create pitfalls for the inattentive or inexperienced interpreter of whole skeletal scans. Urinary bladder activity may obscure bony pathology, and in urinary incontinence even a small drop of radioactive urine on the clothing may distort the images and lead to a problem in interpretation. This situation is unusual and is most often seen in a patient who has had a pelvic exenteration and ureterosigmoidostomy. Poor ureteral drainage[56] or a collecting bag that must be kept clear of bone structures during the imaging procedure interfere with image interpretation.

On rare occasions normal bone scans are obtained in the presence of bone lesions. Such negative scans usually represent instances of very small lesions, failure of the lesions to stimulate osteoblastic activity,[62] or interference by other metabolic conditions with reactive bone formation. Bone scans may be misinterpreted as normal when diffuse, widespread disease completely involves the skeleton or where involvement is incomplete but symmetrical.[20]

Occasionally, metastatic tumor has invaded a bone without causing reactive bone formation (Fig. 8-3). In such instances the scan will be normal while the x-ray film will show the abnormality. Either radiolucent or radiodense x-ray lesions may have increased isotopic concentration; a radiodensity with a normal rate of bone formation may be normal on scan. And even with the proudest bone-imaging and radiograph displays ever shown, tissue studies, usually at autopsy, too often show a wider distribution of marrow metastases than did either method when the patients were being studied and treated.

RADIATION DOSIMETRY

Using 10 mCi of pertechnetate-labeled phosphate for whole skeletal scans, the radiation doses will be as follows: skeleton, 320 mrads; kidneys, 380 mrads; bladder, 910 mrads; ovaries and testes, 120 mrads.[65]

A radiologic skeletal survey (AP, lateral, and Towne films of skull, PA and lateral chest, lateral cervical, lateral dorsal and lumbar spine, AP pelvis, bilateral humeri and femora, bilateral tibiae and fibulae, bilateral radii and ulnae) will deliver about 480 mrads to the ovaries, in addition to a much higher skin dose.[5]

There is little doubt that, for the radiation dosimetry involved, the patient who receives a whole skeletal radionuclide scan obtains a thorough and sensitive survey for skeletal disease, since the procedure frequently detects skeletal disease weeks or months before it becomes evident on x-ray films.

TRAUMA

The prime example of bone trauma is bone fracture. The blood supply at the fracture site is disrupted with some resultant bone necrosis. Bleeding from the broken vessels forms a clot in which rapid ossification takes place. For several weeks calcium and phosphorus concentrations are high at the fracture site. Phosphatase activity is increased within days and continues to be elevated for months. Cartilage grows into the area with rapid osteoid transformation, and trabeculae of new bone covered with proliferating osteoblasts form. This reactive healing response provides intense attraction for imaging agents. The bone scan in this situation is the most intense seen in any disease condition. In the instance of hairline, incomplete, and small bone fractures, bone scintigraphy can provide diagnostic or confirmatory information. Fracture site activity may persist for years. Serial scans of an acute fracture may show increasing retention of activity during the healing phase and a subsequent decrease, whereas a scan of an old injury will reveal the same amount of radionuclide on serial studies.[22]

The bone scan will reflect trauma such as periosteal bruising, surgical procedures that cut or retract bone, tooth disease and extraction, bone or marrow biopsy, bone curettage and transplantation, bone nailing, and limb prosthesis trauma to the site of attachment. Less marked scan changes will occur with alterations in weight bearing that deposit activity along a new weight-bearing axis (Fig. 8-7).

Increasing or decreasing the blood supply to a bone will similarly increase or decrease the intensity of bone tracer localization seen on scan. Injuries that denervate an area tend to increase the blood flow and isotopic concentration (Fig. 8-7). Those which disrupt the circulation tend to decrease the activity. Weeks or months later there will be reversal of the scan appearance with decreased activity in the denervated limb and increased activity in the region of the aseptic necrosis.[18]

Radiation therapy will produce a field of decreased activity within a short time following its delivery[7] (Fig. 8-8). Bone scan evaluation of the treatment field will not be possible for about 3 months.

TUMORS

The most common bone tumor is metastatic carcinoma.[37] Its overall incidence at autopsy in cancer patients was more than 25%, and more than two thirds of breast carcinoma patients had skeletal metastases in one series.[1] The data quoted in this autopsy study are an indication of the number of cancer patients who ultimately develop skeletal metastases. Obviously the patient has no metastases when the disease first develops. The longer one lives with cancer, the greater the chances of having such bone involvement.

Surprisingly, very few metastatic bone lesions produce clinical manifestations. Bone pain or swelling, compression fracture of a vertebra, and pathologic fracture of a long bone sometimes lead to the diagnosis of metastases in bone, but most osseous lesions are asymptomatic. X-ray examination increases the diagnostic yield of late lesions. For a lesion to be detected radiologically, 50% to 75% of the cancellous bone thickness must be destroyed.[14] Bone scintigraphy detects the osteoblastic response to the presence of invading tumor and therefore may improve the diagnostic yield by detecting metastatic, invasive, or primary bone tumor at an earlier stage.

In some leading medical institutions, bone scintigraphy is already a routine part of the initial medical workup for malignancy. These early scans are then referred to at regular intervals for comparison with successive imaging to help

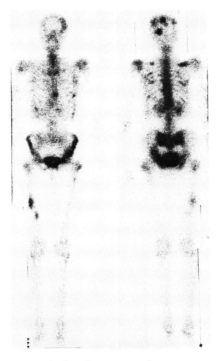

Fig. 8-14. A technetium 99m polyphosphate scan of a woman with progressive metastatic breast carcinoma, which mainly involves the marrow-bearing bones and spares the distal bones, except for the midfemur.

assess the progress of the tumor and the efficacy of therapy. Advance or regression of malignancy as shown on the bone scan is a valuable guideline to the oncologist managing the patient's treatment (Fig. 8-14).

Skeletal distribution of carcinoma metastases favors the bones that contain red marrow and have the greatest blood supply. These are the vertebral column, the ribs, the pelvis, and the skull.[29] Radiographic skeletal surveys include these bones and generally omit the bones of the extremities. Many scintigraphic surveys are similarly limited, except when the patient directs attention to an extremity or where whole skeletal scans are routinely performed.

Since the earliest metastatic tumor sites are frequently located in the bone marrow, they provoke no reactive bone formation until the tumor nodules have grown large enough to involve the surrounding bone. No current methods other than skeletal (marrow) biopsy will detect these lesions.

FUTURE DIRECTIONS

Although bone scintigraphy must be applied with considerable thought and care to each patient's problem, it is a valuable and extremely useful method that deserves wide application. Since it rarely produces false negative results (most of which are in instances readily delineated by x-ray study), considerable attention should be directed to resolving abnormal bone image findings. The patient will benefit from this pursuit, and the physician will gain familiarity with the reliability of the method and its limits.

At this stage the rapidly growing list of useful isotopic bone-imaging agents (Table 8-1) along with the wide variety of devices for imaging has created some confusion. For example, the recent use of the technetium 99m–tagged phosphate compounds, poly-, di-, and pyro-, with gamma camera imaging has provided such highly resolved images that nuclear physicians have been tempted occasionally to overinterpret the results and have caused some clinical distrust.

The direction that must be taken is clear. Bone scintigraphy is innocuous, easily and rapidly produced, and inexpensive. It should by all means become a part of the cancer patient's initial workup, particularly for those tumors which are notorious for their early spread to bone. As skeletal scintigraphy becomes a more rapid and simple test, nuclear medical thoroughness and responsibility may ulti-

Table 8-1. Current and clinically useful bone-seeking tracers for skeletal imaging*

	Strontium 85	Strontium 87m	Fluorine 18	Technetium 99m (phosphates)
Physical half-life	64 days	2.8 hours	110 minutes	6 hours
Primary energy (mev)	0.513	0.388	0.513	0.140
Chemical form	Nitrate	Chloride	Fluoride	Phosphate
Activity (mCi)	0.1	1.0	1.0	10.0
Dose to bone (rads)	4.0	0.14	0.26	0.32 (pyrophosphate) (3)

*From Weber, D. A., et al.: J. Nucl. Med. **10:**8, 1967, with permission of publisher.

mately require head to toe skeletal scans for detection of bone disease. Following is an incomplete list of lesions producing positive skeletal scans.

1. Metastases to bone
2. Metastases to soft tissue (occasional)
3. Primary bone and joint tumors
4. Irradiation defect
5. Osteomyelitis (pyogenic)
6. Arthritis
7. Fracture (injury or surgery)
8. Radiation
9. Paget's disease
10. Epiphyses (normal)
11. Chronic sinusitis
12. Dermatomyositis (myositis ossificans)
13. Histiocytosis X
14. Hyperparathyroidism
15. Hyperostosis frontalis interna
16. Acro-osteolysis
17. Aseptic necrosis of the femoral head
18. Surgical incision of soft tissue
19. Brain tumor[26]
20. Breast—physiologic (lactating and occasionally nonlactating) or pathologic
21. Supraorbital fibrous dysplasia[49]

Positive studies should be confirmed by x-ray study and tomography and, where feasible, by biopsy. The nuclear medicine practitioner should be willing to assume the role of a consultant in oncology and be instrumental in directing the confirmation or correction of his suspicions by correlating x-ray and pathologic findings with the scintigraphic findings. This approach will help establish the true value of nuclear medicine and radionuclide bone imaging and make it meaningful in the diagnosis and follow-up study of each patient.

In addition to static imaging in bone disease, there appears to be a role for dynamic bone studies, perhaps computer assisted, in bone tumor and trauma and in metabolic bone disease. Furthermore, there are instances of soft tissue calcification that may be amenable to study by these methods, both initially and in response to therapy.

References

1. Abrams, H. C., Spiro, R., and Goldstein, N.: Metastases in carcinoma: analysis of one thousand autopsied cases, Cancer 3:74, 1950.
2. Anderson, J., Emery, E. W., McAlister, J. M., and Osborn, S. B.: The metabolism of a therapeutic dose of calcium-45 in a case of multiple myeloma, Clin. Sci. Mol. Med. 15:567, 1956.
3. Bauer, G. C. H., and Wendeberg, B.: External counting of Ca-47 and Sr-85 in studies of localized skeletal lesions in man, J. Bone Joint Surg. 41B:558, 1959.
4. Blau, M., Nagler, W., and Bender, M. A.: Fluorine-18: a new isotope for bone scanning, J. Nucl. Med. 3:332, 1962.
5. Brown, M. L., and Segal, P.: Population dose from x-rays, U.S. 1964, Radiation bio-effects summary report, Jan.-Dec. 1969, BRH/DBE, Publication no. 70-1, Rockville, Md., 1970, Department of Health, Education, and Welfare, Public Health Service, Bureau of Radiological Health.
6. Castronovo, F. P., and Calletron, R. J.: New bone scanning agent: 99m Tc-labelled 1-hydroxy-ethylidene-1, 1-disodium phosphonate, J. Nucl. Med. 13:823, 1972.

7. Castronovo, F. P., Jr., Potsaid, M. S., and Pendergrass, H. P.: Effects of radiation therapy on bone lesions as measured by 99m Tc-diphosphonate, J. Nucl. Med. **14**:604, 1973.

8. Charkes, N. D., and Sklaroff, D. M.: Early diagnosis of metastatic bone cancer by photoscanning with strontium-85, J. Nucl. Med. **5**:168, 1964.

9. Charkes, N. D., Sklaroff, D. M., and Young, I.: A critical analysis of strontium bone scanning for detection of metastatic cancer, Am. J. Roentgenol. Radium Ther. Nucl. Med. **96**:647, 1966.

10. Charkes, N. D., Young, I., and Sklaroff, D. M.: The pathologic basis of the strontium bone scan: studies following the administration of strontium chloride Sr-85 and strontium nitrate Sr-85, J.A.M.A. **206**:2482, 1968.

11. Cohn, S. H., Spencer, H., Samachson, J., and Robertson, J. S.: The turnover of strontium-85 in man as determined by whole-body counting, Radiat. Res. **17**:173, 1962.

12. DeNardo, G., and Volpe, J. A.: Detection of bone lesions with the strontium-85 scintiscan, J. Nucl. Med. **7**:219, 1966.

13. Dudley, H. C., Imrie, G. W. J., and Istock, J. T.: Deposition of radiogallium (^{72}Ga) in proliferating tissues, Radiology **55**:571, 1950.

14. Edelstyn, G. A., Gillespie, P. J., and Grebbell, F. S.: The radiological demonstration of osseous metastases: experimental observations, Clin. Radiol. **18**:158, 1967.

15. Faber, D. D., et al.: An evaluation of the strontium-85 scan for the detection and localization of bone metastases from prostatic carcinoma: a preliminary report of 93 cases, J. Urol. **97**:526, 1967.

16. Fleming, W. H., McIlraith, J. D., and King, E. R.: Photoscanning of bone lesions utilizing strontium-85, Radiology **77**:635, 1961.

17. Folkman, J.: Tumor angiogenesis: therapeutic implications, N. Engl. J. Med. **18**:1182, 1971.

18. Fordham, E. W., and Ramachandran, P. C.: Radionuclide imaging of osseous trauma, Semin. Nucl. Med. **4**:411, 1974.

19. Francis, M. D.: The inhibition of calcium hydroxyapatite crystal growth by polyphosphonates and polyphosphates, Calcif. Tissue Res. **3**:151, 1969.

20. Frankel, R. S., Johnson, K. W., Mabry, J. J., and Johnston, G. S.: "Normal" bone radionuclide image with diffuse skeletal lymphoma, Radiology **111**:365, 1974.

21. Frankel, R. S., Jones, A. E., Johnson, K. W., and Johnston, G. S.: The significance of urinary bladder displacement noted on whole-body 18-F bone scintigraphy, Radiology **109**:397, 1973.

22. Freedman, G. S.: Radionuclide imaging of the injured patient, Radiol. Clin. North Am. **11**:461, 1973.

23. French, R. J., and McCready, V. R.: The use of 18-F for bone scanning, Br. J. Radiol. **40**:655, 1967.

24. Galasko, C. S. B.: Skeletal metastases and mammary cancer, Ann. R. Coll. Surg. Engl. **50**:3, 1972.

25. Genant, H. K., et al.: Bone-seeking radionuclides: an in vivo study of factors affecting skeletal uptake, Radiology **113**:373, 1974.

26. Gottschalk, A.: Bone scanning. In Proceedings of the Symposium in Nuclear Medicine—Its Current Status in Medical Practice. Cleveland, Ohio, USAEC, Division of Nuclear Training and Nuclear Medicine Institute, Cleveland, Ohio, 1967.

27. Grames, G. M., Jansen C., Carlsen, E. N., and Davidson, T. R.: The abnormal bone scan in intracranial lesions, Radiology **115**:129, 1975.

28. Greenberg, E. J., Rothschild, E. O., DePalo, A., and Laughlin, J. S.: Bone scanning for metastatic cancer with radioactive isotopes, Med. Clin. North Am. **50**:701, 1966.

29. Hait, G., Hoerr, S. O., and Hughes, C. R.: Detection of bone metastasis from breast cancer: an accurate, four-film roentgenographic survey, Cleve. Clin. Q. **38**:1, 1971.

30. Ham, A. W.: Histology, ed. 7, Philadelphia, 1974, J. B. Lippincott Co.

31. Hopkins, G. B., Kristensen, K. A. B., and Blickenstaff, D. E.: Fluorine-18 bone scans in the detection of early metastatic bone tumors, J.A.M.A. **222**:813, 1972.

32. Jones, A. G., Francis, M. D., and Davis, M. A.: Bone scanning: radionuclide reaction mechanisms, Semin. Nucl. Med. **6**:1, 1976.

33. Jung, A., Bisaz, S., and Fleisch, H.: The binding of pyrophosphate and two diphosphonates by hydroxyapatite crystals, Calcif. Tissue Res. **11**:269, 1973.

34. Krishnamurthy, G. T., et al.: Comparison of 99mTc-polyphosphate and 18-F. II. Imaging, J. Nucl. Med. **15**:837, 1974.

35. Krishnamurthy, G. T., et al.: Kinetics of 99mTc-labeled pyrophosphate and polyphosphate in man, J. Nucl. Med. **16**: 109, 1975.

36. Lee, W. R., Marshall, J. H., and Sissons, H. A.: Calcium accretion and bone formation in dogs: an experimental comparison between the results of calcium-45 kinetics analysis and tetracycline labelling, J. Bone Joint Surg. **47-B**:157, 1965.

37. Lichtenstein, L.: Bone tumors, ed. 4, St. Louis, 1972, The C. V. Mosby Co.

38. Mall, J. C., Bekerman, C., Hoffer, P. B., Gottschalk, A.: A unified radiological approach to the detection of skeletal metastases, Radiology **118**:323, 1976.

39. Milch, R. A., and Changus, G. W.: Response of bone to tumor invasion, Cancer **9**:340, 1956.

40. Mulry, W. C., and Dudley, H. C.: Studies of radiogallium as a diagnostic agent in bone tumors, J. Lab. Clin. Med. **37**:239, 1951.

41. Neuman, W. F., and Neuman, M. W.: The chemical dynamics of bone material, Chicago, 1958, University of Chicago Press.

42. Nilsson, A., and Ullberg, S.: II. Uptake and retention of strontium-90 in strontium-90–induced osteosarcomas, Acta Radiol. **58**:168, 1962.

43. Pearson, O. H., Solaric, S., Lafferty, F. W., and Storaasli, J. P.: Calcium-47 and strontium-85 tracer studies as a guide to isotope therapy of bone metastases, Radiology **79**:446, 1962.

44. Pecher, C.: Biological investigations with radioactive calcium and strontium, Proc. Soc. Exp. Biol. Med. **46**:86, 1941.

45. Pecher, C.: Biological investigations with radioactive calcium and strontium: preliminary report on the use of radioactive strontium in the treatment of metastatic bone cancer, U. of Calif. Publ. Pharmacol. **2**(11):117, 1942.

46. Pendergrass, H. P., Potsaid, M. S., and Castronovo, F. P., Jr.: The clinical use of 99mTc-diphosphonate HEDSPA: a new agent for skeletal imaging, Radiology **102**:557, 1973.

47. Pistenua, D. A., McDougall, I. R., and Kriss, J. P.: Screening for bone metastases: Are only scans necessary? J.A.M.A. **231**:46, 1975.

48. Rasmussen, H.: Parathyroid hormone, calcitonin, and the calciferols. In Williams, R. H., editor: Textbook of endocrinology, ed. 5, Philadelphia, 1974, W. B. Saunders Co.

49. Rosenthall, L.: The role of strontium-85 in the detection of bone disease, Radiology **84**:75, 1965.

50. Samachson, J., and Lederer, H.: The uptake of calcium-45 and strontium-85 by bone in vitro, Arch. Biochem. Biophys. **88**:355, 1960.

51. Sante, L. R., and Fischer, H. W.: Manual of roentgenological techniques, ed. 20, Ann Arbor, Mich., 1962, Edwards Brothers, Inc.

52. Schaer, L.: Supraorbital fibrous dysplasia demonstrated by fluorine-18 and the scintillation (positron) camera, Radiology **86**:506, 1966.

53. Silberstein, E. B., et al.: Imaging of bone metastases with 99m Tc-Sn-EHDP (diphosphonate), 18 F, and skeletal radiography, Radiology **107**:551, 1973.

54. Simpson, W. J., and Orange, R. P.: Total body scanning with strontium-85 in the diagnosis of metastatic bone disease, Can. Med. Assoc. J. **93**:1237, 1965.

55. Sklaroff, D. M., and Charkes, N. D.: The value of strontium-85 bone scanning in radiation therapy, Am. J. Roentgenol. Radium Ther. Nucl. Med. **99**: 415, 1967.

56. Solway, M. S., Myers, G. H., Jr., Johnston, G., and Ketcham, A. S.: Renography in the evaluation of patients with ileal conduits, Surg. Gynecol. Obstet. **135**:521, 1972.

57. Spencer, H., Laszlo, D., and Brothers, M.: Strontium-85 and calcium-45 metabolism in man, J. Clin. Invest. **36**:680, 1957.

58. Subramanian, G., and McAfee, J. G.: A new complex of 99mTc for skeletal imaging, Radiology **99**:192, 1971.

59. Thrall, J. H., et al.: Pitfalls in Tc99m polyphosphate skeletal imaging, Am. J. Roentgenol. Radium Ther. Nucl. Med. **121**:739, 1974.

60. Thrall, J. H., Geslien, G. E., Corcoran, R. J., and Johnson, M. C.: Abnormal radionuclide deposition patterns adjacent to focal skeletal lesions, Radiology **115**:659, 1975.

61. Treadwell, A. de G., Low-Beer, B. V. A., Friedell, H. L., and Lawrence, J. H.: Metabolic studies on neoplasm of bone with the aid of radioactive strontium, Am. J. Med. Sci. 204:521, 1942.

62. Vieras, F., and Herzberg, D. L.: Focal decreased skeletal uptake secondary to metastatic disease, Radiology 118:121, 1976.

63. Weber, D. A., et al.: Kinetics of radio-nuclides used for bone studies, J. Nucl. Med. 10:8, 1969.

64. Weber, D. A., Keyes, J. W., Benedetto, W. J., and Wilson, G. A.: 99mTc pyrophosphate for diagnostic bone imaging, Radiology 114:131, 1974.

65. Weber, D. A., Keyes, J. W., Jr., Landman, S., and Wilson, G. A.: Comparison of Tc99m polyphosphate and F18 for bone imaging, Am. J. Roentgenol. Radium Ther. Nucl. Med. 121:184, 1974.

66. Williams, D. F., Blahd, W. H., and Wetterau, L., Jr.: Radioactive fluorine-18 photoscanning: a diagnostic evaluation in carcinoma of the prostate, J. Urol. 100:675, 1968.

67. Wirtanen, G. W., Cameron, J. R., and Briggs, R. C.: Pre-radiographic demonstration of bone metastases with strontium-85 photoscanning, Wis. Med. J. 65:469, 1966 (abstract).

Suggested readings

Allen, J. F., and Pinajian, J. J.: A Sr-87m generator for medical applications, Int. J. Appl. Radiat. and Isot. 16:319, 1965.

Bauer, G. C. H., and Scoccianti, P.: Uptake of strontium-85 in non-malignant vertebral lesions in man, Acta, Orthop. Scand. 31:90, 1961.

Briggs, R. C., and Wegner, G. P.: Osseous metaplasia in soft tissue: demonstration of metastasis by Sr-85 scintiscanning, J.A.M.A. 195:185, 1966.

Brower, A. C., and Teates, C. D.: Positive 99mTc-polyphosphate scan in case of metastatic osteogenic sarcoma and hypertrophic pulmonary osteoarthropathy, J. Nucl. Med. 15:53, 1974.

Charkes, N. D.: Bone scanning: principles, technique, and interpretation, Radiol. Clin. North Am. 8:259, 1970.

Chaudhuri, T. K., et al.: Extraosseous noncalcified soft-tissue uptake of 99mTc-polyphosphate, J. Nucl. Med. 15:1054, 1974.

Danigelis, J. A., Fisher, R. L., Ozonoff, M.

B., and Sziklas, J. J.: 99m-to-polyphosphate bone imaging in Legg-Perthes disease, Radiology 115:407, 1975.

Davis, M. A., and Jones, A. G.: Comparison of 99mTc-labeled phosphate and phosphonate agents for skeletal imaging, Semin. Nucl. Med. 6:19, 1976.

Donnelly, B., and Johnson, P. M.: Detection of hypertrophic pulmonary osteoarthropathy by skeletal imaging with 99mTc-labeled diphosphonate, Radiology 114:389, 1975.

DuSault, L. A., Shaw, R. A., and Eyler, W. R.: 99mTc sulfide colloid scanning for bone lesions, Radiology 94:161, 1970.

Fleisch, H., Russell, R. G. G., and Francis, M. D.: Diphosphonates inhibit hydroxyapatite dissolution *in vitro* and bone resorption in tissue culture and *in vivo*, Science 165:1262, 1969.

Gilday, D. L., and Ash, J. M.: Benign bone tumors, Semin. Nucl. Med. 6:33, 1976.

Gilday, D. L., Eng, B., Paul, D. J., and Paterson, J.: Diagnosis of osteomyelitis in children by combined blood pool and bone imaging, Radiology 117:331, 1975.

Handmaker, H., and Leonards, R.: The bone scan in inflammatory osseous disease, Semin. Nucl. Med. 6:95, 1976.

Hayes, A. W.: Radioisotopes of gallium. In Andrews, G. A., Kniseley, R. M., and Wagner, H. N., Jr., editors: Radioactive pharmaceuticals, AEC Symposium Series No-6, CONF-651111, 1966.

Hayes, R. L., Carlton, J. E., and Byrd, B. L.: Bone scanning with gallium-68: a carrier effect, J. Nucl. Med. 6:605, 1965.

Hoffman, H. C., and Marty, R.: Bone scanning. Its value in the preoperative evaluation of patients with suspicious breast masses, Am. J. Surg. 124:194, 1972.

Lichtenstein, L.: Diseases of bone and joints, ed. 2, St. Louis, 1975, The C. V. Mosby Co.

Marty, R., Denney, J. D., McKamey, M. R., and Rowley, M. J.: Bone trauma and related benign disease: assessment by bone scanning, Semin. Nucl. Med. 6:107, 1976.

Meckelenburg, R. L.: Clinical value of generator-produced 87-m strontium, J. Nucl. Med. 5:929, 1964.

Metzger, A. L., Singer, B. R., Bluestone, R., and Pearson, C. M.: Failure of disodium etidronate in calcinosis due to dermatomyositis and scleroderma, N. Engl. J. Med. 291:1294, 1974.

Okuyama, S., et al.: Tumor and skeletal imaging in bone carcinoma: an experimental demonstration, Radiology 113:681, 1974.

Probert, J. C., and Parker, B. R.: The effects of radiation therapy on bone growth, Radiology, 114:155, 1975.

Richards, A. G.: Metastatic calcification detected through scanning with 99mTc-polyphosphate, J. Nucl. Med. 15:1037, 1974.

Robbins, G. F.: The rationale for the treatment of women with potentially curable breast carcinoma, Surg. Clin. North Am. 54:793, 1974.

Robbins, G. F., et al.: Metastatic bone disease developing in patients with potentially curable breast carcinoma, Cancer 29:1702, 1972.

Rubin, P., and Ciccio, S.: Status of bone scanning for bone metastases in breast cancer, Cancer 24:1338, 1969.

Russell, R. G. G., et al.: Treatment of myositis ossificans progressiva with a diphosphonate, Lancet, 1:10, 1972.

Scharma, S. M., and Quinn, J. L.: III. Significance of 13-F-fluoride renal accumulation during bone imaging, J. Nucl. Med. 13:744, 1972.

Slager, U. T., and Reilly, E. B.: Value of examining bone marrow in diagnosing malignancy, Cancer 20:1215, 1967 (Abstract).

Suzuki, Y., Hisaca, K., and Takeda, M.: Demonstration of myositis ossificans by 99mTc pyrophosphate bone scanning, Radiology 111:663, 1974.

Tow, D. E., and Wagner, H. N., Jr.: Scanning for tumors of brain and bone. Comparison of sodium pertechnetate Tc 99m and ionic strontium 87m, J.A.M.A. 199:104, 1967.

Whalen, J. P.: The resorption of bone and its control: its roentgen significance, Radiology 113:257, 1974.

Woeltgens, J. H. M., Bonting, S. L., and Bijovet, O. L. M.: Inorganic pyrophosphatase in mineralizing hamster molars. III. Influence of diphosphonates, Calcif. Tissue Res. 13:151, 1973.

9 Comparative radiology: dysplasias of the canine forelimb

Colin B. Carrig

Dysplasias of the canine forelimb are common clinical problems in veterinary medicine. Several of these dysplasias mimic the appearance of similar dysplasias that affect the human skeleton and so are of interest from a comparative viewpoint. Investigations into the pathogenesis of skeletal dysplasias in man are often compromised by the difficulty of obtaining suitable tissue samples to permit complete investigation of the disease process. The availability of suitable animal models in the investigation of human bone dysplasias has obvious advantages, and investigators in the field of skeletal development should be aware of dysplasias that affect the various species. However, variations in anatomy, growth rates, physiology, and methods of locomotion dictate caution in directly applying results obtained in animal experimentation to the human patient. A knowledge of how the skeletal structures develop in the species used for experimental investigations is essential for meaningful interpretation of results.

Developmental skeletal anomalies in the dog can be difficult to characterize because of the wide range of normal phenotypes occurring in the various breeds. The mature weight of the dog varies from less than 1 kg in the toy breeds (e.g., Chihuahua and Pomeranian) to over 100 kg in the giant breeds (e.g., Great Dane, Irish wolfhound, and Saint Bernard). In addition to great variations in weight, several distinctive morphologic types are recognized (Fig. 9-1). In certain breeds, because of selection over many years, abnormal-appearing skeletal conformation is accepted as being within the breed standard. Most miniature breeds are examples of proportionate dwarfism and result from selection for smaller animals within specific breeds. In other breeds (e.g., bassett hound, bulldog, and dachshund) disproportionate dwarfism is part of the normal conformation for the breed, and they have been termed chondrodystrophied.[1]

Congenital anomalies involving the skeletons of dogs often are isolated occurrences, and frequently no attempt to accurately characterize the deformity is made. Breeders often disguise the presence of deleterious genes in their animals by destroying obviously deformed puppies at an early age. Only rarely are these deformed offspring made available for precise characterization of the defect. However, some breed societies have been successful in reducing the inci-

217

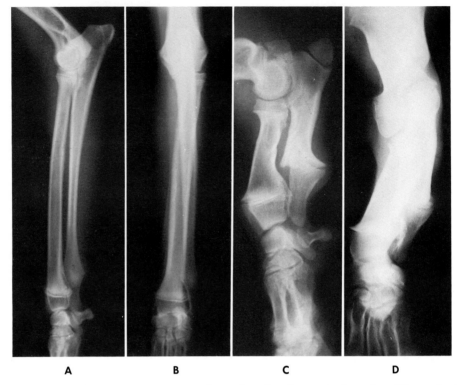

Fig. 9-1. Lateral and anteroposterior radiographs of radius and ulna of a 7½-month-old collie cross (**A** and **B**) and a 3-month-old bassett hound (**C** and **D**). Marked variation in morphology of normal bassett hound compared to that of a longer-legged breed is apparent.

dence of deleterious genes by selective breeding following detection of a hereditary disease in their stock (e.g., chondrodysplasia in the Alaskan malamute).

The forelimb of the dog is important because it is the main weight-bearing apparatus. Canine skeletal structures have usually completed their growth by 8 to 12 months, depending on the size of the dog. Because of this rapid growth rate, marked remodelling changes are necessary to accomplish normal development of the skeletal structures. Slight errors of skeletal development can lead to marked growth abnormalities. This is particularly evident at sites of conversion of cartilage to bone. Paired bones such as the radius and ulna in the forelimb are also susceptible to asynchronous development. Interference with normal growth of either of these bones can lead to marked changes in the adjacent bone as well as in the elbow and carpal joints. This chapter reviews selected acquired and developmental abnormalities of the canine forelimb.

ACQUIRED DYSPLASIAS OF RADIUS AND ULNA

Dogs frequently experience traumas that result in fractures, epiphyseal separations, and soft tissue injuries of varying degrees of severity. Every major fracture of the long bone in an immature animal produces some temporary alteration to the rate of growth of the affected bone, but the changes are usually too insignificant to be recognized clinically. The metaphyseal-epiphyseal junction in immature animals is more susceptible to partial or even complete disruption by shearing or compression forces than are the ligamentous structures supporting the joint[36] and so is frequently injured. When injury occurs within the epiphyseal growth plate of the long bone, the possibility of permanent growth alteration exists. This can lead to angular deformity due to diminished growth of part of the growth plate[5] or to retarded growth of one of a pair of parallel bones such as the radius and ulna.[20, 45, 67] The degree of growth alteration will depend on whether the chondrogenic cells remain attached to the epiphysis and so maintain their blood supply.[74] Crushing injuries to the growth plate have the most profound effect on epiphyseal vessels and are usually associated with more profound interruptions to longitudinal growth of the bone.[74]

The radius and ulna, a pair of bones closely related to one another, have to grow in a synchronized manner to prevent malalignment of their common articular surfaces and to allow unrestricted growth of the individual bone members. Alterations of normal growth in either the radius or the ulna can result in marked morphologic changes in the adjacent bone, together with abnormalities in the elbow and carpal joints. Dysplasias resulting from abnormal growth of the radius and/or ulna are common orthopedic problems. It will be seen from the consideration of normal growth of the canine radius and ulna that abnormal development related to asynchronous growth of these bones will result following retarded growth in the proximal radial growth plate, the distal radial growth plate, or the distal ulnar growth plate. Restriction of the normal movement of the two bones in relation to one another during growth will also result in abnormal development.

Normal development of canine radius and ulna

The radius grows in length from a proximal and distal growth plate. It articulates proximally with the *capitulum humeri* of the humerus and the radial notch of the ulna. Distally it articulates with the proximal row of carpal bones and the styloid process of the distal ulna. The radius bears practically all the weight transmitted from the arm to the forearm. The ulna grows from the distal ulnar growth plate and the ossification center for the olecranon. In some breeds, particularly the German shepherd and greyhound, an additional ossification center is present in the anconeal process.[21, 85, 86] Proximally the trochlear notch of the ulna articulates with the *trochlear humeri* of the humerus and the radial notch of the ulna articulates with the *articular circumference* of the head of the radius. Distally the ulna articulates with the ulnar notch of the radius, the ulnar carpal bone, and the accessory carpal bone. The radius and ulna are united by the proximal and distal radioulnar synovial joints, the interosseous ligament close to the middle of the radius and ulna, and the radioulnar ligament, which attaches the distal radial epiphysis to the styloid process of the ulna. A much thinner osseous membrane extends proximally and distally from the interosseous ligament.

The age at which radiographic closure of the growth plates occurs in the radius and ulna varies by breed. Small breeds generally mature at an earlier age than do larger breeds. The age of radiographic closure of the proximal radial growth plate, the distal radial growth plate, and the distal ulnar growth plate has been determined to range between 222 and 250 days in the beagle.[15]

Reports on the contribution of the proximal and distal radial growth plates to longitudinal growth of the canine radius indicate that variation exists among individual animals. Estimates of the growth contribution of the proximal radial growth plate vary—30%,[38, 72] 40%,[55] or 43% to 50%.[44] The distal ulnar growth plate accounts for 85% of the overall length of the ulna[44, 72, 78] and 100% of the length of the ulna distal to the elbow joint (Figs. 9-2 and 9-3). Since the radius grows in length from both the proximal and distal growth plates and the ulna grows in length below the elbow joint only from its distal growth plate, it is apparent that some change in the relationships between the radius and ulna is necessary during growth to maintain alignment between their articular surfaces

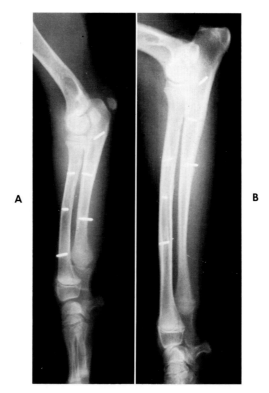

A   **B**

Fig. 9-2. Lateral radiographs of radius and ulna of an Australian shepherd dog at 83 days of age (**A**) and 227 days of age (**B**). Marker pins were inserted into diaphysis of radius and ulna when dog was 60 days of age. Note that distance between pins in each bone remains unchanged. There is a marked alteration of the relationships between pins in ulna compared with those in radius over period of growth.

at the elbow joint. This can be illustrated by placing marker pins in the diaphyseal region of the bones and serially radiographing them over a period of growth (Fig. 9-3). This movement between the radius and ulna as well as the absence of interstitial growth in the diaphyseal region of these bones is demonstrated in Fig. 9-4.

Retardation of longitudinal growth

Abnormal growth of the radius and ulna has been described secondary to delayed growth in the proximal and distal radial growth plates and distal ulnar growth plate.[17, 50, 58]

Deformities due to premature closure of the distal ulnar growth plate are the most common complications of epiphyseal injury in the dog.[45, 50, 57, 58, 78] The conical shape of the distal ulnar growth plate appears to be unique to the dog; thus the apex of the ulnar metaphysis tends to be forced down toward the epiphysis regardless of the type of injury sustained.[78] This frequently results in a crushing type of injury to the chondrogenic layer of cells of the growth plate. Retardation of growth of the distal ulnar growth plate results in a shortened ulna, which acts as a restraint on the radius, producing cranial bowing of the radius and other deformities. These include shortening of the limb, valgus deformation and external rotation of the carpus and metacarpal bones (Fig. 9-5), elbow subluxation, and subsequent osteoarthrosis of the carpal and elbow joints.* The bassett hound frequently develops a forelimb lameness that is due to a retarda-

---

*References 10-12, 43, 45, 53, 58, 78.

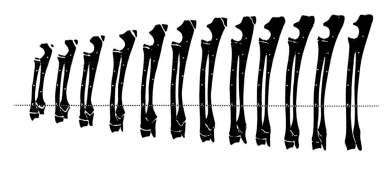

69 83 101 125 142 156 177 186 200 227 242 261

Age (days)

Fig. 9-3. Drawings of lateral radiographs of radius and ulna of same dog shown in Fig. 9-2. Radiographs were taken over period of growth from 69 days of age. Positions of marker pins in radius and ulna are indicated. Drawings have been arranged so that bottom marker pin in radius lies on dotted horizontal line. Relationship of pins in radius and ulna changes over period of growth. Note also that position of proximal pin in ulna maintains a constant relationship with trochlear notch of ulna, indicating that longitudinal growth in ulna distal to trochlear notch comes exclusively from distal ulnar growth plate.

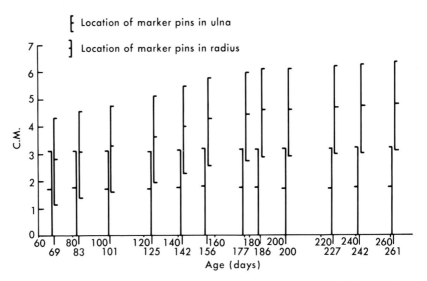

Fig. 9-4. Graphic representation of positions of markers in radius and ulna of dog shown in Fig. 9-2 over period of growth. No interstitial growth in either radius or ulna is indicated by constant distance between pins in each bone. Over period of growth, pins in ulna move proximally compared to those in radius.

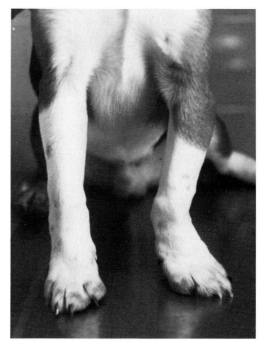

Fig. 9-5. Five-month-old beagle with abnormal development of left forelimb caused by retardation of longitudinal growth of ulna. Shortening of forelimb is seen along with a varus deformity of the elbow, valgus deformity of the carpus, and outward rotation of the paw. Note that normal right forelimb is bearing more weight than normal. This has resulted in digits being somewhat splayed.

tion of the growth of the ulna as compared to that of the radius and results in marked degenerative changes in the elbow joint.[10] This condition is developmental and unrelated to epiphyseal injury.

The early radiographic changes in the canine forelimb following 40% retardation of longitudinal growth of the ulna have been described by Carrig and Morgan.[10] The radiographic changes in the forelimb that occur subsequent to varying degrees of growth retardation in the ulna have been defined by Carrig, Merkley, and Mostosky.[8] Retardation of longitudinal growth of the ulna by approximately 10%, 35%, and 50% was produced experimentally in dogs by the application of x-irradiation to the distal ulnar metaphyseal-epiphyseal region. In the dogs with 10% retardation it was found that considerable adjustment in the growth of the adjacent radius followed. This resulted in a limb that was shorter than the opposite, control limb, but apart from the reduction in length, the morphology of the radius and ulna appeared radiographically similar to the control limb (Fig. 9-6.). In the dogs with 35% retardation, marked morphologic changes

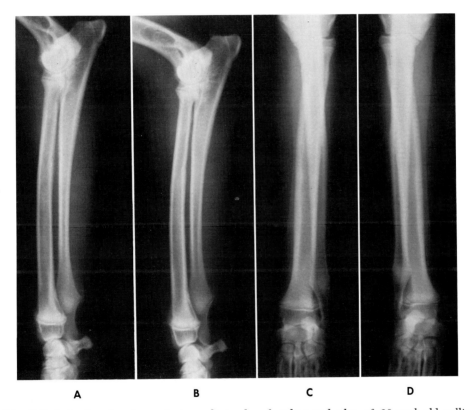

A   B   C   D

Fig. 9-6. Lateral and anteroposterior radiographs of radius and ulna of 30-week-old collie cross. **B** and **D,** Approximately 10% retardation of longitudinal growth of ulna was produced in one forelimb when dog was 10 weeks of age. Only minor morphologic alterations have occurred in treated limb (**B** and **D**) compared with normal forelimb (**A** and **C**). Reduction in longitudinal growth of ulna was compensated for by a reduction in longitudinal growth of radius.

in the forelimb resulted. Changes noted included subluxation at the elbow joint, curvature of the radius, and valgus deformity at the carpus (Fig. 9-7). In the dogs with 50% retardation the morphologic changes were more severe, and clinical lameness was more pronounced. The severity of the morphologic changes in the latter group appeared to be more pronounced at the level of the distal radius, where there was extreme curvature of the distal radius and disruption of the distal radial growth plate (Fig. 9-8, *A* and *B*). The degree of subluxation in the elbow joints of these dogs was also more than that seen in the dogs with 35% retardation. It appears that following minor growth retardations in the ulna the radius has the ability to adjust its growth so that marked deformity does not result. However, when growth retardation of the ulna exceeds the inherent ability of the radius to adjust to this abnormal situation, marked deformity of both the elbow joint and distal radius results. As the degree of growth retardation in the ulna becomes more severe, the major effect is seen in the distal radius. Marked curvature of the distal radius occurs, and disruption of the growth plate results from abnormal stresses placed on this region of the bone (Fig. 9-9).

Changes in elbow joint following retardation of longitudinal growth of ulna. Alteration in the relationships of the elbow joint can be observed radiographically

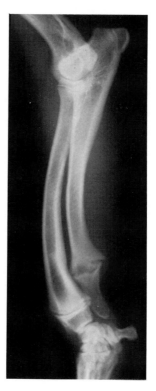

Fig. 9-7. Lateral radiograph of a 30-week-old collie cross following approximately 35% retardation of longitudinal growth in ulna at 10 weeks of age. Reduced longitudinal growth of ulna has resulted in subluxation of elbow joint, curvature of radius, and instability in carpus.

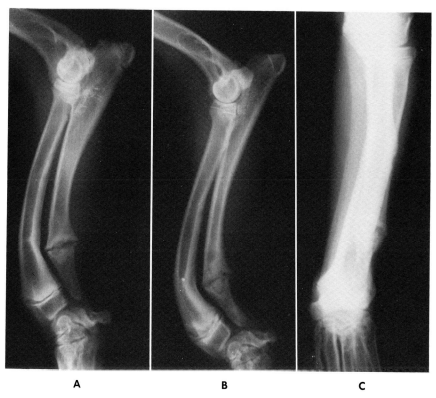

A　　　　　　　　**B**　　　　　　　　**C**

Fig. 9-8. Lateral (**A** and **B**) and anteroposterior (**C**) radiographs of 30-week-old collie cross dogs following approximately 50% retardation of longitudinal growth of ulna at 10 weeks of age. **A,** Changes noted in dog in Fig. 9-7 are more exaggerated with marked subluxation of elbow joint and increased curvature of radius. **B,** Subluxation of elbow joint is not as pronounced and major deformity is marked curvature of distal radius. Distal radial growth plate is becoming disrupted because of abnormal stresses placed on this part of bone. **C,** Varus deformity of elbow and valgus deformity of carpus are seen.

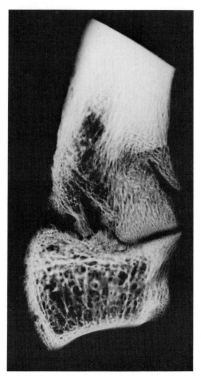

Fig. 9-9. Fine detail radiograph of 1 mm sagittal section of distal radius of dog shown in Fig. 9-8, *B*, at 30 weeks of age. Marked disruption of anterior two thirds of growth plate is seen.

as early as 2 weeks following reduction in ulnar growth. The most sensitive sign of altered relationships between the articular surfaces in the elbow joint is a separation between the subchondral bone of the lateral condyle of the humerus and the subchondral bone of the distal half of the trochlear notch.[11, 12] On the normal extend limb view of the elbow joint, an overlapping of these two bony plates is present and is represented on the radiograph by a thin, crescentic, radiodense zone (Fig. 9-10, *A*). A loss of this radiodense zone indicates that a degree of subluxation caused by the upward displacement of the humeral condyles by the relative overgrowth of the head of the radius is present (Fig. 9-10, *B*). As the amount of subluxation increases, the separation between the distal humeral condyle and the distal half of the trochlear notch becomes more prominent. A decrease in the subchondral bony density in this part of the trochlear notch can be seen. As much as 50% reduction in longitudinal growth of the ulna can occur without major alteration to the radiographic appearance of the anconeal process. When anconeal process disruptions are present in association with premature closure of the distal ulnar growth plate, as they are occasionally in clinical cases, reductions of ulnar growth of over 50% are probably present, or some other influence on the growth of the bones is present.

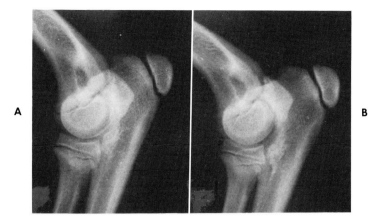

Fig. 9-10. Lateral radiographs of elbow joints of normal limb (**A**) and treated limb (**B**) 49 days after approximately 40% retardation of longitudinal growth of ulna in treated forelimb. Note that in normal limb the radiodense, semilunar shadow caused by superimposition of lateral condyle of the distal humerus and trochlear notch of proximal ulna can be identified. In treated limb this radiodense line is not seen, indicating subluxation of elbow joint. Humeroradial joint space is narrowed in treated limb. (From Carrig, C. B., Morgan, J. P., and Pool, R. R.: J. Am. Anim. Hosp. Assoc. **11**:560, 1975.)

In dissected specimens evidence of degeneration of articular cartilage in the elbow joint is seen as early as 4 weeks following reduction in ulnar growth. The area of articular cartilage most sensitive to degeneration is the lateral articular surface of the distal half of the trochlear notch. The earliest changes observed are thinning and irregularity of the articular cartilage. By 8 weeks after disturbance of ulnar growth, marked thinning and erosion of the cartilage is seen in this predilection site (Fig. 9-11). With severe displacements the area of cartilage erosion extends over to involve the medial articular surface of the distal half of the trochlear notch. Histologically, degenerative changes in the articular cartilage can be detected 2 weeks following altered growth in the ulna. After 8 weeks profound changes are present. The surface layers of cartilage are disrupted, and disorganization of chondrocytes is seen. Thinning of the articular cartilage occurs, and evidence of disruption of the cartilage along a plane parallel to the articular surface is present. Invasion of the cartilage by blood vessels and granulation tissue results, and ossification occurs in association with the invasion of the vascular mesenchyma. Subsequently there is disruption of the articular cartilage, and an area of subchondral bone completely denuded of articular cartilage results (Fig. 9-12).

The degenerative changes in the cartilage are associated with marked changes in the microcirculation at that point. Vascular invasion of the degenerating articular cartilage occurs, and by 8 weeks following altered growth in the ulna extension of blood vessels to a level approximately halfway between the articular surface and the tide mark occurs. Widespread anastomosis between these vessels occurs in a plane parallel to the articular surface. These changes are accompanied

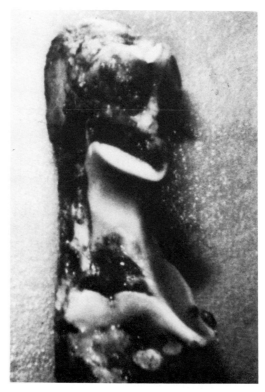

Fig. 9-11. Trochlear notch of ulna 56 days after approximately 40% retardation of longitudinal growth of ulna. There is extensive erosion of cartilage from lateral articular surface of distal half of trochlear notch. Tissues appear dark as vasculature in forelimb was perfused with India ink. (From Carrig, C. B., Morgan, J. P., and Pool, R. R.: J. Am. Anim. Hosp. Assoc. **11**:560, 1975.)

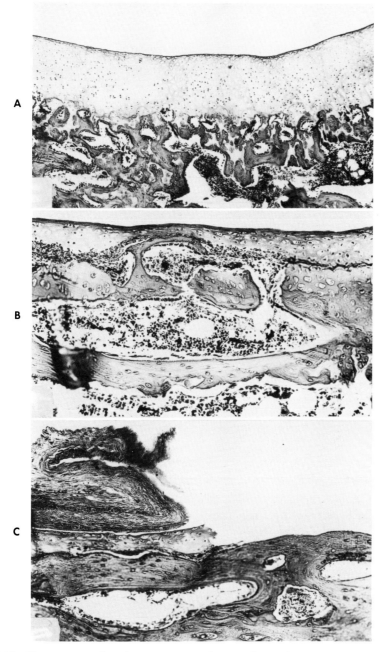

Fig. 9-12. Photomicrographs of tissue section from midsagittal plane of trochlear notch of ulna. **A,** 28 days after approximately 40% retardation of longitudinal growth of ulna at 10 weeks of age. Radial zones of nonviable chondrocytes are separated by zones of viable, dividing chondrocytes. **B,** 56 days after approximately 40% retardation of longitudinal growth of ulna. Extensive invasion of cartilage by vascular mesenchyme has occurred. There is a bony plate extending from subchondral area along path of vascular invasion. Note compression of the superficial zones of cartilage at this site. **C,** 84 days after approximately 40% retardation of longitudinal growth of ulna. Superficial fibrous zone and remaining cartilage are separated from underlying trabecular bone. Bone is completely denuded of cartilage on right side. (6 mµ; H & E; **A** and **B** ×40, **C** ×100) (From Carrig, C. B., Morgan, J. P., and Pool, R. R.: J. Am. Anim. Hosp. Assoc. **11**:560, 1975.)

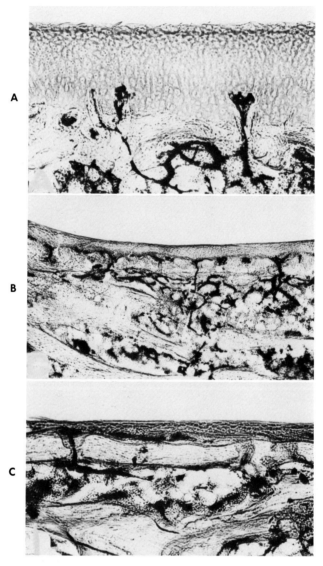

Fig. 9-13. Photomicrographs of tissue section from midsagittal plane of trochlear notch of ulna. **A,** 28 days after approximately 40% retardation of longitudinal growth of ulna. Early invasion of lower zone of articular cartilage by vessels originating from subchondral bone is seen. **B,** 56 days after approximately 40% retardation of longitudinal growth of ulna. Lateral extensions of invading vessels are seen, and these are forming an anastamosing network of vessels within the degenerating articular cartilage. **C,** 84 days after approximately 40% retardation of longitudinal growth of ulna. Vessel penetrating subchondral bone plate is extending between the layer of altered cartilage and the subchondral bone. (India ink perfusion; 72 mμ; **A** and **C** ×100, **B** ×40.) (From Carrig, C. B., Morgan, J. P., and Pool, R. R.: J. Am. Anim. Hosp. Assoc. **11**:560, 1975.)

by hemorrhage, invasion by granulation tissue, and collapse of underlying trabecular bone. At sites where complete denuding of the articular cartilage occurs this vascular anastomotic network becomes exposed to the joint surface (Fig. 9-13).

The location of these degenerative changes in the articular cartilage of the lateral aspect of the distal half of the trochlear notch represents that area of cartilage which loses contact with the opposing surfaces of the humeral condyle. This fact supports observations in man that the most common site of degenerative cartilage lesions is in the area of a joint exposed to little or no stress and strain during joint function.[19, 35, 54, 83] It has been shown not only that nutrient materials pass into immature articular cartilage from both its articular and subchondral surfaces, but also that joint function materially increases this passage.[25, 26, 42] This intermittent pumping action of alternate pressure and rest is essential for adequate nutrition of articular cartilage. It would appear that the lack of an adequate and alternating pressure on the articular cartilage is the cause of degenerative changes noted in the trochlear notch. This is probably related to the necessity of compressive forces on the cartilage for adequate diffusion of nutrients. The subsequent changes seen in the articular cartilage are an attempt by the animal's repair processes to support a tissue that is undernourished from underwork. The lack of degenerative changes in the proximal half of the trochlear notch supports this conclusion, since articular contact is not lost in this area of the joint, and indicates that increased pressure between articular cartilage is less damaging to the cartilage than loss of joint contact.

Restriction of movement between radius and ulna

Considerable movement of the radius in relation to the ulna occurs during normal growth of the canine forelimb (Figs. 9-2 to 9-4). The morphologic changes occurring after restriction of this movement have been studied[55] by introducing Steinmann pins from the radius to the ulna to effectively prevent a change in the relationship between the diaphyses of the radius and ulna. Severe changes in the relationships between the radius and ulna at the elbow joint resulted. Considerable overgrowth of the proximal radial epiphysis in relation to the trochlear notch of the proximal ulna forced the distal humeral condyles in a proximal direction, and severe damage to the anconeal process of the ulna and the distal humeral condyle resulted (Fig. 9-14, *A* and *B*). Marked degenerative changes occurred in the distal half of the trochlear notch as well. These changes were similar to, but more profound than, those occurring in association with retardation of longitudinal growth of the ulna and were also related to the lack of normal joint contact between the trochlear notch and the trochlear humeri of the distal humerus. The severity of the changes in the elbow joint was related to the age at the time of cross-pinning the radius to the ulna (Fig. 9-15). The younger the animal (and with more growth potential remaining in the proximal growth plate of the radius), the greater the displacement of the articular surfaces at the elbow joint and the changes in the joint. In dogs cross-

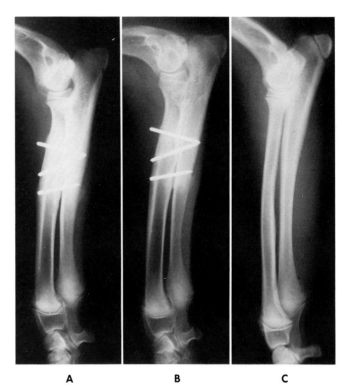

A   **B**   **C**

Fig. 9-14. Lateral radiograph of forelimb of an Australian shepherd 10½ weeks (**A**) and 15 weeks (**B**) after cross-pinning of the radius to the ulna at 12 weeks of age. **C**, Normal forelimb of this dog at 27 weeks of age. Restriction of movement between radius and ulna caused an overgrowth of radius in relation to trochlear notch, and severe changes result in elbow joint. Subchondral density of distal half of trochlear notch is decreased, and disruption of anconeal process of proximal ulna is seen. Lengths of radius and ulna in treated forelimb (**B**) are similar to those in normal forelimb (**C**), indicating that an increased growth rate occurred in the distal radial growth plate.

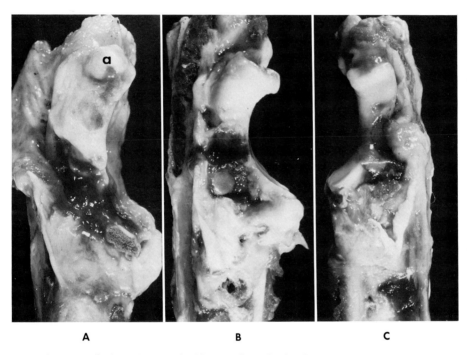

A   B   C

Fig. 9-15. Proximal ulna of 40-week-old Australian shepherds after cross-pinning of radius to ulna at 12 weeks of age (right forelimb, **A**), 20 weeks of age (right forelimb, **B**), and 24 weeks of age (left forelimb, **C**). Severe degenerative changes in trochlear notch have occurred, and severity of change is related to growth potential remaining in radius and ulna at time of cross-pinning. When radius and ulna were cross-pinned at an early age (**A**) marked changes occurred in distal half of trochlear notch where destruction of cartilage and subchondral bone resulted. In proximal half of trochlear notch, marked degenerative changes were noted in articular cartilage and a loose ossicle was present in the region of the anconeal process *(a)*. When limbs were cross-pinned at a later age, changes in trochlear notch were less marked. Most severely affected area was in distal half of trochlear notch.

pinned at 12 to 16 weeks of age severe degenerative changes were seen affecting the entire trochlear notch (Fig. 9-15, *A*). In dogs cross-pinned at 20 to 24 weeks of age marked changes were noted in the trochlear notch, but they were less extensive than in those cross-pinned at an earlier age. In these latter dogs the degenerative changes associated with the anconeal process were also less obvious, and the major degenerative changes were seen in the lateral aspect of the distal half of the trochlear notch (Fig. 9-15, *B* and *C*).

It was noted in the cross-pinned limbs that the overall length of the radius and ulna was not appreciably altered, compared to the normal control limb. The fact that the relationships of the distal radius and ulna were not appreciably altered (Fig. 14, *B* and *C*) indicated that stimulation of longitudinal bone growth from the distal radial growth plate had occurred. This was possibly associated with traction on the distal radius by the strong radioulnar ligament as the ulna continued to grow distally. Measurements of the percentage contribution of the distal growth plate to longitudinal growth of the radius indicated an alteration from approximately 60% in the control radius to approximately 80% in the cross-pinned radius.

It is apparent that restriction of movement between the radius and ulna during the period of growth can result in marked alterations to the growth characteristics and morphology of the bones. Surgical procedures on the radius or ulna in the immature patient should minimize factors that could contribute to the limitation of this movement. Researchers using the canine radius and ulna for the study of skeletal development should ensure that no interference of movement between these bones is produced (e.g., by marker pins crossing from the radius to the ulna), since this would influence results obtained.

DISTURBED ENDOCHONDRAL OSSIFICATION IN FORELIMB

Several skeletal diseases affecting the canine forelimb have been related to faulty development of cartilage to bone. This error in development has been termed osteochondrosis—a generalized, noninfectious disturbance of endochondral ossification in growth cartilage. Articular cartilage and the cartilage of the epiphyseal growth plate are affected. The frequency and severity of osteochondrosis increase with increasing growth rate, and clinical and experimental evidence in dogs, pigs, and cattle indicates that the frequency and severity of this disease process can be lessened if growth is held back by reduced food intake.[2, 33, 37, 61] Mechanical factors are thought to determine the location of the various types of lesions occurring in the skeleton that can be ascribed to faulty endochondral ossification. Lesions in the canine forelimb that can be considered manifestations in the joint of the generalized condition osteochondrosis include osteochondritis dissecans of the humeral head, ununited anconeal process of the ulna, ununited coronoid process of the ulna, and retained hypertrophied endochondral cartilage in the distal ulnar metaphysis.[61]

Osteochondritis dissecans of humeral head

Canine osteochondritis dissecans occurs mainly in the proximal articular surface of the humerus in the large breeds, especially the Great Dane and Saint Bernard.* However, lesions also occur in the lateral femoral condyle, the medial condyle of the humerus, and the hock joint. Osteochondritis dissecans of the humeral head is characterized by shoulder lameness, pain on extension of the leg, and atrophy of the shoulder musculature. The disease affects both humeral heads in approximately 40% to 50% of cases.[24, 79] The lesions are located in the central portion of the caudal aspect of the developing humeral head and are best visualized on the lateral projection of the shoulder joint. The major radiographic finding is a discontinuity or irregularity of the subchondral bone of the humeral head. The lesions vary greatly in size and in severe cases assume the shape of an inverted, radiolucent cone whose apex extends deep into the bony epiphysis (Fig. 9-16, A). The radiolucent defect is usually surrounded by sclerotic bone. Fissures occur in the thickened cartilage and extend to the surface of the articular cartilage. Synovial fluid extends into the fissure defect, and severe clinical signs usually result. The visualization on the plain radiograph of the cartilage flap within a lesion depends on whether calcification has occurred in the flap. If it has occurred, the flap appears as a linear opacity over the lesion (Fig. 9-16, B). The presence of a noncalcified, radiolucent fragment of articular cartilage within a lesion can be identified by positive contrast arthrography. It is not uncommon for the cartilage flap to detach and lie free in the ventral portion of the joint space where the joint capsule attaches to the humeral epiphysis. A loose piece of cartilage often grows in size following detachment from the articular surface. Secondary degenerative joint disease results from longstanding, severe lesions, and erosion of the glenoid cavity of the scapula often is an accompanying lesion. Pathologically enhanced growth of cartilage dominates the picture histologically. It is followed by degeneration of the cartilage in the depths of the lesion, and pathologic endochondral ossification around the lesion results in markedly thickened surrounding bone trabeculae. Osteonecrosis is not a prominent feature of the lesion in the dog.[47]

In man osteochondritis dissecans is considered to be the result of a vascular disturbance, possibly following microfracture of the bone.[31, 32] In the dog the cause is unknown, although growth rate and local mechanical factors appear to be involved in the occurrence of the disease. Abnormal development of the vascular supply to the areas of abnormal cartilage can be demonstrated (Fig. 9-17), but its role in the formation of this lesion is not understood. The normal appearance of the blood supply to the canine humeral head has been described.[9]

Ununited anconeal process of ulna

Detachment of the anconeal process from the proximal ulna is associated with clinical lameness and the development of degenerative joint disease in the

---

*References 52, 61, 62, 65, 66, 79.

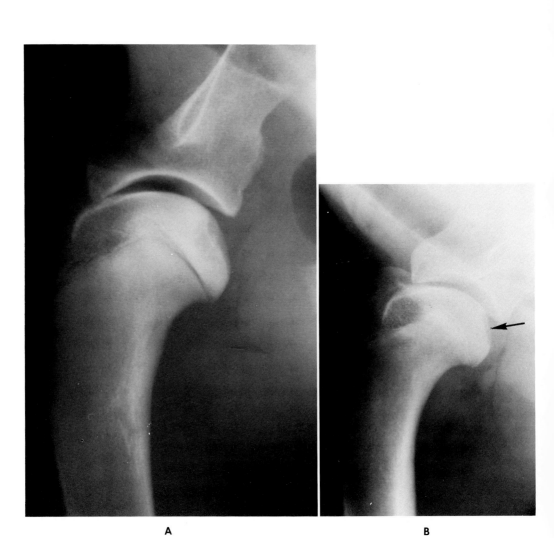

A   **B**

Fig. 9-16. Lateral radiographs of shoulder joint of 9-month-old Great Dane (**A**) and 8-month-old Labrador retriever (**B**) with osteochondritis dissecans. **A,** A large conical-shaped lucent zone is present in posterior aspect of humeral head. Lesion is surrounded by a zone of increased bone density. **B,** A loose calcified cartilaginous flap can be identified overlying lesion in humeral head (arrow).

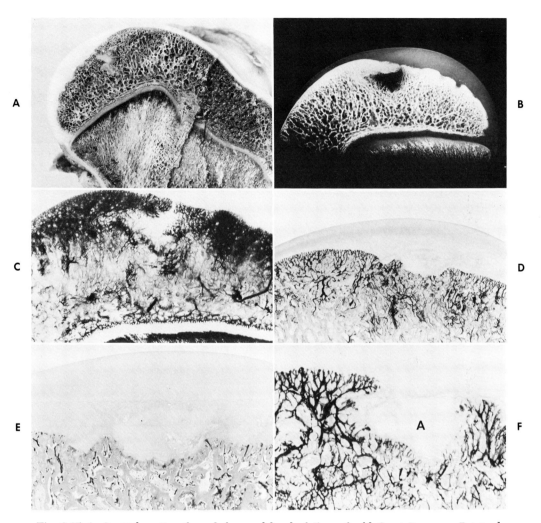

Fig. 9-17 A, Sagittal section through humeral head of 5-month-old Great Pyrenees. Retained cartilage can be recognized within depths of humeral head. Cartilaginous epiphysis has not fully ossified at this time. **B,** Fine detail radiograph of 1 mm thick sagittal section of humeral head of 5-month-old Great Pyrenees. Abnormal ossification of epiphysis has resulted in a zone of retained cartilage within humeral head. **C,** Same section of humeral head as shown in **B.** Vasculature has been perfused with India ink and tissue cleared in xylene. Abnormal-appearing blood vessels can be recognized in depths of zone of retained cartilage. **D,** Humeral head of 5-month-old Great Pyrenees. Vasculature has been perfused with India ink. Vascular supply to developing bony epiphysis is normal except in an area adjacent to a zone of altered cartilage. In this region blood vessels are of uneven caliber, and normal anastomosis between vessels appears reduced. (200 mμ; celloidin embedded.) **E,** Histologic section of humeral head shown to be associated with abnormal vascular supply in **D.** Areas of degenerating cartilage are seen in the predilection zone for osteochondritis dissecans. (8 mμ; H & E; ×40.) **F,** Humeral head of 5-month-old Great Pyrenees. Blood vessels have been perfused with India ink. Abnormal vessels can be seen associated with area of degenerating cartilage (*A*).

elbow joint. The condition has been referred to as elbow dysplasia, and the clinical syndrome has been described.* The anconeal process of the proximal ulna in most breeds does not develop from a separate ossification center, but rather ossifies along with the ulnar diaphysis. However, in some breeds (e.g., German shepherd and greyhound) the anconeal process appears to develop from a separate ossification center, which normally unites to the ulnar diaphysis by the age of 4½ months.[21, 85, 86] In some dogs this fails to occur, and instability of the elbow joint results in degenerative joint disease. The condition can occur unilaterally or bilaterally with varying degrees of severity. Ununited anconeal process is most frequently encountered in the German shepherd, but other breeds can be affected, including the Saint Bernard, basset hound, Labrador retriever, Great Dane, and bloodhound. It is most easily detected on the lateral projection of the flexed elbow joint. This position projects the cleavage line between the anconeal process and the proximal ulna in such a manner that it is free from overlying shadows of the distal humerus (Fig. 9-18).

Treatment consists of surgically removing the ununited ossicle and is usually

---

*References 6, 21, 22, 39, 46, 61, 87.

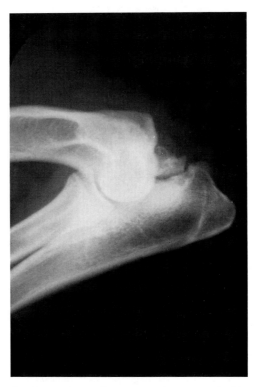

Fig. 9-18. Flexed lateral radiograph of elbow joint of a 7-month-old German shepherd with ununited anconeal process, which is seen along with cleavage line between it and the proximal ulna.

performed when the affected animal is between 5 and 8 months of age. Once severe osteoarthritis is present in the elbow joint, removal of the ossicle usually does not alleviate the clinical lameness.

Ununited coronoid process of ulna

Ununited coronoid process has only recently been recognized as a factor causing degenerative joint disease in the canine elbow joint. It is not clear at this time whether the lesion results from a failure of a separate ossification center to unite to the adjacent ulna or whether the ossicle results from trauma to, and fragmentation of, the developing cartilaginous coronoid process, with subsequent ossification occurring in the detached cartilage. The lesion has been observed most frequently in the golden and Labrador retriever but is also seen in the Rottweiler, German shepherd, Saint Bernard, and other large- or medium-sized dogs.[60] The presence of the loose bony bodies is difficult to detect radiographically because of their close proximity to the head of the radius. The

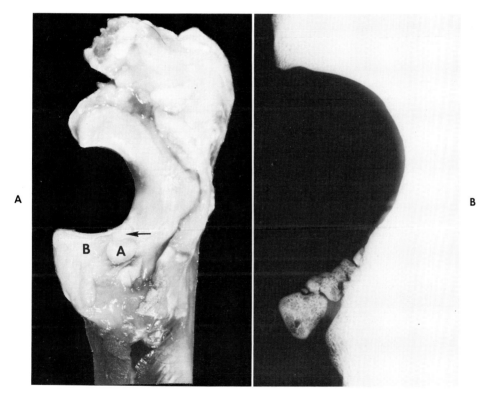

Fig. 9-19. A, Tissues from elbow joint of a 10-month-old Australian shepherd with ununited coronoid process. Loose ossicle *(A)* can be identified lying in region of coronoid process on medial aspect of radial head *(B)*. Adjacent areas of degenerating cartilage can be identified (arrow). Joint capsule is thickened, and degenerative changes are present in articular margins of trochlear notch. **B,** Lateral radiograph of trochlear notch of ulna shown in **A.** Area of altered cartilage contains bony tissue, and separation from coronoid process is present over a large area. Several of the ossified bodies appear to contain microfractures.

osseous body is usually composed of trabecular bone covered by articular cartilage (Fig. 9-19) and is usually attached to the ulna by either connective tissue or by fibrocartilage. Generally there is increased synovial fluid, thickening of the synovial membrane, and erosive lesions in the opposing surface of the trochlear humeri. It has been suggested that removal of the loose bony bodies will minimize the secondary joint disease that often accompanies the condition.[61]

Retained hypertrophied endochondral cartilage in distal ulnar metaphysis

A core of retained, radiolucent cartilage in the distal ulnar metaphysis of the growing dog has been described.[72] It is seen most frequently in the giant breeds. The retained cartilage can be seen radiographically in the metaphyseal region of the ulna as a radiolucent strip or core, which can extend as far as 4 or 5 cm into the metaphysis (Fig. 9-20, *A*). The radiolucent core is surrounded by a thin, dense shell of thickened trabecular bone that creates a sclerotic

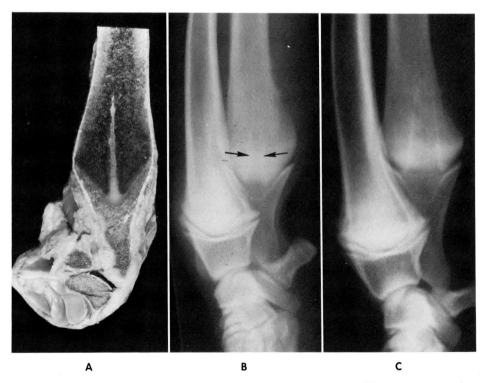

A   **B**   **C**

Fig. 9-20. A, Midsagittal section through distal ulna of a 6-month-old Doberman pinscher demonstrating gross appearance of narrow retained core of cartilage present in metaphyseal region of the bone. **B,** Lateral radiograph of distal radius and ulna from same dog as **A.** Thin cartilage core can be seen extending into metaphyseal region of ulna (arrows). It is surrounded by a thin zone of increased bone density. **C,** Lateral radiograph of distal radius and ulna in 4½-month-old Great Dane. A large cartilage core is present in distal ulna. Interference with longitudinal growth in ulna is suggested by a slight degree of curvature in distal radius. As animal matured, curvature of radius became more exaggerated.

shadow on the radiograph (Fig. 9-20, *B* and *C*). Histologically the core is composed of hypertrophied hyaline cartilage cells piled in long columns (Fig. 9-21). The clinical significance of the retained cartilage core depends on the size of the structure. Smaller cores of cartilage are often observed in the distal ulnar metaphyseal region, and no interference with normal ulnar growth is apparent. When the core is large, interference with longitudinal growth of the ulna occurs, resulting in shortening of the ulna and cranial bowing of the radius (Fig. 9-20, *C*).[43, 58] The etiology of the lesion is unknown, but a vascular disturbance has been postulated.[58] Interference with the blood supply from the metaphyseal arteries to the growth plate can result in hypertrophy of the cartilage cells in the growth plate.[83, 84]

GENERALIZED SKELETAL DYSPLASIAS INVOLVING FORELIMB
Chondrodysplasia in Alaskan malamute

A short-limbed, disproportionate dwarfism has been observed in Alaskan malamutes and classified as a canine chondrodysplasia.[28] Clinically affected animals show a bilateral stunting of the forelimbs, variable in its severity. The hind limbs are affected less than the forelimbs, so the top line of the animal is slanted. The stunting of the forelimb is accompanied by deviation of the forepaw, enlargement of the carpal joints, and lateral bowing of the forelimbs (Fig.

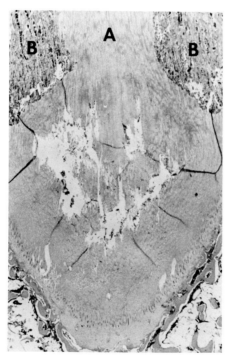

Fig. 9-21. Histologic section of base of cartilage core illustrated in Fig. 9-20, *A*. Hypertrophied cartilage cells *(A)* extend into bony metaphysis *(B)*. Fragmentation in cartilaginous growth plate is considered artifact. (8 mμ; H & E; ×10.)

9-22). The severity of clinical signs depends on the degree of growth retardation. Some severely affected puppies cannot walk properly, but less affected ones will show intermittent lameness. In the mature animal, lameness is rarely observed. Radiographically the skeletal defect is generalized and symmetrical in bones that grow by endochondral ossification. Affected animals can be recognized radiographically as early as 3 weeks of age.[76] Evidence of impaired ossification may be seen at sites of endochondral bone development in all long bones and at the costochondral junction. The most striking characteristic lesion is found in the distal ulnar growth plate. The normal conical shape of the distal ulnar metaphysis fails to develop, and the metaphyseal region is irregular in outline and density (Fig. 9-23). Similar, less obvious changes are present in the distal radial metaphyseal border. Delayed ossification of the carpal bones and the epiphyses of the long bones is seen. Differential growth rate of the radius and ulna is present in the dwarf, with the ulna developing in length at a slower rate than the radius. This differential growth rate results in curvature of the radius and ulna with accompanying lateral bowing of the forelimbs, medial deviation

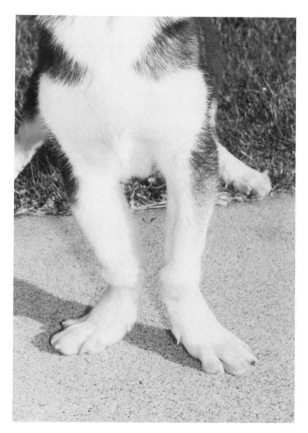

Fig. 9-22. Seven-month-old chondrodysplastic Alaskan malamute demonstrating forelimb deformity associated with this condition. Forelimbs are shorter than normal, and outward rotation of paws is present.

of the carpus, and lateral deviation of the forepaws. The diaphyses of the radius and ulna are wider in the dwarf than in the normal animal[76] (Fig. 9-24).

The mode of inheritance of chondrodysplasia in the Alaskan malamute is a single autosomal recessive gene with complete penetrance, variable expression of dwarfness, and no intermediate phenotypes. A hypochromic, macrocytic, hemolytic anemia has been demonstrated as a pleiotropic effect of the dwarfism gene.[27] Because chondrodysplasia in the Alaskan malamute has been determined to be inherited as a mendelian recessive gene, an attempt has been made to eliminate the gene from the breeding pool by selected matings. The mating of phenotypically normal animals with known dwarfs allows detection of the heterozygous state.

Chondrodysplasia in the Alaskan malamute appears to be similar to some forms of metaphyseal dysostosis described in human patients, particularly resembling the Spahr type, which is an inherited disease in man transmitted by an autosomal recessive gene.[75]

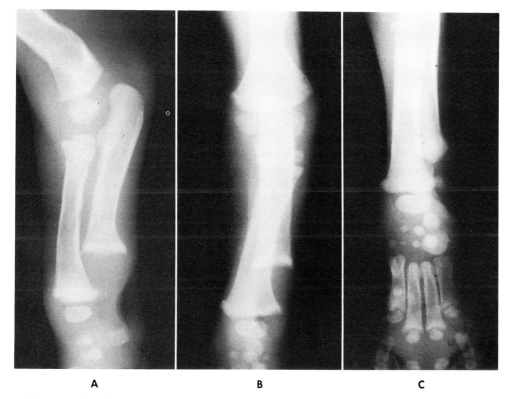

| A | B | C |

Fig. 9-23. **A** and **B**, Lateral and anteroposterior radiographs of radius and ulna of a 4-week-old Alaskan malamute with chondrodysplasia. Abnormal development of distal ulnar metaphysis is present along with delayed ossification of distal radial and ulnar epiphyses and carpal bones. **C**, Anteroposterior radiograph of a normal littermate.

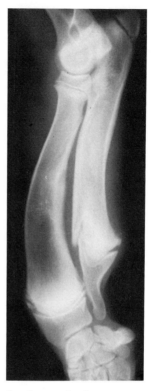

Fig. 9-24. Lateral radiograph of radius and ulna of 7-month-old Alaskan malamute with chondrodysplasia. Abnormal remodeling of bones is evident as well as subluxation of elbow joint, curvature of radius, and abnormal relationships of bones at carpus.

Retinal dysplasia associated with skeletal abnormalities in Labrador retriever

A syndrome characterized by severe retinal dysplasia and multiple skeletal dysplasias has been observed in the Labrador retriever.[7, 77] The first evidence of abnormal skeletal development is seen at approximately 8 weeks of age. Visual deficiencies are also recognized at this time. Obvious retardation of growth of the forelimbs, adduction at the elbow joint, and a valgus deformity at the carpus are seen (Fig. 9-25). Abnormalities observed in the radiographs of the skeletal system include reduction in length of the radius, ulna, and tibia, asynchronous growth of the radius and ulna, ununited anconeal process of the proximal ulna, ununited and hypoplastic coronoid process, hypoplasia of the medial epicondyle of the distal humerus, delayed development of the distal humeral and femoral condyles, osteoarthrosis of the elbow joint, and hip dysplasia (Figs. 9-26 to 9-28). Ocular abnormalities include severe retinal dysplasia with retinal detachment (Fig. 9-29) and cataract formations. A prominent retained remnant of the hyaloid vascular system is occasionally seen. In one dog no evidence of abnormal mucopolysaccharide excretion was detected. Cytogenetic evaluation of the bone marrow samples in two dogs showed autosome morphology and number to be nor-

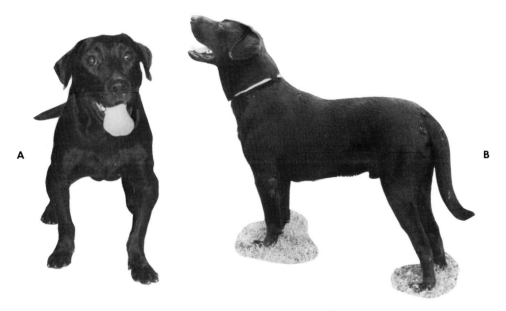

Fig. 9-25. Front view (**A**) and side view (**B**) of 2-year-old male Labrador retriever with retinal dysplasia and skeletal abnormalities. A varus deformity at the elbow joint and a valgus deformity at the carpus is seen. Pupil size is increased. Side view shows forelimbs much shorter than hind limbs and overextension of hock joints. (Courtesy Dr. G. Schmidt.)

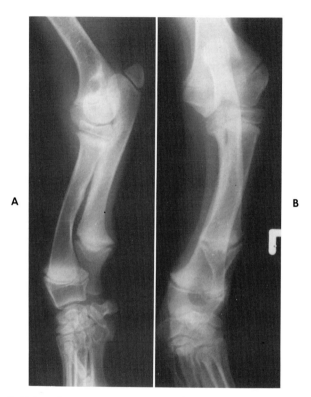

Fig. 9-26. Lateral (**A**) and anteroposterior (**B**) radiographs of radius and ulna of 3-month-old Labrador retriever with retinal dysplasia and skeletal abnormalities. Radius and ulna are shorter than normal, and curvature of radius is present. Delayed development of anconeal and coronoid processes of ulna is evident. A varus deformity at the elbow and valgus deformity at the carpus are appreciated on anteroposterior radiograph.

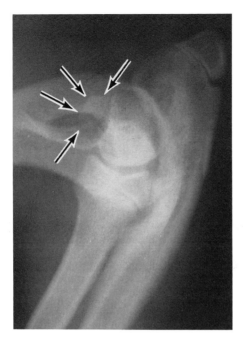

Fig. 9-27. Flexed lateral radiograph of left elbow of a 5-month-old Labrador retriever with retinal dysplasia and skeletal abnormalities. Delayed development of coronoid process of ulna is appreciated, and a detached ossification center for anconeal process is visualized in olecranon fossa of distal humerus (arrows).

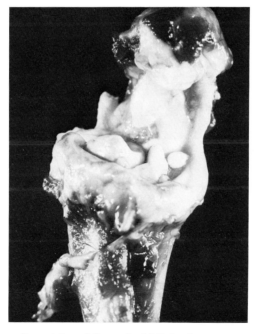

Fig. 9-28. Tissues from elbow joint of 9-month-old Labrador retriever with retinal dysplasia and skeletal abnormalities. Free bony fragments are seen in region of coronoid process of ulna just medial to radial head. A defect can be noted in lateral half of distal articular surface of trochlear notch. Cartilage of trochlear notch is showing degenerative changes, and thickening of joint capsule is present.

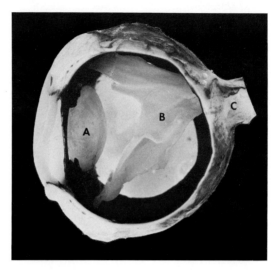

Fig. 9-29. Left eye of 9-month-old Labrador retriever with retinal dysplasia and skeletal abnormalities. Lateral calottes have been removed. Complete detachment of retina is present. Lens *(A)*, detached retina *(B)*, and optic nerve *(C)*.

mal. A normal XY chromosome complement was also present. The changes noted in these dogs appear similar to those reported to occur in hereditary arthro-ophthalmopathy in man.[80-82]

Multiple epiphyseal dysplasia

Multiple epiphyseal dysplasia in the dog has been reported infrequently and only in beagles and poodles.[23, 34, 48, 68, 69] It has been reproduced in three generations of beagles,[69] indicating a hereditable disease similar to the condition in man.[1]

In the dog abnormal movement of the hind limbs is a prominent sign of the disease and is recognized shortly after birth. After 6 months of age evidence of lameness is rarely present and is usually noted only after exercise. Radiographically the disease is first recognized at 3 weeks of age as multiple areas of punctate calcification in the epiphyses. By 4 to 6 months of age the areas of increased density in the epiphyses are uncommon because they become incorporated into the developing epiphyses. In adult dogs the epiphyses are shallow, and the metaphyseal regions of the bones are broader than normal. A few punctate, sclerotic zones are seen in the epiphyses at this time.

Histologically abnormalities of chondrogenesis in the epiphyses can be detected prenatally. Increased production of intercellular ground substance leads to the formation of cystic cavities, the linings of which become calcified at about

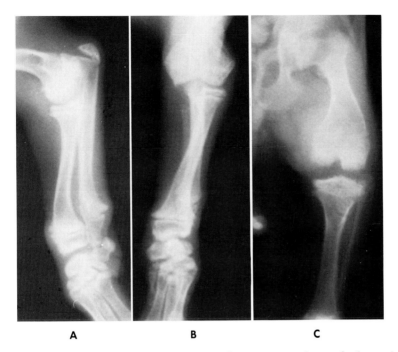

A   B   C

Fig. 9-30. Lateral (**A**) and anteroposterior (**B**) radiographs of radius and ulna and anteroposterior radiograph of femur and tibia (**C**) of a 3-month-old miniature poodle with multiple epiphyseal dysplasia. Irregular development of the epiphyses, which have a mottled radiographic appearance, is seen. (Courtesy Dr. U. V. Mostosky.)

the same time that the epiphyseal ossification centers develop. At this time the disease is recognized radiographically as stippled areas where the calcification of smaller cystic areas becomes condensed into small clumps or mottled areas dispersed throughout larger cystic areas (Fig. 9-30).

Osteochondroma

Osteochondromas occur singly or as multiple lesions. In the latter case they are referred to as hereditary multiple exostoses. Osteochondromas are formed by endochondral growth. They occur adjacent to the epiphyseal growth plate and protrude at right angles to the long axis of the host bone (Fig. 9-31). The bone produced by an osteochondroma is normal, and the lesion should be regarded as an endochondral hamartomatous hyperplasia.[1] Multiple osteochondromas in dogs have been reported.[3, 16, 29, 63] They also occur in horses and cats. A hereditary pattern has been observed in dogs[16] and horses.[51] Usually no clinical signs are seen except when the lesion grows and exerts pressure on overlying soft tissue structures. Malignant transformation into osteosarcoma and chondrosarcoma has been observed in the dog.[3]

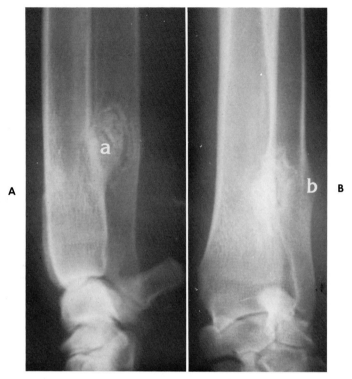

Fig. 9-31. Lateral (**A**) and anteroposterior (**B**) radiographs of distal radius and ulna of 3-year-old Saint Bernard. Osteochondromas are present in metaphyseal regions of radius (*a*) and ulna (*b*). Radial lesion has grown into metaphyseal region of ulna, and remodeling of ulna around osteochondroma is present.

Cystic bone lesions

Cystic bone lesions have been reported infrequently in the dog. Monostotic forms (involving only one bone)[14, 56, 64, 70, 73] and polyostotic forms (involving more than one bone)[13, 14, 30, 41] have been reported (Figs. 9-32 and 9-33). Polyostotic cystic bone lesions have been reported in five Doberman pinschers, and there could be a breed predisposition.[13, 14] The cystic changes occur in the metaphyseal region of the long bones and are first noted at approximately 4 months of age. By 6 or 7 months of age the cystic nature of the disease process is well established and is characterized by expansion of the bone and thinning of the cortices (Fig. 9-33). Cystic lesions have been noted in the distal metaphyseal regions of the radius and ulna, the proximal metaphyseal region of the tibia, and the distal metaphyseal region of the femur. Pseudofractures (Looser's zones) have been noted in association with several of the cystic lesions and in some cases have predisposed the affected bone to fracture (Fig. 9-34).[13, 41, 56] The

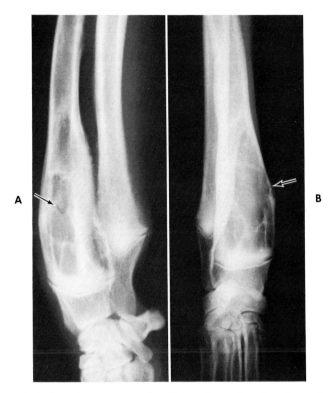

Fig. 9-32. Lateral (**A**) and anteroposterior (**B**) radiographs of a 7-month-old Doberman pinscher with monostotic cystic bone lesion in distal radius. Expansion of cortex of bone is present and a pseudofracture can be seen (arrows). (From Carrig, C. B., and Seawright, A. A.: J. Small Anim. Pract. **10**:397, 1969.)

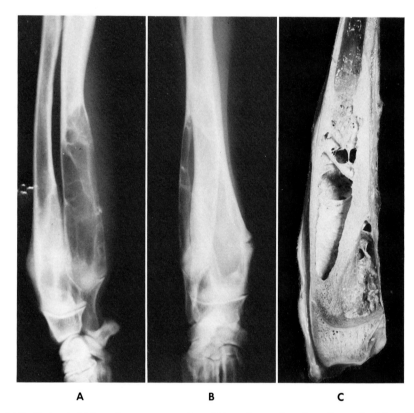

Fig. 9-33. Lateral (**A**) and anteroposterior (**B**) radiographs of a 7-month-old Doberman pinscher with polyostotic cystic bone lesions. Radius and ulna in both forelimbs contained cystic lesions. **C,** Sagittal section through distal radius of 9-month-old Doberman pinscher with polyostotic cystic bone lesions. Cystic lesions, which were filled with straw-colored fluid, are lined with a delicate fibrillar material. (From Carrig, C. B., Pool, R. R., and McElroy, J. M.: J. Small Anim. Pract. **16:**495, 1975.)

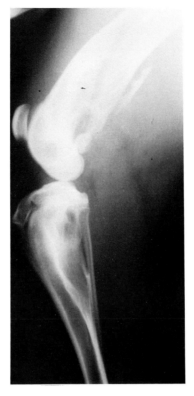

Fig. 9-34. Lateral radiograph of distal femur and proximal tibia of 9-month-old Doberman pinscher with polyostotic cystic bone lesions. A pathologic fracture is present in the femoral lesion.

cystic cavities contain clear, straw-colored fluid and are lined by flesh-colored delicate fibrillar material, which forms a lacy network within them (Fig. 9-33, C). Occasionally blood-tinged fluid is found in the cystic lesions. This is probably related to recent trauma, as it has been reported that only minimal trauma is necessary to cause hemorrhage in cystic structures in bone.[18] Many cystic lesions have multiple compartments partially separated by prominent bony ridges. Pathogenesis of the cystic lesions has not been resolved, but it seems from histologic examination of affected tissues that the secondary spongiosa in the metaphyseal periosteum is the major tissue site that appears abnormal. The growth plate and the primary spongiosa are not affected. In the bones in which cystic structures completely or partially bridge the metaphyseal cortex, the periosteum covering this site is effectively nonosteogenic or produces a meager fibro-osseous periosteal response in which cystic degeneration occasionally is seen. A thin, delicate collagenous membrane lined by large multinucleated giant cells forms the walls of the cystic structures. An intermediate zone of thin osseous trabeculae with plentiful fibrous marrow is seen, and a fibrous subperiosteal region completes the cyst walls (Fig. 9-35). The metaphyses in all bones ex-

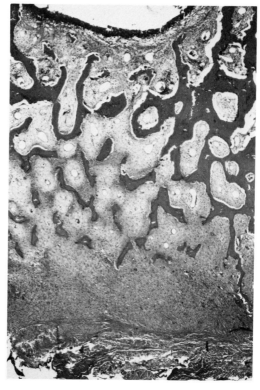

Fig. 9-35. Histologic section of cyst wall of 7-month-old Doberman pinscher with monostotic cystic bone lesions. Dark stained cyst lining and thin, fragile bone trabeculae forming the cyst wall are seen. (From Carrig, C. B., and Seawright, A. A.: J. Small Anim. Pract. **10**:397, 1969.)

amined histologically have shown thickened fibrous periosteums. These periosteal changes appear to be an exaggeration of normal remodelling activity that is often pronounced in the metaphyses of immature bones in breeds with long, slender limbs. Treatment consisting of osteotomy and drainage of the cystic cavity has been successful in resolving the lesions.[14]

Hypertrophic osteodystrophy

Hypertrophic osteodystrophy results from an error in bone growth and is noted in larger breed puppies at age 3 to 5 months. The cause of the disease is not known. Theories have included failure of vitamin C utilization,[49] hypervitaminosis D,[71, 72] and overnutrition.[37] Clinically the disease is characterized by sudden onset of high fever, swelling of the metaphyseal regions, and severe pain. The distal radius and ulna are usually most severely involved, but the metaphyses of all long bones are affected. The disease usually subsides after a few days, only to recur after about a week. It is usual to see two or three relapses before permanent recovery results. In severe cases, marked disruption of the metaphyseal regions of the long bones can result in permanent growth de-

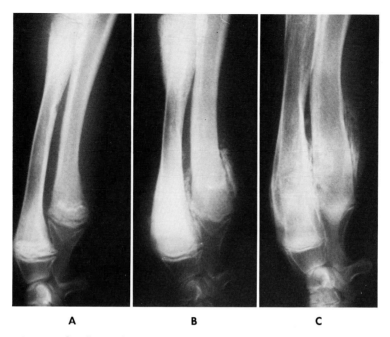

A   **B**   **C**

Fig. 9-36. A, Lateral radiograph of distal radius and ulna of 4-month-old Irish setter with hypertrophic osteodystrophy. Early changes noted in this animal include irregular density in metaphyseal regions of bones and a radiolucent zone in metaphyseal region running parallel to growth plate. **B,** Radiograph taken 2½ weeks later. There is now considerable periosteal bone formation present. **C,** Radiograph taken 12 weeks later. Extraperiosteal bone formation has now remodeled and smoothed out, leading to thickening of diaphyseal and metaphyseal regions of bone. Interference with growth of bones is indicated by curvature of distal radius.

formities. Often the affected animal will exhibit clinical signs of a mild respiratory infection, and thoracic radiographs will show an enhancement of peribronchial and interstitial densities. The early radiographic changes noted in the skeleton include the presence of a radiolucent band within the metaphysis adjacent to and parallel with the growth plate (Fig. 9-36, *A*). The metaphyseal region of the bone is generally increased in density but also contains areas of rarefaction. Later in the course of the disease a cuff of ossified tissue forms in the soft tissues peripheral to the periosteum, adjacent to the metaphysis (Fig. 9-36, *B*). This extraperiosteal new bone formation is initially irregular in outline, but as the disease process subsides, remodelling occurs and the ossified cuff becomes incorporated into the metaphyseal cortex. This results in a marked widening of the metaphyseal region of the bone (Fig. 9-36, *C*).

Histologically the growth plate and the adjacent primary spongiosa are normal. Bone further away from the growth plate becomes replaced with fibrous tissue in a band parallel to the growth plate. Evidence of hemorrhage and necrotic bone can be identified on the distal side of the fibrous band. Woven bone is formed on the diaphyseal side of the fibrous band. This process of re-

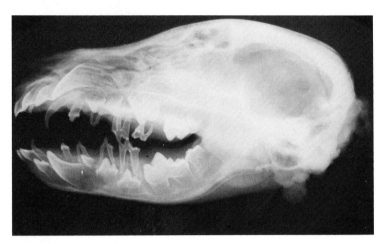

Fig. 9-37. Lateral radiograph of sagittal section of skull of a 5-month-old Airedale terrier with congenital renal disease. Density of bone in mandible is markedly decreased with resorption of lamina dura dentis.

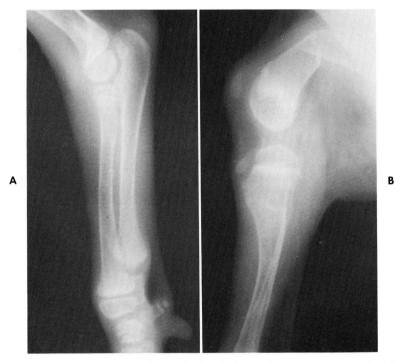

Fig 9-38. Lateral radiographs of radius and ulna (**A**) and femur and tibia (**B**) of 2-month-old Afghan hound with nutritional secondary hyperparathyroidism. There is overall lack of density of bony structures and extreme thinning of cortices. A folding fracture of the femur is present.

sorption and formation continues for weeks, and there is no apparent correlation between the morphologic changes and the episodes of exacerbation of the clinical signs. The fibrous band contains a large number of cells resembling polymorphonuclear leukocytes, and the appearance is one of a severe inflammatory reaction. The microscopic appearance of the extraperiosteal bone is normal.[59]

Secondary hyperparathyroidism

Two types of secondary hyperparathyroidism are seen in the dog—renal and nutritional. Nutritional secondary hyperparathyroidism is usually seen in the period of most active growth, and renal secondary hyperparathyroidism most often is a disease of adolescence (cortical hypoplasia of the kidneys) or adulthood (chronic nephritis).

Nutritional secondary hyperparathyroidism develops when there is an imbalance between dietary calcium and phosphorus. Hypocalcemia can occur following the feeding of a diet with a low calcium content or one containing excessive phosphorus with normal or low calcium levels. Nutritional secondary hyperparathyroidism is frequently seen associated with the chronic feeding of a predominantly meat diet. Most meats contain a most unfavorable calcium-phosphorus ratio (approximately 1:20).

In renal hyperparathyroidism the hyperfunction of the parathyroid gland is caused by a decreased excretion of phosphate, which increases the plasma phosphorus level. This leads to a decrease in the calcium plasma level, which in turn stimulates the parathyroid gland to increase bone resorption, removing calcium from the skeleton in an attempt to restore normal plasma calcium levels.

Secondary hyperparathyroidism manifests itself radiographically as a loss of bone density. In the renal form the lamina dura dentis is the site where bone density is most severely affected, and these structures usually disappear radiographically early in the disease process (Fig. 9-37). Other parts of the skeleton are generally only mildly involved. In nutritional secondary hyperparathyroidism the jaws are usually less affected than the vertebra and long bones. In these areas thinning of the cortices, folding fractures of the long bones, and compression fractures of the vertebrae are most frequently encountered. (Fig. 9-38).

References

1. Aegerter, E., and Kirkpatrick, J. A., Jr.: Orthopedic diseases, ed. 3, Philadelphia, 1968, W. B. Saunders Co.
2. Andreae, von U., and Dämmrich, K.: Über die Beeinflussung der Skelettentwicklung durch energetisch unterschiedliche Fütterung bei einengen Zwillingsbullen, Berl. Munch. Tieraerztl. Wochenschr. **85**:261, 1972.
3. Banks, W. C., and Bridges, C. H.: Multiple cartilaginous exostoses in a dog, J. Am. Vet. Med. Assoc. **129**:131, 1956.
4. Beachley, M. C., and Graham, F. H., Jr.: Hypochondroplastic dwarfism (enchondral chondrodystrophy) in a dog, J. Am. Vet. Med. Assoc. **163**:283, 1973.
5. Campbell, C. J., Grisolia, A., and Zanconato, G.: The effects produced in the cartilaginous epiphyseal plate of immature dogs by experimental surgical traumata, J. Bone Joint Surg. **41A**:1221, 1959.
6. Carlson, W. D., and Severin, G. A.: Elbow dysplasia in the dog: a preliminary report, J. Am. Vet. Med. Assoc. **138**:295, 1961.

7. Carrig, C. B., et al.: Retinal dysplasia associated with skeletal abnormalities in Labrador retrievers, J. Am. Vet. Med. Assoc. **170**:49, 1977.

8. Carrig, C. B., Merkley, D., and Mostosky, U. V.: Asynchronous growth of the canine radius and ulna following 10, 35, and 50 percent retardation of longitudinal growth of the ulna, J. Am. Vet. Radiol. Soc., 1977. (In press.)

9. Carrig, C. B., and Morgan, J. P.: Microcirculation of the humeral head in the immature dog, J. Am. Vet. Radiol. Soc. **15**:28, 1974.

10. Carrig, C. B., and Morgan, J. P.: Asynchronous growth of the canine radius and ulna—early radiographic changes following experimental retardation of longitudinal growth of the ulna, J. Am. Vet. Radiol. Soc. **16**:121, 1975.

11. Carrig, C. B., Morgan, J. P., and Pool, R. R.: The study of degenerative joint disease. Proceedings of the Twenty-fourth Gaines Veterinary Symposium "The Newer Knowledge About Dogs," New York State Veterinary College, Cornell University, Ithaca, N. Y., Oct., 1974.

12. Carrig, C. B., Morgan, J. P., and Pool, R. R.: Effects of asynchronous growth of the radius and ulna on the canine elbow joint following experimental retardation of longitudinal growth of the ulna, J. Am. Anim. Hosp. Assoc. **11**:560, 1975.

13. Carrig, C. B., Pool, R. R., and McElroy, J. M.: Polyostotic cystic bone lesions in a dog, J. Small Anim. Pract. **16**:495, 1975.

14. Carrig, C. B., and Seawright, A. A.: A familial canine polyostotic fibrous dysplasia with subperiosteal cortical defects, J. Small Anim. Pract. **10**:397, 1969.

15. Chapman, W. L., Jr.: Appearance of ossification centers and epiphyseal closures as determined by radiographic techniques, J. Am. Vet. Med. Assoc. **147**:138, 1965.

16. Chester, D. K.: Multiple cartilaginous exostoses in two generations of dogs, J. Am. Vet. Med. Assoc. **159**:895, 1971.

17. Clayton-Jones, D. G., and Vaughan, L. C.: Disturbance in the growth of the radius in dogs, J. Small Anim. Pract. **11**:453, 1970.

18. Cohen, J.: Simple bone cysts: studies of cyst fluid in six cases with a theory of pathogenesis, J. Bone Joint Surg. **42A**:609, 1960.

19. Collins, D. H.: Osteoarthritis. In Collins, D. H.: The pathology of articular and spinal diseases, London, 1949, Edward Arnold & Co.

20. Compere, E. L.: Growth arrest on long bones as the result of fractures that include the epiphysis, J.A.M.A. **105**:2140, 1935.

21. Corley, E. A.: Elbow dysplasia in the German shepherd dog, doctoral dissertation, Colorado State University, 1966.

22. Corley, E. A., and Carlson, W. D.: Radiographic, genetic, and pathologic aspects of elbow dysplasia. Scientific proceedings of the 102nd Annual Meeting of the American Veterinary Medical Association, J. Am. Vet. Med. Assoc. **147**:1651, 1965.

23. Cotchin, E., and Dyce, K. M.: A case of epiphyseal dysplasia in a dog, Vet. Rec. **68**:427, 1956.

24. Craig, P. H., and Riser, W. H.: Osteochondritis dissecans in the proximal humerus of the dog, J. Am. Vet. Radiol. Soc. **6**:40, 1965.

25. Ekholm, R.: Articular cartilage nutrition: how radioactive gold reaches cartilage in rabbit knee joints, Acta Anat., Supp. **15**:1, 1951.

26. Ekholm, R., and Norback, B.: On the relationship between articular changes and function, Acta Orthop. Scand. **21**:81, 1951.

27. Fletch, S. M., and Pinkerton, P. H.: An inherited anemia associated with hereditary chondrodysplasia in the Alaskan malamute, Can. Vet. J. **13**:270, 1972.

28. Fletch, S. M., Smart, M. E., Pennock, P. W., and Subden, R. E.: Clinical and pathologic features of chondrodysplasia (dwarfism) in the Alaskan malamute, J. Am. Vet. Med. Assoc. **162**:357, 1973.

29. Gee, B. R., and Doige, C. E.: Multiple cartilaginous exostoses in a litter of dogs, J. Am. Vet. Med. Assoc. **156**:53, 1970.

30. Gourley, J., and Eden, C. W.: Bone cysts in a dog, Vet. Rec. **66**:63, 1954.

31. Green, J. P.: Osteochondritis dissecans of the knee, J. Bone Joint Surg. **48B**:82, 1966.

32. Green, W. T., and Banks, H. H.: Osteochondritis dissecans in children, J. Bone Joint Surg. **35A**:26, 1953.

33. Grøndalen, T.: Osteochondrosis, arthro-

sis, and leg weakness in pigs, Nord. Vet. Med. **26**:534, 1974.

34. Hanlon, G. F.: Normal and abnormal bone growth in the dog, J. Am. Vet. Radiol. Soc. **3**:13, 1962.

35. Harrison, M. H. M., Schajowicz, F., and Trueta, J.: Osteoarthritis of the hip: a study of the nature and evolution of the disease, J. Bone Joint Surg. **35B**:598, 1953.

36. Harsha, W. N.: Effects of trauma upon epiphyses, Clin. Orthop. **10**:140, 1957.

37. Hedhammar, A., et al.: Overnutrition and skeletal disease. An experimental study in growing Great Dane dogs. Cornell Vet. **64**(Supp. 5):53, 1974.

38. Henschel, E.: Zur Anatomie und Klinik der wachsenden Unterarmknochen, Arch. Exp. Veterinaermed. **26**:741, 1972.

39. Herron, M. R.: Ununited anconeal process in the dog, Vet. Clin. North Am. **1**:417, 1971.

40. Hitz, D.: Ulnadysplasie beim Bassethound, Schweiz Arch. Tierheilkd. **116**:285, 1974.

41. Huff, R. W., and Brodey, R. S.: Multiple bone cysts in a dog—a case report, J. Am. Vet. Radiol. Soc. **5**:40, 1964.

42. Ingelmark, B. E.: The nutritive supply and nutritional value of synovial fluid, Acta Orthop. Scand. **20**:144, 1950.

43. Kasström, H., Ljunggren, G., and Olsson, S.-E.: Growth disturbances of the ulna in dogs—a radiographic study. Abstracts of the Third International Conference of Veterinary Radiologists, J. Am. Vet. Radiol. Soc. **14**:6, 1973.

44. Kleine, L. J.: A radiographic study of experimental premature epiphyseal plate closure of the distal radius and ulna in dogs, M.S. Thesis, Purdue University, 1967.

45. Kleine, L. J.: Radiographic diagnosis of epiphyseal plate trauma, J. Am. Anim. Hosp. Assoc. **7**:290, 1971.

46. Ljunggren, G., Cawley, A. J., and Archibald, J.: The elbow dysplasias in the dog, J. Am. Vet. Med. Assoc. **148**:887, 1966.

47. Ljunggren, G., Olsson, S.-E., and Gustafsson, P. O.: Idiopathic osteonecrosis in the dog. In Zinn, W. M., editor: Idiopathic ischemic necrosis of the femoral head in adults, Baltimore, 1971, University Park Press.

48. Lodge, D.: Two cases of epiphyseal dysplasia, Vet. Rec. **79**:136, 1966.

49. Meier, H., Clark, S. T., Schnelle, G. B., and Will, D. H.: Hypertrophic osteodystrophy associated with disturbance of vitamin C synthesis in dogs, J. Am. Vet. Med. Assoc. **130**:483, 1957.

50. Morgan, J. P.: Radiology in veterinary orthopedics, Philadelphia, 1972, Lea and Febiger.

51. Morgan, J. P., Carlson, W. D., and Adams, O. R.: Hereditary multiple exostosis in the horse, J. Am. Vet. Med. Assoc. **140**:1320, 1962.

52. Mostosky, U. V.: Osteochondritis dissecans of the canine shoulder. Proceedings of the Thirteenth Gaines Veterinary Symposium "The Newer Knowledge about Dogs," School of Veterinary Medicine, Athens, Ga. Jan., 1964.

53. Newton, C. D.: Surgical management of distal ulnar physeal growth disturbances in dogs, J. Am. Vet. Med. Assoc. **164**:479, 1974.

54. Nichols, E. H., and Richardson, F. L.: Arthritis deformans, J. Med. Research, **21**:149, 1909.

55. Noser, G., Carrig, C. B., Merkley, D., and Brinker, W. O.: Asynchronous growth of the canine radius and ulna: effects of cross-pinning the radius to the ulna, Am. J. Vet. Res., 1977. (In press.)

56. Nutt, P.: Bone cysts in the dog, J. Small Anim. Pract. **8**:649, 1967.

57. O'Brien, T. R.: Developmental deformities due to arrested epiphyseal growth, Vet. Clin. North Am. **1**:441, 1971.

58. O'Brien, T. R., Morgan, J. P., and Suter, P. F.: Epiphyseal plate injury in the dog: a radiographic study of growth disturbance in the forelimb, J. Small Anim. Pract. **12**:19, 1971.

59. Olsson, S.-E.: Radiology in veterinary pathology: a review with special reference to hypertrophic osteodystrophy and secondary hyperparathyroidism in the dog, Proceedings of the Second International Conference of Veterinary Radiologists, Stockholm, 1970, Acta Radiol. [Supp.] **319**:255, 1972.

60. Olsson, S.-E.: En ny typ av armbågsledsdysplasti hos hund?: en preliminär rapport, Särtryck Svensk Veterinärtidning **26**(5):152, 1974.

61. Olsson, S.-E.: Lameness in the dog: a review of lesions causing osteoarthrosis of the shoulder, elbow, hip, stifle, and

hock joints, Proc. Am. Anim. Hosp. Assoc. **1**:363, 1975.

62. Olsson, S.-E.: Osteochondritis dissecans in the dog, Proc. Am. Anim. Hosp. Assoc. **1**:362, 1975.

63. Owen, L. N., and Neilsen, S. W.: Multiple cartilaginous exostoses (diaphyseal aclasis) in a Yorkshire terrier, J. Small Anim. Pract. **9**:519, 1968.

64. Owen, L. N., and Walker, R. G.: Osteitis fibrosa cystica of the radius in an Irish wolfhound: replacement by autologous bone graft, Vet. Rec. **75**: 40, 1963.

65. Paatsama, S., Rokkanen, P., Jussila, J., and Sittnikow, K.: A study of osteochondritis dissecans of the canine humeral head using histological, OTC bone labelling, microradiographic and microangiographic methods. J. Small Anim. Pract. **12**:603, 1971.

66. Paatsama, S., Rokkanen, P., Sittnikow, K., and Jussila, J.: Changes in osteochondritis dissecans of the canine humeral head, Scand. J. Clin. Lab. Invest. **27**:(Supp. 116), 1971.

67. Phemister, D. B.: Operative arrestment of longitudinal growth of bones in the treatment of deformities, J. Bone Joint Surg. **15**:1, 1933.

68. Rasmussen, P. G.: Multiple epiphyseal dysplasia in a litter of beagle puppies, J. Small Anim. Pract. **12**:91, 1971.

69. Rasmussen, P. G.: Radiographic and histomorphologic structures in multiple epiphyseal dysplasia. Abstracts of the Third International Conference of Veterinary Radiologists, J. Am. Vet. Radiol. Soc. **14**:5, 1973.

70. Riser, W. H.: Proceedings of the Ninth Annual Seminar of the American College of Veterinary Pathology, Chicago, 1958.

71. Riser, W. H.: Radiographic differential diagnosis of skeletal diseases of young dogs, J. Am. Vet. Radiol. Soc. **5**:15, 1964.

72. Riser, W. H., and Shirer, J. F.: Normal and abnormal growth of the distal foreleg in large and giant dogs, J. Am. Vet. Radiol. Soc. **6**:50, 1965.

73. Rothman, M., and Schnelle, G. B.: Brodie's abscess in a Great Dane, North Am. Vet. **30**:591, 1949.

74. Salter, R. B., and Harris, W. R.: Injuries involving the epiphyseal plate, J. Bone Joint Surg. **45A**:587, 1963.

75. Sande, R. D.: Pathogenesis of dwarfism in Alaskan malamutes, doctoral dissertation, Washington State University, 1975.

76. Sande, R. D., Alexander, J. E., and Padgett, G. A.: Dwarfism in the Alaskan malamute: its radiographic pathogenesis, J. Am. Vet. Radiol. Soc. **15**:10, 1974.

77. Schmidt, G.: Personal communication, 1976.

78. Skaggs, S., DeAngelis, M. P., and Rosen, H.: Deformities due to premature closure of the distal ulna in fourteen dogs: a radiographic evaluation, J. Am. Anim. Hosp. Assoc. **9**:496, 1973.

79. Smith, C. W., and Stowater, J. L.: Osteochondritis dissecans of the canine shoulder joint: a review of 35 cases, J. Am. Anim. Hosp. Assoc. **11**:658, 1975.

80. Spranger, J.: Hereditary arthro-ophthalmopathy, Ann. Radiol. (Paris), **11**:359, 1968.

81. Stickler, G. B., et al.: Hereditary progressive arthro-ophthalmopathy, Mayo Clin. Proc. **40**:433, 1965.

82. Stickler, G. B., and Pugh, D. G.: Hereditary progressive arthro-ophthalmopathy. II. Additional observations on vertebral anomalies, a hearing defect, and a report of a similar case, Mayo Clin. Proc. **42**:495, 1967.

83. Trueta, J.: Studies of the development and decay of the human frame, Philadelphia 1968, W. B. Saunders Co.

84. Trueta, J., and Amato, V. P.: The vascular contribution to osteogenesis. III. Changes in the growth cartilage caused by experimentally induced ischaemia, J. Bone Joint Surg. **42B**:571, 1960.

85. VanSickle, D. C.: A comparative study of the postnatal elbow development of the greyhound and the German shepherd. Scientific proceedings of the 102nd Annual Meeting of the American Veterinary Medical Association, J. Am. Vet. Med. Assoc. **147**:1650, 1965.

86. VanSickle, D. C.: The relationship of ossification to canine elbow dysplasia, Anim. Hosp. **2**:24, 1966.

87. Vaughan, L. C.: Congenital detachment of the processus anconeus in the dog, Vet. Rec. **74**:309, 1962.

10 Radiologic diagnosis of pleural effusions

John H. M. Austin and Gregory M. Carsen

Accumulation of excess pleural fluid is an important finding in many diseases—a finding that the radiologist is often the first to identify. As clinical radiologists, we shall emphasize the following major topics in this review of recent developments in the understanding of pleural effusions: pathophysiology, detection, diagnosis by laboratory techniques, pleural fluid in the pediatric age-group, diagnosis of massive pleural effusion, radiologic findings in cardiovascular, neoplastic, infectious, abdominal, and other (including iatrogenic) diseases associated with pleural fluid, and percutaneous needle biopsy in the diagnostic management of patients with pleural effusion.

PATHOPHYSIOLOGY

The membranes of the parietal and visceral pleurae are permeable to the flow of liquid. Normally a few milliliters of fluid are present in each pleural cavity, but as much as 15 ml may be within normal limits.[7, 65] Because as little as 5 ml of pleural fluid is demonstrable by lateral decubitus radiographs,[64] minimal quantities of pleural fluid have been shown in from 4% to 13% of healthy subjects.[41, 65] Approximately 30% of women have small pleural effusions postpartum.[41]

Mechanisms of normal pleural fluid transport.[7] A small quantity of fluid normally exits from pleural capillaries. This filtered fluid in the pleural cavity either reenters capillaries or is drained by the lymphatic system. The quantity of fluid in the pleural space depends on many factors: surface area and vascularity of the pleura, hydrostatic and colloid osmotic pressure in the pleural capillaries and lymphatics, permeability of the capillaries and mesothelium, and movements of the chest wall. In the human the parietal pleura is supplied by systemic vessels and the visceral pleura mainly by pulmonary vessels. Hydrostatic pressure therefore normally causes pleural fluid to flow from the parietal to the visceral surfaces. Pleural lymphatic drainage is mainly through the hila into the mediastinal lymphatic network, but animal experiments suggest that particulate matter and cells also enter the parietal lymphatic system and from there enter intercostal, internal mammary, and mediastinal drainage.[14] The muscular movements of respiration appear to help pump fluid through the lymphatics. A portion of pleural lymphatic flow also is believed to cross the diaphragm through transdiaphragmatic lymphatic channels.[80]

Mechanisms of pleural fluid accumulation in disease. The normal balances among the physiologic and anatomic variables in pleural fluid flow may be altered in various ways. Capillary filtration is increased by local inflammation, including local elevation of temperature. Colloid osmotic pressure normally moves fluid from the protein-poor pleural space to the protein-rich plasma in capillaries, but if plasma albumin is less than about 1.5 gm/100 ml, colloid pressure is no longer available as a mechanism for clearing fluid from the pleural space. Relationships between hydrostatic pressure and pleural fluid transport are complex, but, in summary, pulmonary venous hypertension alone is not believed to significantly increase the quantity of pleural fluid, whereas systemic venous hypertension does.[60] Lymphatic drainage may be disrupted either by increased intralymphatic pressure, as in mediastinal fibrosis or cancer, or by postinflammatory pleural scarring.

Ascites is commonly accompanied by pleural effusion, probably by way of the lymphatic connections across the diaphragm.[47, 80] These connections are larger on the right than on the left, and this fact has been offered as an explanation for the greater incidence of right-sided rather than left-sided effusions in patients with ascites.[50] In those with hepatic cirrhosis, azygous hypertension may also increase filtration pressures in the parietal pleura, and hypoproteinemia may further decrease osmotic absorption of pleural fluid into pleural capillaries.

DETECTION OF PLEURAL FLUID

Diagnostic radiography. The location in the pleural cavity of abnormal quantities of fluid depends on three important considerations: gravity, patency versus obliteration of the pleural space, and elasticity of the various parts of the lungs.

If a patient is upright, gravity causes free pleural fluid to collect at the bottom of the pleural space under the basal segments of the lung. It is generally accepted that free fluid collects in the subpulmonic location until a quantity of about 150 to 500 ml is present.[21, 41] Frontal radiographs may show the base of the lung to be elevated and the dome of the apparent hemidiaphragm laterally displaced by the supradiaphragmatic fluid. On the left the stomach bubble may appear separated from the base of the lung.

Accumulation of excess pleural fluid around the sides of the lung is also common. On frontal views the radiologic sign of a meniscus effect appears laterally and sometimes medially. On lateral view the meniscus appears in the most dependent portion of the chest, the posterior costophrenic angle.

The lateral decubitus radiograph has been the most widely used radiographic projection for the detection of free pleural fluid since its description by Rigler in 1931.[72] The demonstration of small amounts of free fluid may occasionally be improved by elevating the patient's pelvis, catching the fluid in the upper thorax.[41, 65]

When the patient is in the supine position, pleural fluid is often difficult to detect. When effusion overlies the posterior hemithorax, on frontal views only a generalized hazy increase in density may be seen. If the quantity of fluid is at least moderately large, regardless of position or projection, the space between the periphery of the lung and the adjacent ribs may widen, indicating pleural effusion wrapping around the sides of the lung. Similarly, medial accumulations of fluid may cause apparent widening of the mediastinal shadows or of the para-spinal pleural reflection.[76, 87] Oblique views also may help define the position and quantity of fluid either in the fissures or around the sides of the lungs; the left posterior oblique view is particularly helpful for evaluating fluid in the left major fissure.

Fluid in the interlobar fissures may be radiographically evident as widening of the fissure shadows or as fusiform densities (so-called pseudotumor). Fluid in the fissures may or may not be associated on plain chest radiographs with other evidence of pleural fluid (Figs. 10-1 and 10-2).

Radiographic visibility of the parenchyma of the lower lungs may be impaired by pleural fluid. To enhance visibility, two views may be employed to occasional advantage—the lateral decubitus in the Trendelenburg position[41] and

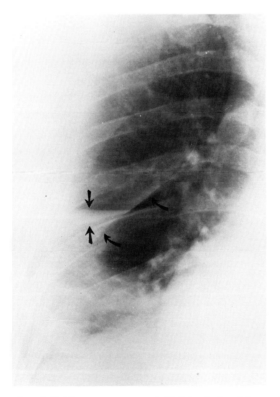

Fig. 10-1. Interlobar pleural fluid as seen on a right lateral decubitus radiograph. Fluid in the minor fissure (between vertical arrows) is a common finding on frontal radiographs, but fluid in the major fissure (curved arrows) is not commonly seen.

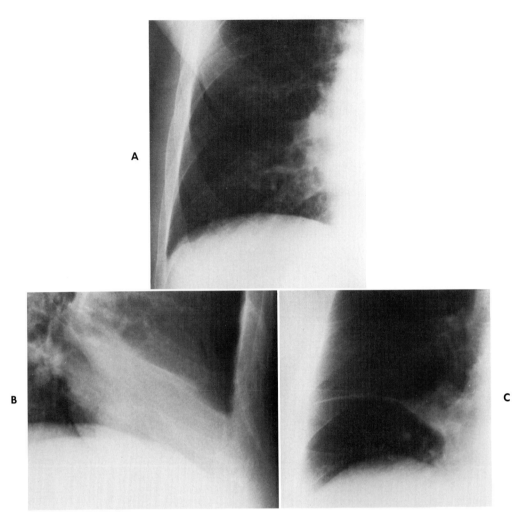

Fig. 10-2. Atypical distribution of pleural fluid—medial accumulation in minor fissure (best seen on lordotic view). **A,** Frontal radiograph. Right heart border is blurred. **B,** Lateral radiograph. Hazy increased density appears inferior to posterior aspect of minor fissure. **C,** Lordotic view discloses medial widening of minor fissure. Sharp definition of superior and inferior margins of this widening indicates interlobar pleural fluid rather than pulmonary disease. Opacity disappeared after therapy with a diuretic agent.

the prone lateral chest radiograph.[79] Another advantage of these two projections is that they also can be used to evaluate the mobility of pleural fluid.

Pleural fluid frequently loculates and does not move freely within the pleural cavity.[21] Adhesions are the most common cause of loculated fluid and therefore of atypical accumulations of pleural fluid as seen on chest radiographs (Figs. 10-3 and 10-4). In active inflammatory disease, fibrinous reaction often contains fluid in the region of active inflammation. Loss of elasticity in the lung may also prevent fluid from freely moving in the pleural space; wherever pleural fluid is present, adjacent pulmonary parenchyma loses volume (so-called compression

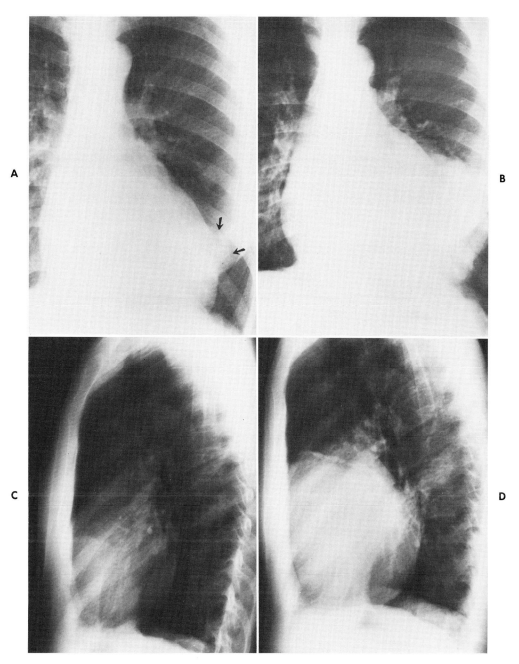

Fig. 10-3. Atypical distribution of pleural effusion—effect of pleural adhesions. **A,** Frontal radiograph in a patient with cardiomegaly and lingular pleural-parenchymal adhesions (arrows). **B,** Lobulated opacities appeared along left heart border in conjunction with an episode of cardiac decompensation and fluid retention. Opacities represent anteriorly loculated pleural fluid. **C,** Lateral radiograph corresponding to **A. D,** Lateral radiograph corresponding to **B.** Following diuresis and cardiotonic regimen, appearance of subsequent radiographs returned to that of **A** and **C.**

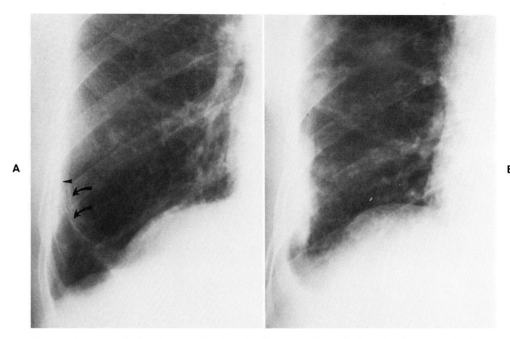

Fig. 10-4. Atypical distribution of pleural effusion—effect of pleural adhesions. **A,** Erect frontal radiograph. Pleural thickening is evident along lateral aspect of right lung (arrowhead). Arcuate linear opacities (curved arrows) represent either pleural-parenchymal scars or pleural thickening extending around convexity of lung. **B,** During an episode of congestive heart failure, localized pleural opacity is evident in same region. Following a cardiotonic and diuretic regimen, appearance of frontal radiographs returned to that of **A.**

atelectasis). Pleural-parenchymal adhesions, interstitial scarring, pulmonary emphysema, active infection, and neoplasia may all limit the ability of the lung to compress under the pressure of fluid in the adjacent pleura.

Nuclear medicine. Scintigraphic images of the lung are abnormal in the presence of pleural effusion. The pleural fluid displaces and compresses adjacent lung, which appears on pulmonary radionuclide studies as locally decreased perfusion or ventilation.

When a patient with a known pleural effusion is to be studied by a pulmonary perfusion scan, it is advisable for the patient to be in the erect position as the radioisotope is injected.[23, 86] Assuming the fluid is freely mobile, a localized defect of perfusion in the posterior costophrenic gutter is to be expected. If at the time of injection the patient is in any other position (e.g., supine), mobile fluid may be expected to compress the parenchyma of the lung at sites other than the posterior costophrenic gutter. Interpretation of the significance of focal abnormalities of pulmonary perfusion then becomes difficult.

Subpulmonic effusion on the right increases the distance between the base of the right lung and the top of the liver. In a patient with pleural fluid at the base of the right hemithorax, combined scintigraphic imaging of pulmonary perfusion and the liver (liver-lung scan) shows an abnormal separation of the pul-

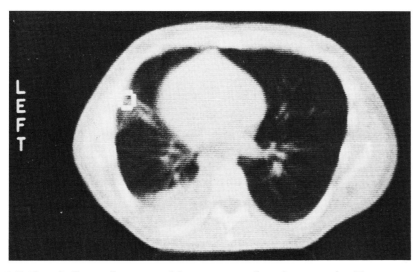

Fig. 10-5. Pleural effusion demonstrated by computerized axial tomography. Transverse section of chest at level of pulmonary hila in a supine patient shows a posterior collection of fluid in left hemithorax. (Courtesy Ralph J. Alfidi, M.D.)

monary and the hepatic images. This finding is not specific. Subdiaphragmatic disease such as subphrenic abscess may be indistinguishable on liver-lung scan from subpulmonic pleural fluid.

When pleural fluid is in an interlobar fissure, a linear or bandlike zone of decreased perfusion in the position of the fissure may be apparent on pulmonary perfusion scan ("fissure sign"). This sign also is not specific.[45] A similar pattern of decreased perfusion may be caused by fibrosis thickening the fissure, pulmonary microemboli, or emphysema in the periphery of the lung adjacent to the fissure.

After thoracentesis, scintigraphic studies have shown pulmonary perfusion does not immediately return to normal in the zones of lung formerly compressed by the fluid.[23, 63] When a large effusion totally surrounds the lung, imaging of the pulmonary perfusion shows greatest activity centrally in the lung and progressive, rather uniform diminution of activity toward the periphery.

Ultrasound. Pleural effusion appears as an internal echo-free zone on ultrasonic studies of the chest wall. In the normal subject, acoustical interference in the air-containing lung produces a fuzzy pattern at the junction of the chest wall and lung.[48] In a patient with pleural fluid the pleural space on echo study appears sharply marginated, especially at its internal margin. Fibrosis of the pleura, however, produces a pattern of multiple, weak, interrupted echos and therefore a poorly defined internal border.[55] If the entire hemithorax is opacified by fluid, ultrasound may be used to detect position and motion of the diaphragm.[84]

Computerized axial tomography. Still in infant stages of clinical development, computerized tomography has successfully demonstrated a posterior pleural effusion in a patient in the supine position (Fig. 10-5).[2]

LABORATORY DIAGNOSIS OF PLEURAL FLUID

During the past few years the diagnostic capability of laboratory examination of pleural fluid has greatly expanded. Although this chapter is radiologically oriented, we believe that some of these advances should be discussed briefly.

In an appropriate clinical setting, after a pleural effusion has been demonstrated to be large enough to tap safely, a thoracentesis may be required for further evaluation of the fluid. The routine examination of the fluid considers its gross appearance, protein content, specific gravity, cell count and differential, bacterial studies, cytology, and possible pleural biopsy.[12]

It is useful to know if pleural fluid is a transudate or an exudate because transudative effusions indicate pleural edema and exudative effusions indicate pleural inflammation. Generally, if the specific gravity is less than 1.016 and the protein content less than 3.0 gm/100 ml, the fluid is considered a transudate. If the specific gravity and protein levels are higher, the fluid is considered an exudate; however, it has been demonstrated that a protein level of 3.0 gm/100 ml is not infallible for separating exudates from transudates.[11] In a recent study of 103 exudative pleural effusions Light and Ball[52] made the following observations:

1. The ratio of pleural fluid protein to serum protein was greater than 0.5.
2. The lactic dehydrogenase (LDH) level in the pleural fluid was greater than 200 I.U.
3. The ratio of pleural fluid LDH to serum LDH was greater than 0.6.

At least one of these criteria was present in all but one exudate studied. Of the 47 transudates studied, only one met any of the three criteria.

Funahashi and Sarkar[26] and Light, MacGregor, Ball, and Luchsinger[54] have investigated the diagnostic use of pH, Pco_2, and Po_2 levels in pleural fluid. They found that the Po_2 and Pco_2 levels were too variable to be reliable in the diagnosis of specific diseases. However, pH values showed fairly acceptable consistency. If the pH of the fluid was less than 7.29, there was a definite association with nonhemorrhagic, nonmalignant disease, whereas a pH greater than 7.29 was associated with congestive heart failure, cirrhosis, or malignancy. In differentiating a malignant pleural effusion from one caused by tuberculosis, a pH of less than 7.3 was found to be suggestive of tuberculosis and one greater than 7.4 of malignancy.[54] Of particular diagnostic import was the finding that if a parapneumonic effusion had a pH of less than 7.20, tube drainage was necessary to produce resolution of the process.[54]

Cytogenetic studies. The role and accuracy of cytologic studies for detection of malignant pleural disease have been well established. However, it is known that in cases of suspected malignancy, standard cytologic techniques do not always yield a definite diagnosis. Since 1956 it has been known that malignant cells contain chromosomal aberrations not found in normal cells on cytogenetic studies using routine cytogenetic techniques.[37] Numerical and structural chromosomal deviations are very rare in benign mesothelial cells obtained by thoracentesis, but rather common in pleural malignancy. Malignant cells in pleural fluid are also very well suited for cytogenetic studies.[44] It has been demonstrated that the cytogenetic diagnosis of malignancy can be achieved somewhat earlier in the course of disease than with routine cytologic studies.[38] When routine cytologic studies of pleural effusions fail to yield a definite diagnosis, particularly in cases highly suspicious for malignancy, cytogenetic analysis appears to be a valuable and complementary examination with a high diagnostic yield.

PEDIATRIC DISEASES ASSOCIATED WITH PLEURAL EFFUSION

In the neonate the most common cause of pleural fluid in quantities large enough to cause respiratory distress is chylothorax or hydrothorax. Wesenberg refers to this entity as "lymphothorax."[90] Although very rare when compared to neonatal chylothorax, nonchylous spontaneous pleural effusion in the newborn has been reported.[46] It is of obscure etiology, and if untreated, may be fatal.[18] Neonatal pleural fluid is usually straw-colored and nonchylous, but it may still represent the earliest manifestation of the syndrome of idiopathic chylothorax of the newborn. The syndrome with true chylous fluid in the chest classically appears after the ingestion of milk or formula. The chylous fluid is opalescent, contains fat, protein, and cholesterol, and is milky in appearance.

When chylous fluid accumulates spontaneously in the newborn, it has a slight right-sided predominance, is of variable quantity, and may cause mediastinal shift, compression atelectasis of the ipsilateral and/or contralateral lung, and respiratory distress. If the latter occurs, thoracentesis is required. Although non-chylous pleural effusions are more frequently seen in the older pediatric age-group, they can occur in neonates and very young children with esophageal rupture,[39] hydrops fetalis, congestive heart failure, Turner's syndrome,[13] infantile polycystic disease, polycythemia, iatrogenic hypervolemia, cystic adenomatoid malformation of the lung, and obstructed pulmonary venous return.[90] In the older pediatric age-group, infectious diseases are responsible for the vast majority of pleural effusions, and if parenchymal consolidation and pleural effusion are present, primary tuberculosis and staphylococcal pneumonia should be the first two differential considerations.

Pleural effusion in primary tuberculosis in childhood is so common that Caffey[9] regards it as part of the primary complex rather than a complication of the disease. Fraser and Paré[22] state that in the absence of detectable parenchymal disease tuberculosis is the most common cause of pleural effusion. In staphylococcal pneumonia during childhood, pleural fluid as empyema has been reported in as many as 90% of cases.[77] Because many other bacterial infections may cause pleuropulmonary reactions and pleural effusions, the presence of pleural fluid does not help establish which organism is the offending agent. Particularly in children, pleural effusions associated with pneumonitis can be seen with viral and mycoplasma infections.[34, 85]

Acute glomerulonephritis is not a rare pediatric disease. Because close to 50% of patients with this disease have pleural effusions, it should be considered an important cause of effusion in children.[49] The pathophysiology for the effusion has not been completely elucidated. Children with acute glomerulonephritis may also demonstrate cardiomegaly, pulmonary vascular congestion, and occasional pulmonary edema.

DIAGNOSIS OF MASSIVE PLEURAL EFFUSION

The most common cause of very large pleural effusions is malignancy[56] (Fig. 10-6). The next most common is empyema. Less common causes are (1) hepatic cirrhosis with ascites, (2) congestive heart failure, and (3) hemothorax, which may be either posttraumatic secondary to a ruptured aortic aneurysm or may follow anticoagulant therapy. Although virtually any malignant neoplasm can cause massive pleural effusions, the two most frequent are carcinoma of the lung (approximately 50% of cases) and breast (approximately 25% of cases).[56]

Large pleural effusions can depress the hemidiaphragm. A massive effusion may even invert it, in which case on inspiration the hemidiaphragm actually ascends.[66]

CARDIOVASCULAR DISEASES ASSOCIATED WITH PLEURAL EFFUSION

Congestive heart failure. In cardiac failure, bilateral pleural effusions are common. Unilateral effusion on the right, but not the left, is said to be common

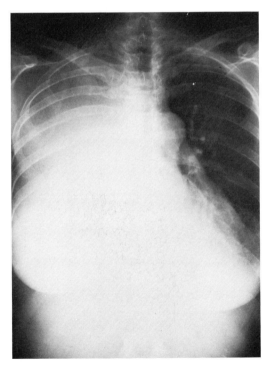

Fig. 10-6. Tension hydrothorax. Complete opacification of right hemithorax and shift of mediastinum to left in a patient with a massive right hydrothorax secondary to ovarian carcinoma metastatic to pleura.

in cardiac failure. This generally accepted view, to our knowledge, has never been studied using decubitus radiographs. In the study usually cited for this view, McPeak and Levine[58] in 1946 analyzed upright chest radiographs of 52 patients with effusions believed to be caused by cardiac failure. Pleural fluid was bilateral in 28 of the patients (54%), unilateral on the right in 20 (38%), and unilateral on the left in 4 (8%). These findings, however, are at variance with the same investigators' analysis of postmortem examinations of 110 patients with effusions believed to be caused by cardiac failure. In that group pleural fluid was bilateral in 99 of the patients, unilateral on the right in 6, and unilateral on the left in 5.[58] Right unilateral pleural effusion in cardiac failure does appear to be more common than unilateral effusion on the left, but the relative rarity of the latter is open to question. As noted earlier in this chapter, the apparent right-sided predominance of pleural effusion may be related to the larger diaphragmatic lymphatic system on that side.[80]

Postinfarction syndrome (Dressler's syndrome). In the days or weeks after a myocardial infarction a syndrome of pericarditis and pleuritis with effusion may develop. The patient is usually febrile and complains of pleuropericardial pain. The syndrome is benign, self-limited, and not uncommon.

Pulmonary embolism. Pleural effusion occurs in approximately one of three patients with pulmonary embolism.[83] The shorter the duration of symptoms (i.e., several hours), the less likely the presence of pleural fluid. Pleural effusion after embolism develops over a time span of many hours, so that radiographs exposed 2 or 3 days after embolization are more likely to show pleural fluid than those exposed a few hours after embolization.[83] The quantity of effusion following pulmonary emboli is almost always small.

Sickle cell anemia. Pulmonary complications (thrombosis, emboli, infarction, and pneumonia) are common in sickle cell disease, but the literature on the disease rarely mentions the frequency of pleural effusion.[1] Pleural effusion, usually small, is found in approximately 30% of the sickle-SS patients who develop pulmonary infection or infarctions.

Recently, cytologic study of pleural fluid in patients with sickle cell disease has revealed abnormally sickled red blood cells in the fluid.[17]

NEOPLASTIC DISEASES ASSOCIATED WITH PLEURAL EFFUSION

Metastatic disease. Although virtually any cancer may metastasize to the pleura, the most common neoplastic cause of pleural fluid is ipsilateral bronchogenic carcinoma. The mechanism of spread is believed to be pulmonary arterial invasion by the primary tumor, followed by tumor emboli to the visceral pleura.[61] Metastatic bronchogenic carcinoma in the parietal pleura without associated visceral pleural involvement is rare. The extent of pleural metastatic disease correlates poorly with the development of fluid. According to Meyer,[61] most patients with pleural metastatic disease and pleural effusion also have neoplastic involvement of mediastinal lymph nodes, obstructing lymphatic drainage from the pleura. The right paratracheal stripe on the posteroanterior chest radiograph is an important marker of mediastinal lymphatic disease and should be closely inspected by the radiologist if a patient has pleural effusion.[76]

Lymphoma. Approximately 10% of patients with lymphoma develop pleural fluid in the course of this illness. Unlike metastatic carcinoma to the pleura, in which the cytologic detection of malignant cells in pleural fluid means the pleura is invaded by the carcinoma, lymphoma cells may simply pass in and out of the pleural cavity as they circulate about the body.[89] Therefore radiation to enlarged or nonenlarged mediastinal or even retroperitoneal lymph nodes may possibly be beneficial in the patient with lymphoma and pleural effusion.[68] Radiologic evidence of enlarged hilar or mediastinal lymph nodes is usually absent in patients with lymphoma and pleural effusion.

Myeloma. Electrophoresis of pleural fluid may be helpful in establishing the rare diagnosis of pleural involvement by myeloma.[4] Cytologic analysis of the fluid may yield plasma cells, but pleural biopsy is advisable to confirm the diagnosis

Malignant pleural mesothelioma. Pleural effusion is a common, but by no means invariant, finding in malignant mesothelioma of the pleura.[40] The quantity of fluid varies, producing little to total hemithoracic opacification. Because the major anatomic pathologic finding is sheets of irregular neoplastic thickening of the pleura, the pleural fluid may be loculated or distributed in an atypical manner (i.e., the lateral margin of the lung is often irregular or even concave). A history of asbestos exposure is frequent.

On frontal radiographs, involvement of the ipsilateral chest wall is occasionally seen in malignant mesothelioma. The soft tissues lateral to the rib cage may be thickened—a finding believed to be caused by neoplastic obstruction of lymphatic drainage of the chest wall.[70]

Benign pleural mesothelioma. Pleural effusion is very rarely associated with these benign fibrous lesions.[43]

INFECTIOUS DISEASES ASSOCIATED WITH PLEURAL EFFUSION

Pneumonias. Any patient with pneumonia may develop ipsilateral pleural effusion in the course of the illness. The quantity of fluid is usually small. A notable exception is *Mycobacterium tuberculosis,* in which the effusion may be small, moderate, or even massive. In tuberculosis presenting as pleural effusion the symptomatic onset may be abrupt and may mimic acute bacterial pneumonia.[5] In this case, only 1 in 3 patients initially demonstrates active pulmonary lesions on chest radiographs. Rupture into the pleural cavity from a subpleural focus of active pulmonary infection is believed to be the pathogenesis of the pleural involvement in tuberculosis. Pleural biopsy and culture are often necessary to obtain the diagnosis.

As a rule, pneumonias caused by gram-negative bacteria are more commonly associated with pleural effusion than those caused by gram-positive organisms. For instance, in one series pleural fluid was present in 16 of 19 patients with pneumonia caused by *Pseudomonas aeruginosa,* in 10 of 15 with pneumonia caused by *Klebsiella* bacilli, and in 5 of 7 with pneumonia caused by *Escherichia coli*.[88] These gram-negative infections characteristically are found in patients with chronic debilitating disease. They usually involve at least one lower lobe and are patchy in distribution. The quantity of pleural effusion is usually small but may be moderately large. Associated empyemas are not rare.

Pleural effusions develop in approximately 20% of patients with viral pneumonias.[19] These effusions are characteristically small and transient. When symptomatically acute pneumonia caused by *Mycoplasma pneumoniae* presents as lobar or segmental pulmonary consolidation, pleural fluid may be associated.[69]

In pneumonia caused by fungi, pleural effusion is not unusual. Approximately 15% of patients with acute pneumonia caused by *Coccidioides immitis* have pleural fluid.[32] The pleura may be involved in disseminated cryptococcosis.[75]

Effusions are not uncommon in paragonimiasis.

Empyema. The quantity of free pleural fluid may vary from none to a large amount. Often the fluid is loculated; multiple attempts at thoracentesis may be required before the probing needle happens to enter a loculus. Oblique chest radiographs are advisable to help locate the areas of greatest pleural widening, which are usually the optimal sites for thoracentesis. We have found fluoroscopic assistance of thoracentesis and pleural biopsy occasionally to be invaluable for obtaining appropriate specimens for laboratory analysis. Ultrasound may also be useful in selecting sites for thoracentesis.[55]

Only 50% of patients with empyema develop the disease secondary to pneumonia.[30] A number of patients develop empyema after chest surgery. A smaller number develop empyema because of transdiaphragmatic passage of infection. Amebiasis may spread across the diaphragm from the liver to the right pleural cavity; less commonly it may spread to the pericardium and the left pleural cavity.[51] Rarely, a pulmonary hydatid cyst may rupture into the pleural space.[71]

Bronchopleural fistula. Small fistulas tend to close spontaneously; large ones usually require surgical intervention. For the patient who is an operative candidate, positive contrast radiographic studies can identify the number, size, and site of fistulas. The usual study is sinography, with the injection of a radiopaque contrast material through a chest tube already placed in the involved pleural cavity. Hsu, Bennett, and Wolff[42] recommend sinography as the procedure of choice to outline small, peripheral bronchopleural fistulas and bronchography to demonstrate the airways and fistulous communication(s) in all other cases. Radionuclide fog inhalation also may demonstrate fistulous communication, but anatomic specificity is limited, compared to positive contrast studies.[33]

INTRA-ABDOMINAL DISEASES ASSOCIATED WITH PLEURAL EFFUSION

Pleural effusions are seen in association with many intra-abdominal diseases. Although a variety of mechanisms have been proposed for the production of pleural fluid in patients with abdominal diseases, common to each theory is the belief that the transdiaphragmatic lymphatic system transports fluid from the abdomen to the thorax. One speculation suggests that in certain pathologic states the negative pressure in the thorax provides a gradient for fluid movement from the abdomen, where the pressures are higher than in the pleural cavities.[7]

Elevation and decreased motion of the diaphragm secondary to an adjacent inflammatory process (e.g., abscess or pancreatitis) may also impede lymphatic absorption of pleural fluid because decreased intercostal and diaphragmatic muscular activity decreases pleural lymphatic flow.[82] This phenomenon may explain why pleural effusion is common after abdominal surgery, especially after an upper abdominal procedure. In a recent prospective series of 200 patients who underwent abdominal exploration,[53] lateral decubitus chest radiographs were exposed 2 or 3 days after the operation. Of these patients 48% showed pleural effusion, usually small. Nearly all the effusions resolved without specific treatment.

Meigs' syndrome. In Meigs' syndrome the pathologic cause of the ascites and pleural fluid is unknown.[59] The currently accepted hypothesis is that fluid weeps from the surface lymphatic network of an ovarian tumor, originally described as a benign solid tumor such as a fibroma, thecoma, or granulosa cell tumor. The term Meigs' syndrome recently has been used to describe any ovarian tumor associated with ascites and hydrothorax. As in hepatic cirrhosis with ascites and pleural effusion, the intra-abdominal fluid of Meigs' syndrome is believed to flow through the diaphragmatic lymphatics into the pleural space.

Subphrenic abscess and pancreatitis. Although subphrenic abscess and pancreatitis are important examples of subdiaphragmatic inflammatory disease in which pleural effusions may develop, the mechanisms of production of the pleural fluid may be different. Pleural effusion is found in approximately 80% of patients with a pyogenic subphrenic abscess.[62] In the absence of a diaphragmatic defect or a thoracoabdominal fistula, the pleural fluid above the abscess is sterile. It probably represents drainage of inflammatory edema fluid through the transdiaphragmatic lymphatic system. Pleural effusion is found in approximately 8% of patients with acute pancreatitis.[20] The fluid is usually on the left because the tail of the pancreas is inferior to the undersurface of the left hemidiaphragm. As in subphrenic abscess, the pleural fluid is believed to represent transdiaphragmatic lymphatic drainage of inflammatory edema fluid. A second mechanism is the direct effect of amylase, lipase, and other lytic enzymes released from the pancreas. These enzymes cause fat necrosis within the diaphragm and disrupt the diaphragmatic lymphatic network. Inflammatory edema fluid containing levels of amylase higher than in the serum then may enter the left pleural cavity. Pancreatic enzymes may also be transported through the thoracic duct to the chest. They may directly injure the lymphatic channels draining the pleura and thereby cause pleural fluid to accumulate.

Amebiasis. In amebiasis, rupture of an hepatic amebic abscess across the right hemidiaphragm may cause a right pleural effusion. Rarely, left pleural effusion may occur in amebiasis, usually by direct extension of the infection from the liver across the diaphragm to the pericardium and from there to the left hemithorax.[51]

MISCELLANEOUS CONDITIONS ASSOCIATED WITH PLEURAL EFFUSION

Asbestosis. Occasionally pleural effusion is associated with asbestosis.[28] Pleural biopsy is usually advisable in a patient with a history of asbestos exposure and cryptogenic pleural fluid to rule out other causes of pleural effusion (e.g., malignant mesothelioma or tuberculosis). Pleural plaques presenting as irregular patches of pleural thickening, with or without calcification, are the most common radiologic sign of asbestosis.

Chylothorax. Lipid in pleural fluid produces a milky appearance, but not all milky effusions contain chyle. Only if the fluid contains high levels of triglycerides and low levels of cholesterol may it be considered chylous. Lipid-laden malignant cells, for instance, may degenerate and cause a milky appearance of pleural fluid.

The causes of chylothorax are varied.[15, 24] Trauma is the most common. Usually the trauma is operative or penetrating, but it may be blunt. Another cause is obstruction to thoracic lymphatic channels that enlarges collateral channels, which may carry chyle into the pleural cavity. Neoplasia involving mediastinal lymphatic channels is the most common cause of such obstruction. Rarer causes include mediastinal inflammation such as tuberculosis and thrombosis of the left subclavian vein. Chylothorax is idiopathic in a number of patients. If a patient with chylothorax has no history of chest trauma, Freundlich[24] advocates lymphangiography to determine the anatomic sites of obstruction and the extent and configuration of lymphatic abnormalities.

Drugs. As the pharmacologic armamentarium continues to expand, increasing numbers of drugs have been implicated in a variety of pulmonary diseases.[73] Only two, however, appear to be associated with the production of pleural effusions. Nitrofurantoin can produce both an acute and chronic pulmonary parenchymal reaction. At present it is the only drug known to produce an acute pleural effusion associated with an acute reaction to the drug. The precise mechanism is unclear, but it is known that nitrofurantoin can cause an idiosyncratic or allergic response.[36] Methysergide (Sansert) occasionally produces a chronic pleural effusion in addition to pleural and pulmonary fibrosis.[73] The mechanism is not known.

Polyserositis and other manifestations of systemic lupus erythematosus, including pleural effusion, have been reported with use of twenty-five drugs.[73] When the drugs are withdrawn, the changes of polyserositis generally regress.

Aminosalicylic acid	Isoquinazepon	Procainamide
Digitalis	Mephenytoin	Propylthiouracil
Diphenylhydantoin	Methyldopa	Reserpine
Ethosuximide	Methylthiouracil	Streptomycin
Griseofulvin	Oral contraceptives	Sulfonamides
Guanoxan	Penicillin	Tetracycline
Gold	Phenylbutazone	Thiazides
Hydralazine	Primidone	Trimethadione
Isoniazid		

Endometriosis. Pleural endometriosis is a rare cause of right-sided hemo-thorax.[92] It has been described only in young nulliparous women with ex-tensive endometriosis in the abdomen. Pneumothorax at the time of menses may also occur. The unilaterality of the disease is believed to be caused by direct communication between the peritoneum and the pleural cavity—an unusual anomaly, which has been described only on the right.[92]

Interstitial pneumonias. Pleural effusion, generally small and of unknown cause, is occasionally found in the "usual" interstitial pneumonias or in des-quamative interstitial pneumonias.[27]

Radiation therapy. When a pleural effusion appears after a course of radia-tion therapy to the chest, it becomes a source of concern because the effusion may herald the recurrence of malignant disease. Radiation therapy alone, how-ever, can induce a benign pleural effusion, which usually resolves spontaneously. In a study of 200 patients treated for breast cancer, Bachman and Macken[3] reported an incidence of 5% of nonmalignant pleural effusion. These patients received an estimated dose of 4000 to 6000 R to the apex of the lung. In each patient who developed pleural fluid, radiation pneumonitis was observed, usu-ally appearing a month or two before the ipsilateral development of the pleural effusion. The effusions resolved spontaneously in 4 to 6 months, although a few persisted for 3 to 4 years. The dose of radiation did not correlate with either the quantity of effusion or the extent of fibrosis of the lung. Three pa-tients also have been reported with benign pleural effusions after mediastinal radiation of 4000 to 6000 R.[91] Radiation pneumonitis was absent in these pa-tients.

Rheumatoid disease. Rheumatoid pleural effusions are found almost ex-clusively in men, usually during middle age.[10] The pleural disease may precede the onset of symptoms in the joints. Indeed, the pleural disease appears often to be independent from either articular or pulmonary involvement.

Biopsy usually shows nonspecific pleuritis, but on occasion characteristic histologic findings of rheumatoid disease are detected.[57] The effusions tend to be chronic and may be bilateral. The quantity of fluid varies from small to moderate. Associated pleural adhesions are common. Glucose levels in the fluid tend to be remarkably low (less than 10 mg/100 ml), secondary to a poorly understood abnormality of active transport across the blood-pleura bar-rier.

Cytodiagnosis of rheumatoid pleural disease has advanced considerably in recent years. Cytologic techniques now can provide the diagnosis in the ma-jority of patients with rheumatoid pleural effusion.[8]

Sarcoidosis. Pleural effusion is an uncommon but well-recognized part of the syndrome of sarcoidosis. Pleural fluid occurs at some time in the course of the disease in 2% to 4% of patients with sarcoidosis.[25, 78] Pleural biopsy, usually advisable to rule out other causes of pleural effusion, shows noncaseating pleural granulomas.[78] Mild pleural thickening is commonly seen on chest radiographs of patients with pleural sarcoidosis and effusion. The fluid is usually unilateral.

Systemic lupus erythematosus. Small pleural effusions are common and may be either unilateral or bilateral.[35] Chemically the effusions are nonspecific; histologically the pleuritis is nonspecific. Fibrosis with two to four times normal thickness of the pleura is occasionally evident on chest radiographs. Various pharmacologic agents, listed on p. 275, have been associated with the development of pleural effusion and other manifestations of systemic lupus erythematosus.

Polyarteritis nodosa is another collagen vascular disease in which pleuritis, either nonspecific or showing necrotizing arteritis, may cause small effusions.

Uremia. Hemorrhagic pleuritis and pleural effusion have recently become recognized as occasional findings in patients undergoing chronic hemodialysis.[29, 31] The pleuritis is fibrinous and chronic. The quantity of effusion may vary from small to large. In 2 patients uremic pleuritis has been reported to cause effusions sufficiently large to cause respiratory distress, which was relieved by pleural decortication.[29, 31]

NEEDLE BIOPSY IN DIAGNOSIS OF PLEURAL EFFUSION

Percutaneous needle biopsy of the pleura is often a useful procedure in the diagnosis of the patient with cryptogenic pleural effusion or thickening. For instance, in a patient with a history of asbestos exposure, unilateral pleural effusion, and pleural thickening over the peripheral aspects of the lung on plain chest radiographs, malignant mesothelioma is a leading diagnostic possibility. The cytologic diagnosis of malignant mesothelioma, however, is usually difficult. In this instance pleural biopsy (with a needle large enough to provide a core of tissue) at the time of initial thoracentesis is advisable. Suspicion of pleural tuberculosis is another common indication for percutaneous biopsy of the pleura because diagnosis may be produced within 24 hours, whereas cultures of the pleural fluid or sputum may yield acid-fast bacilli 8 weeks later. Similarly, suspicion of rheumatoid pleural effusion or pleural sarcoidosis may be confirmed by pleural biopsy.

Needle biopsies and spread of intrathoracic disease. What is the risk of thoracentesis spreading cancer into subcutaneous tissue along the path of the needle track? The risk is exceedingly small; only two instances have been reported.[81]

What is the risk of thoracentesis spreading infection into subcutaneous tissues along the path of the needle track? To the best of our knowledge, no such instances have been reported.

What is the risk that percutaneous needle biopsy of intrapulmonary cancer will spread the cancer along the path of the needle track? The risk is extremely slight. In the few cases reported, nearly all the patients had advanced metastatic disease at the time of appearance of cancer in the needle track.[74] From aspiration needle biopsy of lung cancer, the likelihood of implantation metastasis is about one in every 2000 or 3000 biopsies.[74] There have been reports of 2 patients allegedly developing malignant pleural effusions after percutaneous needle aspiration biopsy of solitary lung lesions,[6] but an eminent cytologist has sharply disputed the diagnosis of malignancy in the cytologic preparations of the pleural fluid from these patients.[67]

What is the risk of transthoracic needle biopsy of intrapulmonary infection spreading infection along the path of the needle track? For this theoretical possibility, no evidence exists.[16, 74]

References

1. Abramson, H., Bertles, J. F., and Wethers, D. L.: Sickle cell disease, diagnosis, management, education and research, St. Louis, 1973, The C. V. Mosby Co.
2. Alfidi, R. J.: Personal communication, 1975.
3. Bachman, A. L., and Macken, K.: Pleural effusion following radiation for breast carcinoma, Radiology **72:**699, 1959.
4. Badrinas, F., Rodriguez-Roisin, R., Rives, A., and Picado, C.: Multiple myeloma with pleural involvement, Am. Rev. Respir. Dis. **110:**82, 1974.
5. Berger, H. W., and Mejia, E.: Tuberculous pleurisy, Chest **63:**88, 1973.
6. Berger, R. L., Dargan, E. L., and Huang, B. L.: Dissemination of cancer cells by needle biopsy of the lung, J. Thorac. Cardiovasc. Surg. **63:**430, 1972.
7. Black, L. F.: The pleural space and pleural fluid, Mayo Clin. Proc. **47:**493, 1972.
8. Boddington, M. M., Spriggs, A. I., Morton, J. A., and Mowat, A. G.: Cytodiagnosis of rheumatoid pleural effusions, J. Clin. Pathol. **24:**95, 1971.
9. Caffey, J.: Pediatric x-ray diagnosis, ed. 6, Chicago, 1972, Year Book Medical Publishers, Inc., p. 412.
10. Carr, D. T., and Mayne, J. G.: Pleurisy with effusion in rheumatoid arthritis, with reference to the low concentration of glucose in pleural fluid, Am. Rev. Respir. Dis. **85:**345, 1962.
11. Carr, D. T., and Power, M. H.: Clinical value of measurement of concentration of protein in pleural fluid, N. Engl. J. Med. **259:**426, 1958.
12. Cecil-Loeb textbook of medicine (Beeson, P., and McDermott, W., editors) ed. 12, Philadelphia, 1967, W. B. Saunders Co., pp. 560-561.
13. Chernick, V., and Reed, M. H.: Pneumothorax and chylothorax in the neonatal period, J. Pediatr. **76:**624, 1970.
14. Courtice, F. C., and Simmonds, W. J.: Physiological significance of lymph drainage of the serous cavities and lungs, Physiol. Rev. **34:**419, 1954.
15. Crosby, I. K., Couch, J., and Reed, W. A.: Chylopericardium and chylothorax, J. Thorac. Cardiovasc. Surg. **65:**935, 1973.
16. Dahlgren, S., and Nordenström, B.: Transthoracic needle biopsy, Chicago, 1966, Year Book Medical Publishers, Inc., p. 68.
17. Dekker, A., Graham, T., and Bupp, P. A.: The occurrence of sickle cells in pleural fluid: report of a case with sickle cell disease, Acta Cytol. **19:**251, 1974.
18. Depp, D. A., Atherton, S. O., and McGough, E.: Spontaneous neonatal pleural effusion, J. Pediatr. Surg. **9:**809, 1974.
19. Fine, N. L., Smith, L. R., and Sheedy, P. F.: Frequency of pleural effusions in mycoplasma and viral pneumonias, N. Engl. J. Med. **283:**790, 1970.
20. Fishbien, R., Murphy, G. P., and Wilder, R. J.: The pulmonary manifestations of pancreatitis, Dis. Chest **41:**392, 1962.
21. Fleischner, F. G.: Atypical arrangement of free pleural effusion, Radiol. Clin. North Am. **1:**347, 1963.
22. Fraser, R. G., and Paré, J. A. P.: Diagnosis of diseases of the chest, Philadelphia, 1970, W. B. Saunders Co., p. 1146.
23. Freeman, L. M., and Johnson, P. M.: Clinical scintillation imaging, ed. 2, New York, 1975, Grune & Stratton, Inc., pp. 512-514.
24. Freundlich, I. M.: The role of lymphangiography in chylothorax, Am. J. Roentgenol. Radium Ther. Nucl. Med. **125:**617, 1975.
25. Freundlich, I. M., Libshitz, H. I.,

Glassman, L. M., and Israel, H. L.: Sarcoidosis; typical and atypical thoracic manifestations and complications, Clin. Radiol. **21**:376, 1970.

26. Funahashi, A., and Sarkar, T. K.: Measurement of respiratory gases and pH of pleural fluid, Am. Rev. Respir. Dis. **108**:1266, 1973.

27. Gaensler, E. A., Carrington, C. B., and Coutu, R. E.: Chronic interstitial pneumonias, Clin. Notes Respir. Dis. **10**:3-16, Spring, 1972.

28. Gaensler, E. A., and Kaplan, A. I.: Asbestos pleural effusion, Ann. Intern. Med. **74**:178, 1971.

29. Galen, M. A., et al.: Hemorrhagic pleural effusion in patients undergoing chronic hemodialysis, Am. Intern. Med. **82**:359, 1975.

30. Geha, A. S.: Pleural empyema: changing etiologic, bacteriologic, and therapeutic aspects, J. Thorac. Cardiovasc. Surg. **61**:626, 1971.

31. Gilbert, L., et al.: Fibrinous uremic pleuritis: a surgical entity, Chest **67**:53, 1975.

32. Greendyke, W. H., Resnick, D. L., and Harvey, W. C.: The varied roentgen manifestations of primary coccidioidomycosis, Am. J. Roentgenol. Radium Ther. Nucl. Med. **109**:491, 1970.

33. Greyson, N. D., and Rosenthall, L.: Detection of postoperative bronchopleural fistulas by radionuclide fog inhalation, Can. Med. Assoc. J. **103**:1366, 1970.

34. Grix, A., and Giammona, S. T.: Pneumonitis with pleural effusion in children due to mycoplasma pneumonia, Am. Rev. Respir. Dis. **108**:665, 1974.

35. Gross, M., Esterly, J. R., and Earle, R. H.: Pulmonary alterations in systemic lupus erythematosus, Am. Rev. Respir. Dis. **105**:572, 1972.

36. Hailey, F. J., Glascock, H. W., and Hewett, W. F.: Pleuropulmonary reactions to nitrofurantoin, N. Engl. J. Med. **281**:1087, 1968.

37. Hansen-Melander, E., Kullander, S., and Melander, S.: Chromosome analysis of human ovarian cystosarcoma in the ascites formed, J. Natl. Cancer Inst. **16**:1067, 1956.

38. Hansson, A., and Korsgaard, R.: Cytogenetical diagnosis of malignant pleural effusions, Scand. J. Respir. Dis. **55**:301, 1974.

39. Harell, G. S., Friedland, G. W., Daily, W. J., and Cohn, R. B.: Neonatal Boerhaave's syndrome, Radiology **95**: 665, 1970.

40. Heller, R. M., Janower, M. L., and Weber, A. L.: The radiological manifestations of malignant pleural mesothelioma, Am. J. Roentgenol. Radium Ther. Nucl. Med. **108**:53, 1970.

41. Hessén, I.: Roentgen examination of pleural fluid: a study of the localization of free effusions, the potentialities of diagnosing minimal quantities of fluid and its existence under physiological conditions, Acta Radiol. (suppl. 86), pp. 1-80, 1951.

42. Hsu, J. T., Bennett, G. M., and Wolff, E.: Radiologic assessment of bronchopleural fistula with empyema, Radiology **103**:41, 1972.

43. Hutchinson, W. B., and Friedenberg, M. J.: Intrathoracic mesothelioma, Radiology **80**:937, 1963.

44. Jackson, J. F.: Chromosome analysis in cells in effusion in cancer patients, Cancer **20**:537, 1967.

45. James, A. E., Jr., et al.: The fissure sign: its multiple causes, Am. J. Roentgenol. Radium Ther. Nucl. Med. **111**: 492, 1971.

46. John, E.: Pleural effusion in the newborn, Med. J. Aust. (suppl.) **1**:102, 1974.

47. Johnston, R. F., and Loo, R. V.: Hepatic hydrothorax: studies to determine the source of the fluid and report of 13 cases, Ann. Intern. Med. **61**:385, 1964.

48. Joyner, C. R., Jr., Horman, R. J., and Reid, J. M.: Reflected ultrasound in the detection and localization of pleural effusion, J.A.M.A. **200**:399, 1967.

49. Kirkpatrick, J. A., and Fleisher, D. S.: The roentgen appearance of the chest in acute glomerulonephritis in children, J. Pediatr. **64**:492, 1964.

50. Lemon, W. S., and Higgins, G. M.: Lymphatic absorption of particulate matter through the normal and paralysed diaphragm: experimental study, Am. J. Med. Sci. **178**:536, 1929.

51. LeRoux, B. T.: Pleuro-pulmonary amoebiasis, Thorax **24**:91, 1969.

52. Light, R. W., and Ball, W. C., Jr.: Lactate dehydrogenase isoenzymes in pleural effusion, Am. Rev. Respir. Dis. **108**:660, 1973.

53. Light, R. W., and George, R. B.: In-

cidence and significance of pleural effusions after abdominal surgery, Am. Rev. Respir. Dis. **111**:904, 1975.

54. Light, R. W., MacGregor, M. I., Ball, W. C., Jr., and Luchsinger, P. C.: Diagnostic significance of pleural fluid pH and pCO_2, Chest **64**:591, 1973.

55. Mahal, G. E.: Ultrasound in the diagnosis of empyema, Ann. Intern. Med. **83**:123, 1975.

56. Maher, G. G., and Berger, H. W.: Massive pleural effusion: malignant and nonmalignant causes in 46 patients, Am. Rev. Respir. Dis. **105**:458, 1972.

57. Mays, E. E.: Rheumatoid pleuritis: observations in eight cases and suggestions for making the diagnosis in patients without the "typical findings," Dis. Chest **53**:202, 1968.

58. McPeak, E. M., and Levine, S. A.: The preponderance of right hydrothorax in congestive heart failure, Ann. Intern. Med. **25**:916, 1946.

59. Meigs, J. V.: Fibroma of the ovary with ascites and hydrothorax: Meigs' syndrome, Am. J. Obstet. Gynecol. **67**:962, 1954.

60. Mellins, R. B., Levine, O. R., and Fishman, A. P.: Effect of systemic and pulmonary venous hypertension on pleural and pericardial fluid accumulation, J. Appl. Physiol. **29**:564, 1970. Cf. Fraser, R. G.: Reviewer's comments, Invest. Radiol. **6**:290, 1971.

61. Meyer, P. C.: Metastatic carcinoma of the pleura, Thorax **21**:437, 1966.

62. Miller, W. T., and Talman, E. A.: Subphrenic abscess, Am. J. Roentgenol. Radium Ther. Nucl. Med. **101**:961, 1967.

63. Mishkin, F. S., and Brashear, R.: An experimental study on the effect of free pleural fluid on the lung scan, Radiology **97**:238, 1970.

64. Moskowitz, H., Platt, R. T., Schachar, R., and Mellins, H.: Roentgen visualization of minute pleural effusion: an experimental study to determine the minimum amount of pleural fluid visible on a radiograph, Radiology **109**:33, 1973.

65. Müller, R., and Löfstedt, S.: Reaction of pleura in primary tuberculosis of the lungs, Acta Med. Scand. **122**:105, 1945.

66. Mulvey, R. B.: The effect of pleural fluid on the diaphragm, Radiology **84**:1080, 1965.

67. Naylor, B.: Letter to the editor, J. Thorac. Cardiovasc. Surg. **64**:324, 1972.

68. Nobler, M. P.: The abscopal effect in malignant lymphoma and its relationship to lymphocyte circulation, Radiology **93**:410, 1969.

69. Putman, C. E., Curtis, A. M., Simeone, J. F., and Jensen, P.: *Mycoplasma* pneumonia: clinical and roentgenographic patterns, Am. J. Roentgenol. Radium Ther. Nucl. Med. **124**:417, 1975.

70. Pyle, I. R.: Personal communication, 1975.

71. Ramos, L., et al.: Radiological characteristics of perforated pulmonary hydatid cysts, Radiology **116**:539, 1975.

72. Rigler, L. G.: Roentgen diagnosis of small pleural effusions: new roentgenographic position, J.A.M.A. **96**:104, 1931.

73. Rosenow, E. C., III: The spectrum of drug-induced pulmonary disease, Ann. Intern. Med. **77**:977, 1973.

74. Sagel, S. S., and Forrest, J. V.: Fluoroscopically assisted lung biopsy techniques. In Sagel, S. S., editor: Special procedures in chest radiology, Philadelphia, 1976, W. B. Saunders Co.

75. Salyer, W. R., and Salyer, D. C.: Pleural involvement in cryptococcosis, Chest **66**:139, 1974.

76. Savoca, C. J., Austin, J. H. M., and Goldberg, H. I.: Widening of the right paratracheal stripe: a useful diagnostic tool. Presented at the Sixty-first Scientific Assembly, The Radiological Society of North America, Chicago, Dec. 2, 1975.

77. Schultze, G.: Unusual manifestations of primary staphylococcal pneumonia in infants and children, Am. J. Roentgenol. Radium Ther. Nucl. Med. **81**:290, 1959.

78. Sharma, O. P., and Gordonson, J.: Pleural effusion in sarcoidosis: a report of 6 cases, Thorax **30**:95, 1975.

79. Simmonds, B., Friedman, P. F., and Sokoloff, J.: The prone chest film, Radiology **116**:11, 1975.

80. Spencer, H.: Pathology of the lung, ed. 2, Oxford, 1968, Pergamon Press, pp. 56-58.

81. Stewart, B. N., and Block, A. J.: Subcutaneous implantation of cancer following thoracentesis, Chest **66**:456, 1974.

82. Stewart, P. B., and Burgen, A. S.: The turnover of fluid in the dog's pleural cavity, J. Lab. Clin. Med. **52**:212, 1958.

83. Szucs, M. M., Jr., et al.: Diagnostic sensitivity of laboratory findings in acute

pulmonary embolism, Ann. Intern. Med. **74**:161, 1971.

84. Taylor, T. K.: Use of ultrasound in the opaque hemithorax, Br. J. Radiol. **47**: 199, 1974.

85. Thombs, D. D.: Cold agglutinin positive pneumonia, a review of 30 cases in children, Ohio State Med. J. **63**:1171, 1967.

86. Tow, D. E., and Wagner, H. N., Jr.: Effect of pleural fluid on the appearance of the lung scan, J. Nucl. Med. **11**:138, 1970.

87. Trackler, R. T., and Brinker, R. A.: Widening of the left paravertebral pleural line on supine chest roentgenograms in free pleural effusions, Am. J. Roentgenol. Radium Ther. Nucl. Med. **96**:1027, 1966.

88. Unger, J. D., Rose, H. D., and Unger, G. F.: Gram-negative pneumonia, Radiology **107**:283, 1973.

89. Weick, J. K., et al.: Pleural effusion in lymphoma, Cancer **31**:848, 1973.

90. Wesenberg, R. L.: The newborn chest, New York, 1973, Harper & Row, Publishers, pp. 199-201.

91. Whitcomb, M. E., and Schwarz, M. I.: Pleural effusion complicating intensive mediastinal radiation, Am. Rev. Respir. Dis. **103**:100, 1971.

92. Yeh, T. J.: Endometriosis within the thorax: metaplasia, implantation, or metastasis? J. Thorac. Cardiovasc. Surg. **53**:201, 1967.

11 Linear shadows in chest radiographs

David H. Trapnell

In this chapter a linear shadow is defined as one that is at least 1 cm long and not more than 2 mm wide. Such a radiographic shadow could be produced either by a cordlike structure with sufficient inherent radiodensity to distinguish it from the surrounding tissues (e.g., a bit of metal wire) or by a sheetlike object of insufficient radiodensity to be visible if it were cordlike but enough to cast a linear shadow when the sheet is projected tangential to the x-ray beam. Nearly all the pulmonary causes of line shadows in chest radiographs are in the latter group. It is apparent therefore that only those which are tangential to the x-ray beam are shown, and that many such structures may be present which are undetected in radiographs simply because they are not tangential.

Pulmonary anatomy does not allow a random distribution of such sheetlike structures (normal or abnormal). Thus linear shadows arising in the lung usually conform to certain anatomic positions and have characteristic radiographic appearances, described later. Lines that do not correspond with these must either be artifacts completely outside the patient or be caused by sheetlike or cordlike structures in the pleura or chest wall. However, in some diseases producing gross disorganization of the lung, such as progressive massive fibrosis complicating pneumoconiosis, long linear shadows may appear in almost any position of the lung.

The key to the accurate diagnosis of any linear shadow is a combined assessment of the following:

1. *Its full extent.* It is necessary to extrapolate beyond its apparent ends to see if, in fact, it continues further on. Fig. 11-1 shows an apparently normal lesser fissure. However, on looking to and beyond the lateral end of the line it is clear that multiple similar lines are present in the axilla. The fact that the line is produced by strapping on the chest wall can be inferred from this alone but is, of course, greatly reinforced by the fact that the right lung has been removed!

2. *Its anatomic position.* A look at the end of the linear shadow may reveal that one or both ends are beyond the edge of the lung, indicating that it cannot be pulmonary. Alternatively, or in addition, the connection between the line and the structure causing it may then be obvious. The dense edge of the spine of the

282

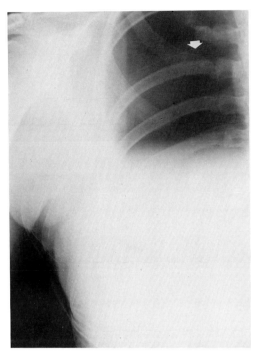

Fig. 11-1. A pseudo-lesser fissure. Line was produced by strapping on chest wall following a total right pneumonectomy.

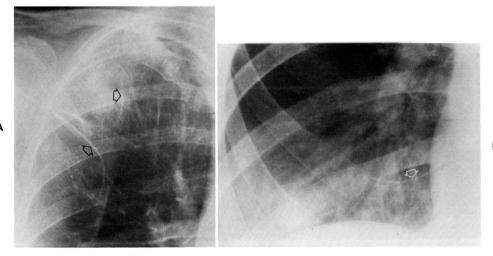

Fig. 11-2. A, Curvilinear shadows produced by spine and upper angle of scapula. B, Curvilinear shadow cast by calcification in upper edge of a costal cartilage. Compare with Fig. 11-20.

scapula (Fig. 11-2, *A*), the lateral edge of the manubrium, the upper and lower borders of a rib, or marginal calcification in a costal cartilage (Fig. 11-2, *B*) may usually be readily identified in this way.

Ideally, of course, localization of any structure casting a linear shadow should be based on two radiographic projections made at right angles to each other, as is usually possible with the lesser fissure. However, this is frequently not possible because the sheetlike structure is tangential to the x-ray beam in one projection only. For example, the main interlobar fissure is normally visible in a lateral projection but, with one unusual exception described later, is never visible in PA or AP projections.

Thus far, these basic principles of interpretation have been applied to lines caused by artifacts, the skeleton, and the main fissure. Such lines have been described in more detail elsewhere[14] and will not be discussed further here. Nonetheless, the same basic principles are fundamental to the accurate diagnosis of all other linear shadows in chest radiographs. Failure to apply these principles has occasionally led to the embarrassment even of great radiologists who thought that appearances were so "typical" that basic rules of interpretation could be shelved. They have diagnosed, for example, a left "lesser fissure" without a lateral projection to prove its anterior position.

FISSURES

The main and lesser fissures of the lung are well known. However, the presence and significance of uncommon, accessory fissures are less often appreciated. The most common is the *inferior accessory fissure*, which occurs on the right in 11% of normal English lungs but in only 0.3% of left lungs.[12] It separates the

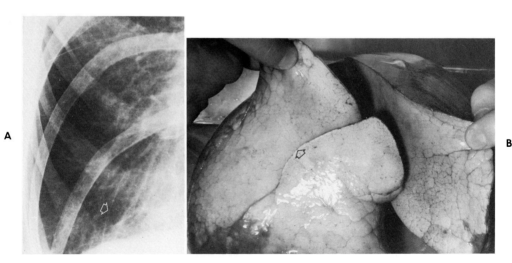

A

B

Fig. 11-3. **A,** Inferior accessory fissure (arrow). **B,** Diaphragmatic surface of same right lung inflated at autopsy to show lower edge of inferior accessory fissure with main fissure aspect of middle lobe lying to right. (From Trapnell, D. H.: Principles of x-ray diagnosis, London, 1967, Butterworth & Co. Publishers Ltd.)

medial basal segment from the other basal segments and varies in position from close to the cardiophrenic angle to close to the costophrenic recess (Fig. 11-3). As other fissures do, it may form a clearly defined boundary separating an area of consolidation in the medial basal segment from adjacent normal lung (Fig. 11-4) or in the adjacent segments from a normal medial segment (Fig. 11-5). Like other fissures, too, the inferior accessory fissure may be the site of a collection of pleural fluid (Fig. 11-6). Failure to recognize the presence of this fissure in such a case may lead to the erroneous conclusion that a wedge of collapse-consolidation is present.

The *superior accessory fissure* occurs in 6% of normal right lungs but less than 0.1% of left lungs.[12] It separates the apical segment of the lower lobe from the basal segments. Like the lesser fissure, it may be complete, extending to the hilum (Fig. 11-7) or incomplete (Fig. 11-8). This fissure is also like the lesser fissure in that it is usually visible in anterior and lateral projections (Fig. 11-7) and like the other fissures, too, in that it may separate consolidated from normal lung or be the site of a collection of pleural fluid. It is obviously important to distinguish such abnormalities involving the uncommon superior accessory fissure (which is posterior in position) from those involving the common lesser fissure anteriorly.

The lesser fissure should never be called "double" unless the two parts of the fissure appear very close to each other (Fig. 11-9). When 1 or 2 cm separates the lines, the lower fissure is nearly always a superior accessory fissure (Fig. 11-7).

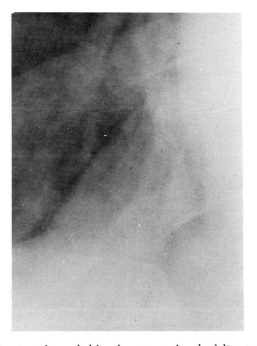

Fig. 11-4. Consolidation in right medial basal segment, sharply delineated on its lateral aspect by inferior accessory fissure.

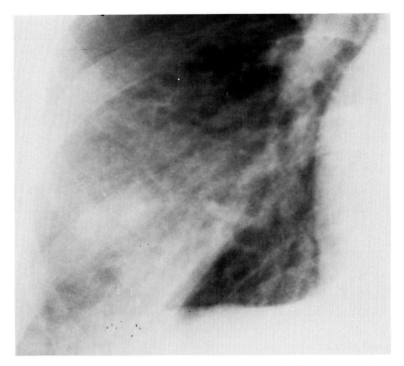

Fig. 11-5. Consolidation in all basal segments except the medial and separated by inferior accessory fissure.

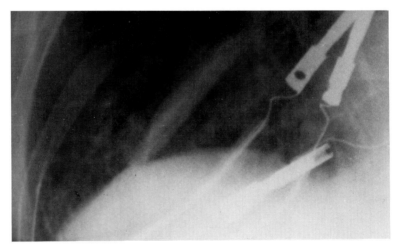

Fig. 11-6. Fluid collected in inferior accessory fissure. (This was shown clearly in a film made the previous day.)

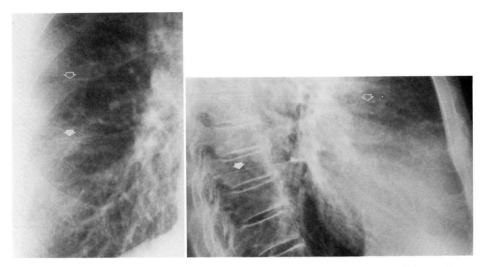

Fig. 11-7. Superior accessory fissure (solid arrows) lying below and behind lesser fissure (open arrows).

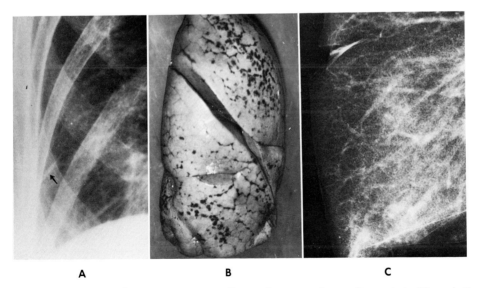

| A | B | C |

Fig. 11-8. A, A partial superior accessory fissure shown in chest radiograph in life and, **B,** in inflated lung at autopsy. **C,** Radiograph of inflated lung. Removal of lung from thorax allowed fissure to gape open. (From Trapnell, D. H.: Radiol. Clin. North Am. **11**:77, 1973.)

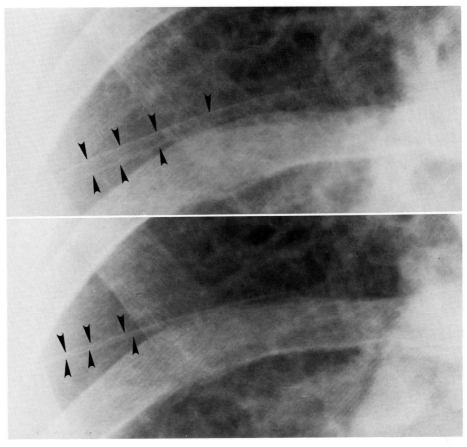

Fig. 11-9. Normal lesser fissure appearing "double" in one phase of respiration. Note that the two lines are very close together.

On the left side the superior accessory fissure may appear in anterior projections of the chest to be an example of a left lesser fissure (between the anterior segment of the upper lobe and the lingula), but a lateral projection will show its true, posterior position. I have yet to see a satisfactorily proved example of a left lesser fissure. They must be extremely rare. (Can anyone send me one?!).

The *azygos* vein fissure must never be diagnosed unless the vein is visible at the lower end of the fissure. Although this is easily recognized in some cases—resembling a drop of water at the lower end of a hair—the variable position of the fissure and the shape of the shadow cast by the vein may sometimes be confusing (Fig. 11-10).

The *upper end of the main fissure* is sometimes visible in anterior radiographs when there is partial collapse of the apical segment of the lower lobe. For this to occur, the segmental shrinkage has to cause the lateral edge of the main fissure to swing backward so that it becomes tangential to the x-ray beam. Because of this, it is sometimes difficult or impossible to see the main fissure in the lateral

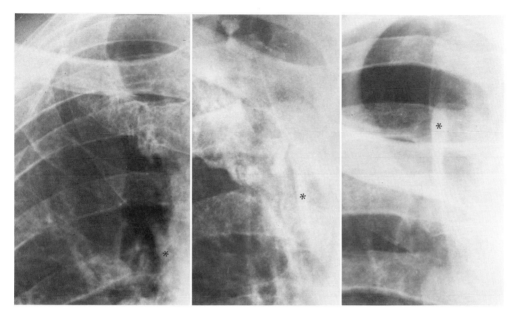

Fig. 11-10. Azygos lobe fissure in different patients. Vein (*) is shown to be in a variety of positions, and lobe varies in size from one patient to another.

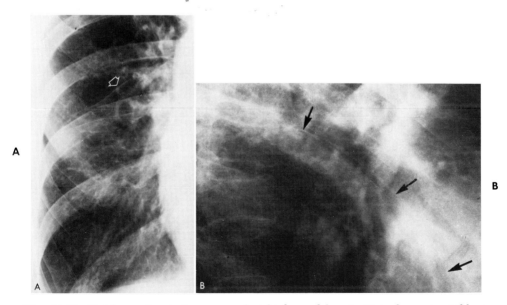

Fig. 11-11. Shrinkage of apical segment of right lower lobe. **A,** Main fissure is visible in PA projection because apical segment collapse has pulled it downward so that it is tangential to the x-ray beam. Line extends above hilum in **A,** and upper end of fissure is less clear than normal in lateral projection, **B.** (From Trapnell, D. H.: Radiol. Clin. North Am. 11:77, 1973.)

projection. The clue to the correct diagnosis in such cases is that the upper end of the line shadow extends above the hilum in the anterior projection (Fig. 11-11).

ANTERIOR MEDIASTINUM

In the adult the anterior mediastinum is normally very thin and consists mainly of the adjacent parietal and visceral pleurae of the two lungs where they touch each other behind the sternum. Low kilovoltage PA films do not show this, but a high kilovoltage technique often does, particularly if the mediastinum is slightly displaced to one side (Fig. 11-12). Of course, it is only seen as a line when the anterior mediastinum is tangential to the x-ray beam.

PLEURA

Apart from those areas which form an interlobar fissure, the pleura is normally indistinguishable from the chest wall with which it is in intimate contact. Although this is always true of the parietal pleura, the visceral layer may be visible when a pneumothorax is present. There is very rarely any difficulty in arriving at the correct diagnosis. However, if a pleural adhesion is present, the shape of the lung surface may be deformed so that an appearance resembling an emphysematous bulla may be produced (Fig. 11-13) in one phase of respiration. A radiograph made in a different phase of breathing, which would not significantly alter the shape of a bulla, reveals the true cause of the line shadow.

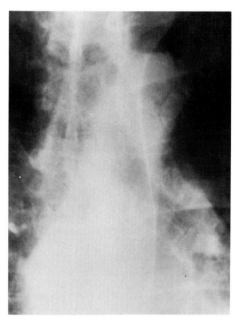

Fig. 11-12. Anterior mediastinum shown in a high kV radiograph (exposed for the mediastinum rather than the lung).

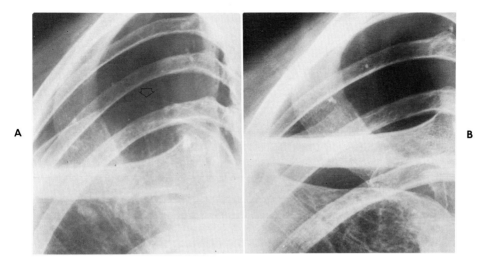

Fig. 11-13. A, Very delicate curved line shadow (arrow) produced by visceral layer of pleura over lung apex and a pneumothorax. A classic appearance causing no diagnostic problem. **B,** Same patient in expiration. Shape of lung surface is now deformed by a pleural adhesion at level of clavicle.

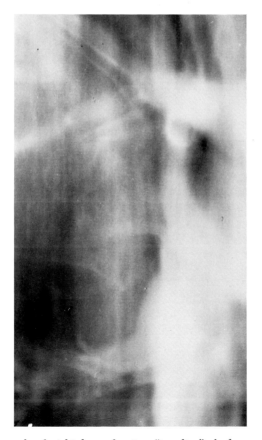

Fig. 11-14. AP tomograph of right lung showing "tramline" shadows produced by walls of bronchi in an emphysematous patient with chronic bronchitis.

BRONCHIAL WALLS

Healthy bronchi are never visible except near the hilum. Here they may commonly be seen in AP tomographs, particularly when a high kilovoltage technique is used (Fig. 11-14). Thickening of the walls of bronchi occurs in some disease processes, but it is usually only in bronchiectasis or mucoviscidosis in children that the increased wall thickness is of a sufficient magnitude to be identified confidently in standard chest films. In chronic bronchitis the thickening known to occur microscopically is too slight to be visible in radiographs except sometimes when a bronchus is projected end-on. Here the summation effect of the longitudinal view of the bronchus may be sufficient to show an increase in the thickness of the bronchial wall when a series of radiographs covering at least a year is available. In my view, it is wiser not to mention this sign, even if its presence is suspected, than to report its presence when there is doubt.

INTERLOBULAR SEPTA

The basic respiratory unit of the lung is called an acinus, each of which is supplied by a terminal bronchiole. Acini are grouped together in clumps of three to five to form a "secondary" lobule. The lobule has been defined in many different ways, but it is best described as that part of the lung supplied by a cluster of three to five terminal bronchioli.[5] Each lobule has a central artery and bronchus and a peripheral venous drainage. In addition, there are lymphatic vessels around the periphery of the lobule and around the central bronchoarterial bundle.[13] Between some, but by no means all, of the lobules are interlobular connective tissue septa. In the surface layers of the lung these septa are generally located at points where the pleural shape is changing (e.g., over the apex or at corners of lobes), but they are rare along the flatter surfaces of the lung (e.g., the parts forming the main fissure).[5] Wherever they occur, the interlobular septa that touch the visceral pleura ("surface septa") are approximately at right angles to it. They normally measure about 1.5 cm in length but may be as long as 2 cm. Occasionally one of the surface interlobular septa is directly continuous with a "deep" septum, particularly anteriorly.

It is in the interlobular septa that the peripheral veins and lymphatics of the lobules run, and they are consequently called "interlobular" lymphatics or veins in this part of their course, even though they are normally the direct continuation of vessels in the pleura (consequently called pleural).[8] The veins and lymphatics of the pleura are actually *in* the pleura histologically (even though to the naked eye they appear to be under it and, consequently but erroneously, have sometimes been called subpleural).

The interlobular veins and lymphatics continue their course to the hilum in sheaths of connective tissue and are, of course, still between lobules. For simplicity, interlobular lymphatics are called perivenous where they leave the interlobular septum and become wrapped in the perivascular connective tissue.

In the human there are anastomotic lymphatic channels that join one group of perivenous lymphatics with another or with a more proximal peribronchial group.[8] Such lymphatics run in sheets that form part of the connective tissue "skeleton" of the lung.[14] These sheets are interlobular in position but are not so regularly arranged as the interlobular septa in the surface of the lung. As an approximation, however, these connective tissue planes in the depth of the lung may be called the deep interlobular septa, and those in contact with the visceral pleura may be called the surface septa.

Neither the surface nor the deep interlobular septa can be demonstrated by radiography in healthy patients, even in the isolated, inflated lung at autopsy. They are too thin. However, when these septa are thickened by disease such as cardiac[6, 14] or "allergic"[4] edema, lymphangitis carcinomatosa[9] (Figs. 11-15 and 11-16), or sarcoidosis[3, 11] (Fig. 11-17) or when, in addition, opaque material is deposited within and adjacent to them (pneumoconiosis,[10] hemosiderosis[2]), they may be visible in chest radiographs made in life when the incident x-ray beam is tangential to them.

The method by which this has been proved is fully described elsewhere,[14] but some examples are included here to illustrate. Alternatively, the technique described by Heitzman[3] may be used. It is only by a complete examination both of radiographs of a whole inflated lung and of individual slices of it and subsequent histologic examination of abnormalities strictly and individually located in the radiographs that a true radiologic-pathologic correlation can be made.

In this way it can be shown that, as might be anticipated from a consideration of their anatomic location, *the pulmonary lymphatics are never visible as such in radiographs.* Each individual lymphatic is a tiny rodlike structure of soft tissue radiodensity too small even when distended to be detected by optimal radiography. Moreover, the lymphatics are surrounded by either the pleura or connective tissue of a radiodensity identical to that of the lymphatic vessels themselves. Many lymphatics are wrapped around pulmonary arteries or veins and, however distended they might be, could only contribute to the apparent size of the vessel along which they run.

Thus from a theoretical point of view, which can be readily proved experimentally, the linear shadows, originally described by Kerley[5a] as "A" and "B" lines, cannot possibly be caused by lymphatics. It is therefore high time that such lines be no longer called lymphatic lines or by any other empirical or eponymous term. They should be known by the structures that cause them—the interlobular septa. The surface septa produce "B" lines and the deep septa "A" lines in the pathologic states just described. It should be noted that this conclusion is at variance with one I published in 1963,[8] which has unfortunately been widely quoted but has since been corrected.[13, 14]

A very rare cause of septal lines is sarcomatous permeation of the interlobular septa (Fig. 11-18). There is gross thickening of the interlobular septa entirely due to the sarcomatous tissue. The lymphatics that presumably had been present in the septa were invisible in multiple histologic sections, and the linear shadows were produced exclusively by the septa. This is very unusual but further proves that lymphatics do not cause septal lines. In most cases in which

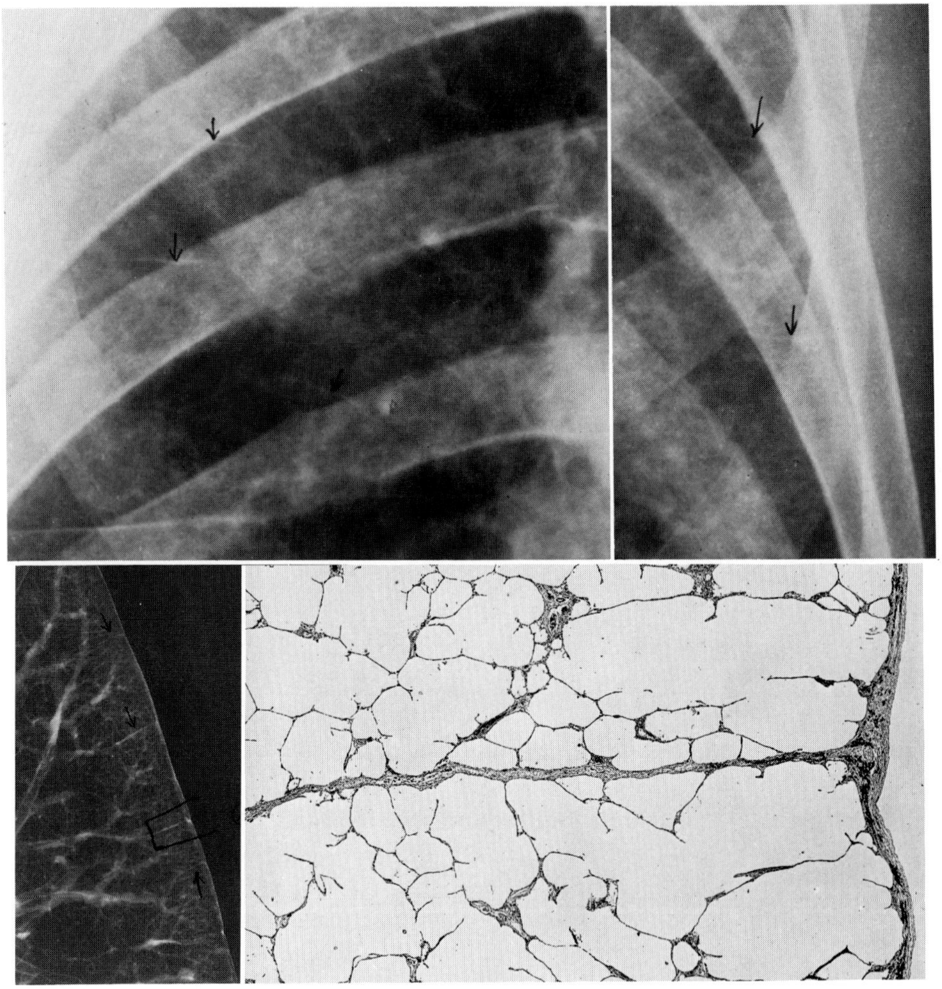

Fig. 11-15. A, Deep septal lines in right upper lobe of a patient with lymphangitis carcinomatosa shortly before his death. B, Surface septa in same patient in left lower lobe. C, Radiograph of a slice of inflated fixed left lung showing a surface septal line. The marked area was removed for histologic examination. D, Photomicrograph (H & E; ×22) of line-causing structure shown to be a surface interlobular septum thickened by a fibrocellular reaction to tumor cells in the interlobular lymphatics. (From Trapnell, D. H.: Thorax 19:251, 1964.)

Fig. 11-16. A, Inflated fixed whole right lung at autopsy. A primary bronchial carcinoma lies in posterior segment of upper lobe. There is extensive lymphangitis carcinomatosa. B, Radiograph of a slice of the upper lobe showing tumor and line shadows extending from it. Marked area was removed for histologic examination. C, Photomicrograph (H & E; ×22) showing a deep interlobular septum. D, Part of same septum (×122) showing tumor cells in lymphatics and blood cells in veins along with a marked fibrous reaction in septum. (A from Trapnell, D. H.: Radiol. Clin. North Am. 11:77, 1973. B to D from Trapnell, D. H.: Thorax 19:251, 1964.)

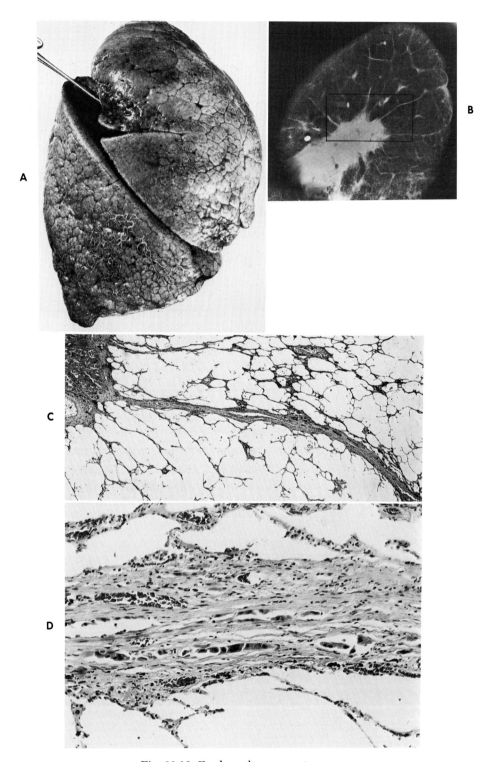

Fig. 11-16. For legend see opposite page.

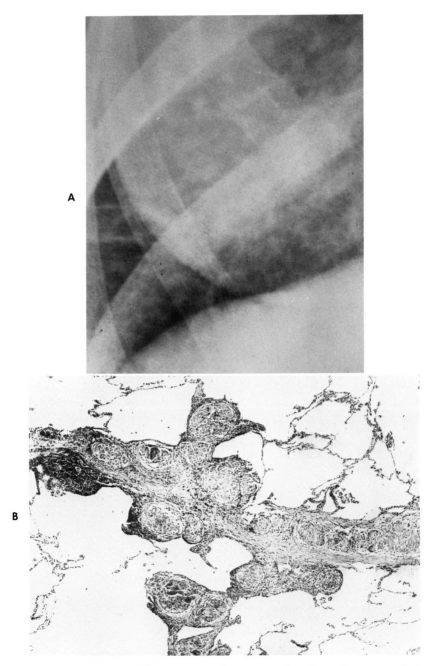

Fig. 11-17. A, Surface septal lines in sarcoidosis. Note that their edges are indistinct. B, Photomicrograph (H & E; ×58) of one of the surface interlobular septa showing sarcoid granulomas in it and extending irregularly into adjacent lung, no doubt producing the indistinct edges of the septal shadows. (B from Trapnell, D. H.: Br. J. Radiol. 37:811, 1964.)

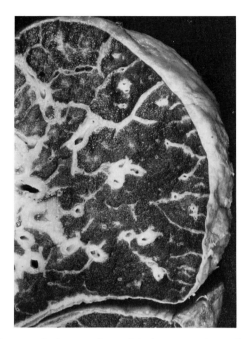

Fig. 11-18. Gross thickening of pleura and interlobular septa of apical part of left upper lobe in a boy whose whole body was permeated by a fibrosarcoma of the thigh. Septal lines in this rare case were produced exclusively by sarcoma cells in the septa.

septal lines are present the interlobular or anastomotic lymphatics contribute a small part to the total thickness of the septum (Figs. 11-15 and 11-16). It is the whole septum (including the edema, tissues, or structures in it) that casts the shadow formerly called an "A" or "B" line.

A number of pathologic processes produce appearances that may be compared with interlobular septa.

Emphysema. Most emphysema starts in the center of the acinus (centriacinar) and may extend to involve the whole acinus or lobule (panacinar, panlobular). Occasionally, however, the process may be most marked beside the interlobular septa (paraseptal emphysema).[5] In such cases the normal interlobular septa are given "edge enhancement" partly by the excess of air beside them and partly by summation of their shadow and that of the edges of small adjoining bullae. The result may thus be that actual septa are visible, although probably "thickened" by adjoining lung tissue (Fig. 11-19). In such a case, however, the curvilinear margins of larger bullae may also be detected, and the other radiographic features of emphysema are present. Infrequently the edge of a single large bulla is approximately straight. In such a case it is the total absence of blood vessels within the bulla that is the clue to its identity. Curved line shadows produced by the margins of large emphysematous bullae and postinfective "cysts" containing air (pneumatoceles) usually present no diagnostic problem. Small bullae must be distinguished from the cystlike spaces of bronchiectasis. A combination of anterior and lateral radiographs usually resolves any doubt.

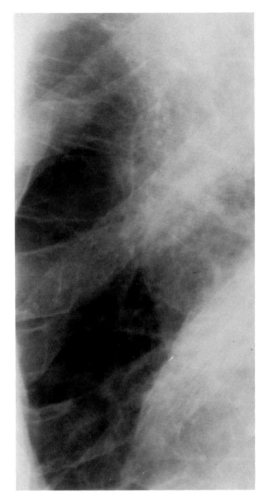

Fig. 11-19. Emphysema, presumed to be paraseptal, producing septal lines. Lateral projection.

Pulmonary infarction and infection. As small areas of infection or infarction in the lung resolve, a linear shadow may occur. In a known case of resolving pneumonia such lines present no diagnostic problem. Sometimes, however, they may be found as an unexpected abnormality in radiographs of symptom-free patients (Fig. 11-20). The presumption often made (probably correct) is that such lines represent old infarcts. However, this view is not supported by much strictly controlled radiologic-histologic evidence (because the patients are symptom-free). Exactly what proportion of the residual line shadow is caused by the infarcted area and how much, if any, by in-drawing of the pleura over an old infarct (a theory suggested by Simon[7]) remains to be shown by more carefully controlled radiologic-histologic studies.

The shadows of resolving pneumonia may be shaggy and ill defined, often so much so that they cannot strictly be called linear shadows (as defined previ-

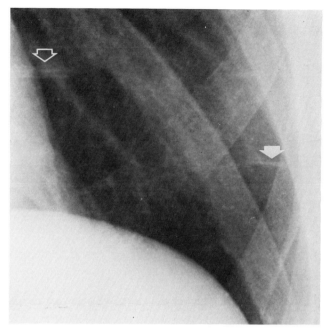

Fig. 11-20. Asymptomatic line shadow (solid arrow), unchanged for 9 years. Presumed to be caused by an old infarct. Open arrow indicates calcification in edge of a costal cartilage.

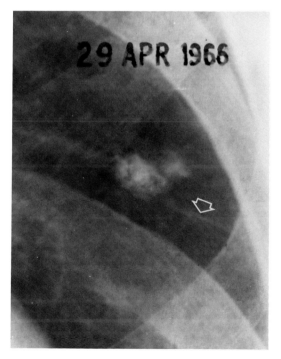

Fig. 11-21. Line shadow that appeared beside an old tuberculous lesion. Line was not present 10 years previously.

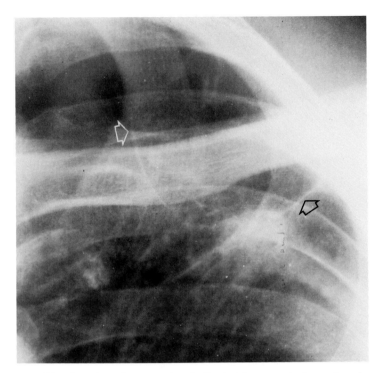

Fig. 11-22. An old tuberculous lesion with a bulla (white arrow) above it and an apparent septal line (black arrow) between lesion and pleura.

ously), but old foci of tuberculous infection may develop sharply defined line shadows adjacent to them (Fig. 11-21). Such lines may only become visible years after the disease has otherwise "healed." They presumably represent bands of fibrous tissue and may, in fact, be thickened interlobular septa. A contributing factor in some cases may be the edge of an adjacent emphysematous bulla which abuts on the fibrous tissue band or thickened interlobular septum (Fig. 11-22).

LONG, STRAIGHT LINE SHADOWS NOT DUE TO ANY NORMAL ANATOMIC STRUCTURE

A study of chest radiographs reveals that long line shadows sometime occur which cannot be attributed to interlobar fissures, interlobular septa, blood vessels, bronchi, or any other structures. Such lines may be classified into two groups in two ways as follows:

A		B
Lines visible in anterior and lateral projections	*or*	Lines visible in one projection only
Approximately horizontal lines (cutting across the bronchi)		Nonhorizontal lines in any position

Horizontal lines are usually visible in anterior and lateral projections. They are generally called Fleischner's plate atelectasis after Fleischner,[1] who originally

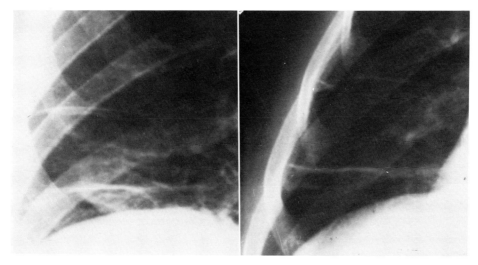

Fig. 11-23. So-called Fleischner's plate atelectasis radiographed at fluoroscopy in different degrees of rotation of patient. (From Trapnell, D. H.: Radiol. Clin. North Am. **11**:77, 1973.)

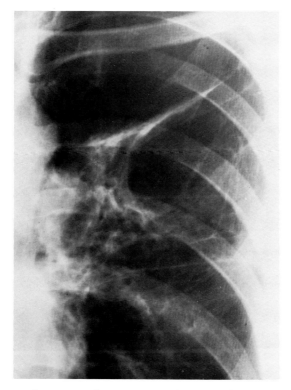

Fig. 11-24. Long irregular line shadows in lung following radiotherapy. Gradual shrinkage later changed the appearances of the shadows.

described them (Fig. 11-23). Nonhorizontal long lines are normally visible in one projection only (Fig. 11-24).

These two classifications record different aspects of the same diagnostic problems. Here is an important area for future research. As far as I know, there has been no exact radiologic-pathologic correlation demonstrating beyond doubt the mechanism by which the long lines in groups A or B are produced. In place of facts, therefore, we must accept (for the time being) current theory to explain the appearances.

Horizontal linear shadows visible in projections at right angles to each other. To cast shadows of this kind there must be sheetlike or platelike zones of airlessness in the lung. In such cases multiple tomographic sections will confirm (although such confirmation is rarely necessary) the three-dimensional shape of the airless zone. Such "plates" usually cut across the path of the bronchi and blood vessels. What process can produce this widely distributed but very thin sheetlike zone of airless lung in such a position has never been explained. Fleischner's[1] suggestion that it is "atelectasis" (i.e., airless lung) seems to fit the clinical observations that there may be no evidence of infection and that as ventilation of the lung is improved, the lines disappear Such lines may be multiple and most commonly occur when diaphragmatic movement is restricted.

Lines visible in one projection only, usually not horizontal. As indicated before, lines that do not conform to normal pulmonary anatomy are often said to arise in the pleura or in grossly disorganized lung. If the pleura is to cast line shadows, it must have a fold or crease in it to produce the sheetlike structure causing the line. This hypothesis is perfectly reasonable but still needs more strictly controlled evidence to support it. In some forms of pulmonary fibrosis such as that associated with progressive massive fibrosis or following radiotherapy to the lung (Fig. 11-24), similar line shadows occur. In this case, too, the cause may be pleural, but sheets of scarred lung may presumably produce identical appearances. Although the distinction may be academic from the management point of view, more factual evidence is urgently needed. In the lung the most likely cause for such sheetlike structures is fibrous thickening of the superficial and deep interlobar septa.

CONCLUSION

Careful observation of linear shadows in chest radiographs is the only valid basis for rational (and thus reliable) radiologic diagnosis. It is surely better to confess, if necessary, that the cause of a line is not understood than carelessly to call it linear atelectasis or some such thing. If this chapter has achieved nothing else, I hope it may be a stimulus to further research along these fascinating lines!

References

1. Fleischner, F. G., Hampton, A. O., and Castleman, B.: Linear shadows in the lung (interlobular pleuritis, atelectasis and healed infarction), Am. J. Roentgenol. Radium Ther. Nucl. Med. **46:** 610, 1941.

2. Fleischner, F. G., and Reiner, L.: Linear x-ray shadows in acquired pulmonary hemosiderosis and congestion, N. Engl. J. Med. **250**:900, 1954.

3. Heitzman, E. R.: The lung: radiologic and pathologic correlations, St. Louis, 1973, The C. V. Mosby Co.

4. Ngan, H., Millard, R. J., Lant, A. F., and Trapnell, D. H.: Nitrofurantoin lung, Br. J. Radiol. **44**:21, 1971.

5. Reid, L.: The pathology of emphysema, London, 1967, Lloyd-Luke, Ltd.

5a. Shanks, S. C., and Kerley, P., editors: A textbook of x-ray diagnosis, ed. 2, London, 1951, H. K. Lewis Ltd., Publishers.

6. Short, D. S.: Radiology of the lung in severe mitral stenosis, Br. Heart J. **17**: 33, 1955.

7. Simon, G.: Principles of chest x-ray diagnosis, ed. 3, London, 1971, Butterworth & Co. Publishers Ltd.

8. Trapnell, D. H.: The peripheral lymphatics of the lung, Br. J. Radiol. **36**: 660, 1963.

9. Trapnell, D. H.: Radiological appearances of lymphangitis carcinomatosa, Thorax **19**:251, 1964.

10. Trapnell, D. H.: Septal lines in pneumoconiosis, Br. J. Radiol. **37**:805, 1964.

11. Trapnell, D. H.: Septal lines in sarcoidosis, Br. J. Radiol. **37**:811, 1964.

12. Trapnell, D. H.: Principles of x-ray diagnosis, London, 1967, Butterworth & Co. Publishers Ltd.

13. Trapnell, D. H.: The blood vessels and lymphatics of the lung. In MacLaren, J. W., editor: Modern trends in diagnostic radiology, London, 1970, Butterworth & Co. Publishers Ltd.

14. Trapnell, D. H.: The differential diagnosis of linear shadows in chest radiographs, Radiol. Clin. North Am. **11**: 77, 1973.

12 Radionuclide imaging
of the myocardium

Frederick J. Bonte and Robert W. Parkey

Imaging of the myocardium with radionuclide tracers is directed toward the estimation of myocardial perfusion and blood flow and the detection of ischemic heart disease. For many years nuclear physicians and their cohorts worked diligently but unsuccessfully to develop imaging procedures for the visualization of the myocardium and its diseases. Recently, however, they have acquired new imaging technologies and equipment and developed new radiopharmaceuticals. This combination has evolved into a group of truly promising diagnostic procedures. Two classes of myocardial imaging tests have emerged: (1) imaging of the perfused, presumably normal, myocardium or its vasculature and (2) imaging of the abnormal or diseased myocardium.

IMAGING OF PERFUSED MYOCARDIUM

The earliest successful efforts at myocardial imaging were achieved using "intracellular" cations such as potassium and its analogs as tracers. Potassium 42, the most readily available radioisotope of potassium, emits photons of an energy too high for imaging purposes. As a result, many analog radionuclides have been investigated as possible tracers, including radioisotopes of rubidium (^{18}Rb,[21] ^{86}Rb[6, 23]), cesium (^{129}Cs,[28] ^{131}Cs[9]), and thallium (^{201}Tl[22]). The most widely used cation tracers to date have been ^{43}K[19] and ^{201}Tl.[31] Potassium 43 has principal gamma energies of 373 and 619 keV that are better suited to the detectors and collimators available with rectilinear scanners than to those of scintillation cameras, the leading family of imaging devices at the present time. More recently ^{201}Tl has become available and is replacing ^{43}K as a cation tracer. With biologic properties similar to potassium, its half-life of 74 hours, gamma photopeaks of 130 to 160 keV, and an x-ray photon of 81 keV make it more suitable for camera imaging.

Fig. 12-1 is a rectilinear scan of the chest of a normal dog, made in the left anterior oblique projection and begun a few minutes after the intravenous administration of 2.0 mCi of ^{43}KCl. The spherical structure visualized (Fig. 12-1, *H*) represents principally the thick musculature of the left ventricular wall. The ring, or "doughnut," configuration is due to the lower radioactivity of blood

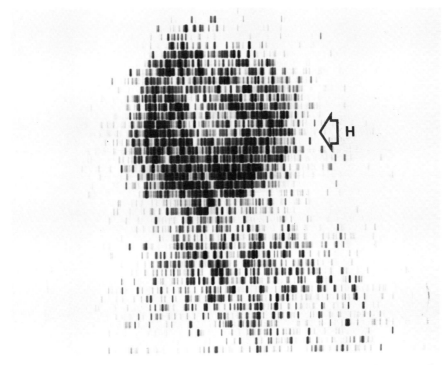

Fig. 12-1. Rectilinear scan of chest and upper abdomen of a normal 20 kg dog begun shortly after intravenous injection of 2.0 mCi of ^{43}KCl. Ring-shaped structure *(H)* principally represents image of thick left ventricular wall. Structure caudad to heart is liver.

in the left ventricular chamber. A myocardial infarct will appear as a defect, or area of low radioactivity, within the normal pattern (Fig. 12-2, *B*).

Strauss and Zaret et al.[30, 35] have used ^{43}K imaging to demonstrate areas of transient myocardial ischemia resulting from exercise. Fig. 12-2, *A*, represents the "resting" ^{43}K scintigram of a young serviceman. His normal ECG appears below the scan. On the following day the authors brought the patient back and injected a second dose of ^{43}KCl after 30 minutes of treadmill exercise, during which angina developed. Fig. 12-2, *B*, shows a defect in the distribution of ^{43}K, indicating impaired perfusion of the myocardium in the area of question. Note also the appearance of the ECG. This remains the method of choice for demonstrating transient areas of myocardial ischemia.

Other families of myocardial imaging tracers have been studied. The most promising seem to be labeled long-chain unsaturated fatty acids. In 1956 Dole[12] and Gordon and Cherkes[15] showed that unsaturated plasma fatty acids serve as a prime energy source for myocardial metabolism.[12, 15] Evans et al.[13] succeeded in obtaining rectilinear scans of the myocardium of experimental animals and volunteer patients with ^{131}I-labeled oleic acid. Several investigators[4, 26] have confirmed Evans' work and have studied other compounds that can be labeled while preserving the unsaturated bond. Presently the most promising of these seems to

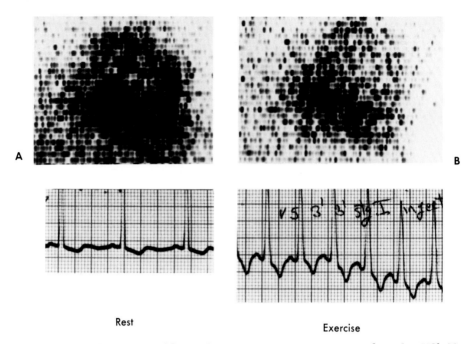

Rest

Exercise

Fig. 12-2. **A,** Rectilinear scan of heart of a young serviceman at rest made with ⁴³KCl. Note relatively normal resting ECG. **B,** Repeat ⁴³KCl scan of same individual following exercise, which produced angina pectoris. Note appearance of a defect in scan pattern of left ventricle superiorly, representing an area of transient myocardial ischemia. ECG has now become markedly abnormal. (Reprinted by permission from N. Engl. J. Med.: Zaret, B. L., et al.: **288:**809, 1973.)

be ¹⁶iodo,9,10-hexadecenoic acid labeled with ¹³¹I or ¹²³I. If this compound could be successfully and reproducibly labeled with ⁹⁹ᵐTc, it might become the agent of choice for imaging the normally perfused myocardium.

Harper et al.[17] have obtained myocardial scintigrams with ¹³N ammonia made in their cyclotron laboratory. Although the 511 KeV annihilation radiation of ¹³N presented collimation problems when they attempted to use a scintillation camera for imaging purposes, they have shown convincing demonstrations of myocardial infarcts, which appeared as defects in the pattern of left ventricular myocardial radioactivity. Tomographic and positron cameras are being developed and show great promise.[32] These have been used with the short-life cyclotron-produced radionuclides.[25] Although this work is interesting, the very short half-lives preclude the use of these tracers in institutions other than those equipped with cyclotrons.

An alternative approach to myocardial imaging was described by Quinn et al.,[27] who injected macroaggregated serum albumin labeled with ¹³¹I into coronary arteries. After the particles had wedged in distal coronary arteries, scintigrams were secured, which in effect showed the distribution of the myocardial arterial vasculature. Other groups[1, 16] have extended Quinn's work to volunteer patients using ⁹⁹ᵐTc-labeled particulates and have demonstrated defects in the vascular distribution pattern that can be equated with coronary artery disease. Problems arise due to incomplete mixing of the particles with blood, "streaming" or laminar flow, and direct injection of the particles into a branch of a coronary artery. Although transient ECG abnormalities have been observed, no serious complications have occurred in patients studied by this method.[16]

Images of the perfused myocardium have also been made following the intra-coronary-arterial injection of a diffusible indicator such as [133]Xe. Xenon injection is usually done in conjunction with roentgen coronary arteriography for the purposes of determining mean and regional myocardial blood flow. Although images of the distribution of the coronary vasculature may be obtained, they are of less value than the quantitative blood flow information that may be generated by computer treatment of the image data.[2, 5]

IMAGING OF ABNORMAL MYOCARDIUM

The end result of coronary vascular disease is myocardial ischemia leading to infarction. As one of the major causes of death in the United States, myo-cardial infarction has engaged the attention of nuclear physicians since the de-velopment of nuclear imaging techniques. Very likely, the earliest successful attempts to image myocardial infarcts were those of Carr et al.[7, 8] employing chlormerodrin labeled with [203]Hg. However, the test was not sufficiently reproducible to be considered reliable, and the search turned to other agents.

Recognizing that myocardial infarction was characterized by necrosis (per-haps the basis for occasional successful labeling with chlormerodrin), we tried unsuccessfully to label infarcts with ^{131}I fluorescein. However, this approach was brought to fruition by Holman et al.,[18] using ^{99m}Tc tetracycline.

Fig. 12-3 shows a study performed by Holman et al.[18] The patient was imaged 26 hours after the administration of 15 mCi of ^{99m}Tc tetracycline. Note the localization of agent in a pattern corresponding to the distribution of a clini-cally proved inferior myocardial infarct. This technique represented a further advance.

The process of myocardial infarction and necrosis frequently features the presence of a macrophage population, suggesting that ^{67}Ga citrate might be use-ful for infarct imaging. Although Kramer et al.[20] have reported encouraging pre-liminary results, this agent is not truly a useful one.

In studying the migration of calcium ion into dying myocardial cells, D'Agos-tino and Chiga[10, 11] observed electron-dense crystals within the mitochondria of the involved cells and identified these as hydroxyapatite. Later, Shen and Jen-nings[29] studied the infarction process and related mitochondrial calcium deposi-tion to irreversible cellular damage. Accordingly, we[3] attempted to label experi-mental canine myocardial infarcts with a family of radiopharmaceuticals utilized for bone imaging. The tracer we initially selected was ^{99m}Tc stannous pyrophos-phate, and extensive animal distribution studies have suggested that this agent may have slightly better distribution features at optimal imaging time than other

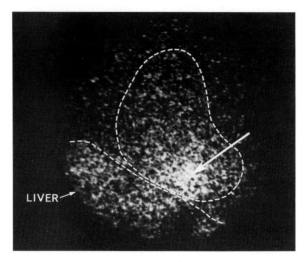

LIVER

Fig. 12-3. Anterior view of thorax and upper abdomen of a patient with evidence of an inferior myocardial infarct. Long arrow indicates focal uptake of ^{99m}Tc tetracycline in the infarct. Dotted lines outline cardiac silhouette and indicate level of diaphragm. (Courtesy B. L. Holman, M.D.)

agents of this family (such as diphosphonate and the polyphosphates) that were available at the time this study was performed.

A representative canine experiment is seen in Fig. 12-4. Fig. 12-4, *A*, is the left lateral scintigram of the thorax of a dog made an hour after the administration of the tracer of ^{99m}Tc stannous pyrophosphate (PYP). The anticipated skeletal distribution is seen. Fig. 12-4, *B*, is the lateral chest radiograph of the same animal made after instillation of 0.1 ml of metallic mercury into branches of the anterior descending coronary artery, an experimental technique utilized to produce myocardial infarction. Fig. 12-4, *C*, made 24 hours after Fig. 12-4, *B*, and an hour after intravenous administration of 3.0 mCi of ^{99m}Tc PYP shows localization of the tracer in a site corresponding to that of the experimental infarct. Fig. 12-4, *D*, represents a left lateral scintigram of the same animal 2 weeks after infarction, showing disappearance of the localization phenomenon as an index of recovery.

Following appropriate animal tissue distribution and toxicologic studies we began to employ infarct imaging in patient volunteers.[24] Initially we worked in the Nuclear Medicine Laboratory, but our most recent 3000 patients were imaged at the bedside in the Coronary Care Unit with a mobile scintillation camera system. We presently administer 15 mCi of ^{99m}Tc in 5 mg of pyrophosphate and obtain images an hour later. Anterior, left anterior oblique, and left lateral views are obtained, to a total of 200,000 to 300,000 counts per image.

We have found that the image of a myocardial infarct becomes detectable within 18 to 24 hours after the occurrence of infarction. The image attains maximum clarity on the second or third day postinfarction and then begins to fade. The pattern often returns to normal by 7 days and certainly should become nor-

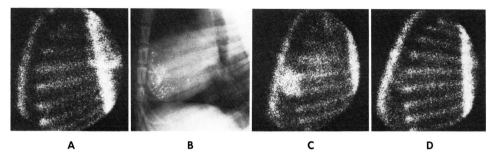

A   **B**   **C**   **D**

Fig. 12-4. **A,** Left lateral scintigram of thorax of a normal 20 kg dog made an hour after administration of ⁹⁹ᵐTc stannous pyrophosphate showing anticipated skeletal distribution. **B,** Lateral chest radiograph of same animal after instillation of 0.1 ml of metallic Hg embolus into branches of anterior descending artery. Procedure resulted in anterior myocardial infarction. **C,** Lateral thoracic scintigram made 24 hours after **B** and an hour after administration of ⁹⁹ᵐTc PYP showing localization of tracer in a site corresponding to experimental infarct. **D,** Left lateral scintigram made 2 weeks after infarction showing disappearance of localization phenomenon. (From Bonte, F. J., et al.: Radiology **110:**473, 1974.)

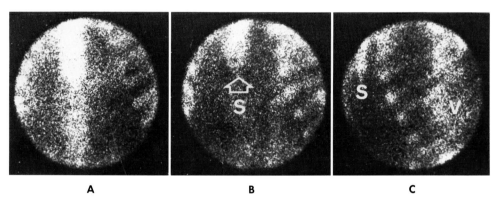

A   **B**   **C**

Fig. 12-5. **A,** Negative scintigram of a patient without acute myocardial infarction made an hour after administration of ⁹⁹ᵐTc PYP. Anterior projection. **B,** 45° left anterior oblique view of same patient. S denotes sternum. **C,** Left lateral view. S denotes sternum and V thoracic spine. (From Parkey, R. W., et al.: Circulation **50:**540, 1974. Reprinted by permission of the American Heart Association, Inc.)

mal within 10 to 14 days. As a matter of fact, the disappearance of localization is evidence of infarct healing. If it does not occur, or if the image of the infarct becomes larger, a diagnosis of extension may be made.

In interpreting myocardial infarct scintigrams, one must first be familiar with the normal PYP image of the thorax, as seen in Fig. 12-5, which shows anterior, oblique, and left lateral views of the thorax of a patient with chest pain who was found not to have had a myocardial infarct. Normal features of this type of image include sternum *(S)*, ribs, and spine *(V)*.

When present, the myocardial infarct appears as a "hot" area, superimposing the normal PYP distribution, as in Fig. 12-6. This is a small transmural infarct, and its anterior location becomes apparent from its position adjacent to the sternum in the lateral view (Fig. 12-6, *C*).

An infarct in a more lateral and posterior position gives the appearance seen in Fig. 12-7. Note that with rotation the sharply defined infarct localization moves away from the sternum. This phenomenon aids in the physical localization of the infarct. Work is now underway to determine whether scintigrams in several projections might be used to estimate infarct size, which, in turn, could aid in predicting the kind of recovery a given patient might expect.

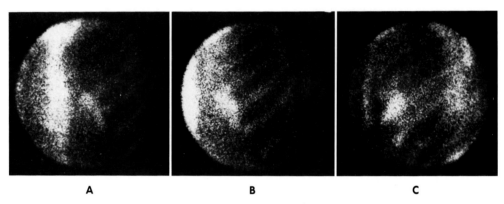

A   **B**   **C**

Fig. 12-6. A, Positive 99mTc PYP scintigram of a patient with proved anterior wall infarct. Anterior projection. **B,** 45° left anterior oblique scintigram shows anterior wall infarct rotating with sternum. **C,** Left lateral scintigram shows anterior location of infarct localization. (From Parkey, R. W., et al.: Circulation **50:**540, 1974. Reprinted by permission of the American Heart Association, Inc.)

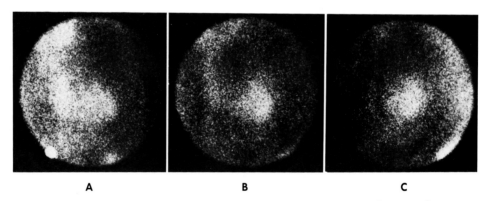

A   **B**   **C**

Fig. 12-7. A, Positive 99mTc PYP scintigram of a patient with proved lateral and posterior wall infarct. Anterior projection. **B,** 45° left anterior oblique view. **C,** Left lateral view showing localization rotating away from sternum, indicating its lateral and posterior position. (From Parkey, R. W., et al.: Circulation **50:**540, 1974. Reprinted by permission of the American Heart Association, Inc.)

Myocardial infarct imaging with TcP agents will probably detect about 95% of transmural infarcts, failing to detect only the very small ones. With thin, flat subendocardial infarcts, however, localizations are sometimes subtle[33] and the chance for error is greater than with the transmural type. False-positive localizations may be obtained in 10% to 15% of all patients, generally caused by diffuse myocardial disease such as that found in patients with "unstable angina pectoris."

The search for other radiopharmaceuticals for myocardial infarct imaging continues,[14] and perhaps the ultimate agent has not yet been described. However, it seems clear that myocardial infarct imaging has considerable merit and will soon become one of the most frequently performed radionuclide imaging studies.

References

1. Ashburn, W. L., Braunwald, E., Simon, A. L., and Gault, J. H.: Myocardial perfusion imaging in man using ^{99m}Tc-MAA, J. Nucl. Med. **11**:618, 1970.
2. Bonte, F. J., et al.: Radionuclide determination of myocardial blood flow, Semin. Nucl. Med. **3**:153, 1973.
3. Bonte, F. J., et al.: A new method for radionuclide imaging of myocardial infarcts, Radiology **110**:473, 1974.
4. Bonte, F. J., Graham, K. D., and Moore, J. G.: Experimental myocardial imaging with ^{131}I-labeled oleic acid, Radiology **168**:195, 1973.
5. Cannon, E. J., Dell, R. B., and Dwyer, E. M.: Measurement of regional myocardial perfusion in man with ^{133}Xe and a scintillation camera, J. Clin. Invest. **51**:964, 1972.
6. Carr, E. A., Beierwaltes, W. H., Wegst, A. V., and Bartlett, J. D.: Myocardial scanning with rubidium-86, J. Nucl. Med. **3**:76, 1962.
7. Carr, E. A., Cafruny, E. J., and Bartlett, J. D.: Evaluation of ^{203}Hg-chlormerodrin in the demonstration of human myocardial infarcts by scanning, Univ. Mich. Med. Cent. J. **29**:27, 1963.
8. Carr, E. A., et al.: The detection of experimental myocardial infarcts by photoscanning, Am. Heart J. **64**:650, 1962.
9. Carr, E. A., Gleason, G., Shaw, J., and Krontz, B.: Direct diagnosis of myocardial infarction by photoscanning after the administration of cesium-131, Am. Heart J. **68**:627, 1964.
10. D'Agostino, A. N.: An electron microscopic study of cardiac necrosis produced by 9α-fluorocortisol and sodium phosphate, Am. J. Pathol. **45**:63, 1964.
11. D'Agostino, A. N., and Chiga, M.: Mitochondrial mineralization in human myocardium, Am. J. Clin. Pathol. **53**:820, 1970.
12. Dole, V. P.: A relation between nonesterified fatty acids in plasma and the metabolism of glucose, J. Clin. Invest. **35**:150, 1956.
13. Evans, J. R., et al.: Use of radioiodinated fatty acid for photoscans of the heart, Circ. Res. **16**:1, 1965.
14. Fink-Bennett, D., Dworkin, H. J., and Lee, Y.-H.: Myocardial imaging of the acute infarct, Radiology **113**:449, 1974.
15. Gordon, R. S., and Cherkes, A.: Unesterified fatty acid in human blood plasma, J. Clin. Invest. **35**:206, 1956.
16. Grames, G. M., et al.: Safety of the direct coronary injection of radiolabeled particles, J. Nucl. Med. **15**:2, 1974.
17. Harper, P. V., et al.: Clinical feasibility of myocardial imaging with ^{13}NH$_3$, J. Nuc. Med. **13**:278, 1972.
18. Holman, B. L., et al.: Detection and localization of experimental myocardial infarction with ^{99m}Tc-tetracycline, J. Nucl. Med. **14**:595, 1973.
19. Hurley, P. J., et al.: ^{43}KCl: a new pharmaceutical for imaging the heart, J. Nucl. Med. **12**:516, 1971.
20. Kramer, R. J., et al.: Myocardial infarct imaging with ^{67}Ga-citrate, J. Nucl. Med. **14**:418, 1973.
21. Lamb, J. S., Khentigan, A., Baker, G. A., and Winchell, H. S.: Rubidium-81 in evaluation of regional myocardial perfusion, J. Nucl. Med. **15**:509, 1974.
22. Lebowitz, E., et al.: Thallium-201 for medical use, J. Nucl. Med. **16**:151, 1975.

23. Nolting, D., et al.: Measurement of coronary blood flow and myocardial rubidium uptake with Rb-86, J. Clin. Invest. **37**:921, 1958.

24. Parkey, R. W., et al.: A new method of radionuclide imaging of acute myocardial infarction in humans, Circulation **50**:540, 1974.

25. Phelps, M. E., Hoffman, E. J., Mullani, N. A., and Ter-Pogossian, M. M.: Application of annihilation coincidence detection to transaxial reconstruction tomography, J. Nucl. Med. **16**:210, 1975.

26. Poe, N. D., et al.: Evaluation of 16-iodo-hexadecenoic acid as an indicator of regional myocardial perfusion, J. Nucl. Med. **15**:524, 1974.

27. Quinn, J. L., Serratto, M., and Kezdi, P.: Coronary artery bed photoscanning using radioiodine albumin macroaggregates (RAMA), J. Nucl. Med. **7**:107, 1966.

28. Romhilt, D. W., et al.: Cesium-129 myocardial scintigraphy to detect myocardial infarction, Circulation **48**:1242, 1973.

29. Shen, A. C., and Jennings, R. B.: Kinetics of calcium accumulation in acute myocardial ischemic injury, Am. J. Pathol. **67**:441, 1972.

30. Strauss, H. W., et al.: Noninvasive evaluation of regional myocardial perfusion with potassium-43. Technique in patients with exercise-induced transient myocardial ischemia, Radiology **108**:85, 1973.

31. Strauss, H. W., et al.: Thallium-201 for myocardial imaging: relation of thallium-201 to regional myocardial perfusion, Circulation **51**:641, 1975.

32. Ter-Pogossian, M. M., Phelps, M. E., Hoffman, E. J., and Mullani, N. A.: Positron-emission transaxial tomograph for nuclear imaging (PETT), Radiology **114**:89, 1975.

33. Willerson, J. T., et al.: Acute subendocardial myocardial infarction in patients; its detection by technetium-99m stannous pyrophosphate myocardial scintigrams, Circulation **51**:436, 1975.

34. Willerson, J. T., et al.: Technetium stannous pyrophosphate myocardial scintigrams in patients with chest pain of varying etiology, Circulation **51**:1046, 1975.

35. Zaret, B. L., et al.: Noninvasive regional myocardial perfusion with radioactive potassium; studies of patients at rest, with exercise, and during angina pectoris, N. Engl. J. Med. **288**:809, 1973.

13 Thrombus detection

R. Edward Coleman, John F. Harwig, and Michael J. Welch

Deep venous thrombosis is a common complication in hospitalized patients. Autopsy series have shown that deep venous thrombosis and pulmonary emboli are common and usually not detected prior to death.[5, 29, 58] In thorough autopsy investigations with careful dissection of the venous system of the lower extremities, antemortem venous thrombosis is found in 50% to 80% of the autopsies.[31, 90, 106] Phlebography and the fibrinogen uptake test have more recently confirmed the high incidence of deep venous thrombosis in various patient groups and have demonstrated the lack of signs and symptoms associated with venous thrombosis, which makes clinical diagnosis difficult.[27, 59, 86] So that early therapy of deep venous thrombosis can be instituted to prevent immediate complications, such as pulmonary embolism, and late sequelae, such as the postphlebitic syndrome, many tests have been evaluated for the early detection of venous thrombosis, including the fibrinogen uptake test,[27, 58, 59, 86] ultrasound,[25, 112] and electrical impedance test.[54, 121] Venography is still the most precise method for demonstrating the presence or absence of venous thrombosis, but repetitive studies are impractical and may be associated with complications.[94, 118] Since the fibrinogen uptake test has been shown to be a safe, accurate method of detecting forming thrombi,[59] it has been used to screen large groups of patients to define the incidence of venous thrombosis in a variety of conditions,[26, 28, 59, 85] to study the natural history of thrombi,[55] and to determine the effects of anticoagulant or thrombolytic therapy.[30, 44, 56] Other radiopharmaceuticals have been tested for detecting venous thrombosis, but none has gained widespread acceptance. Several agents are presently being evaluated as tracers to be used to image venous thrombi,[12, 19, 80] pulmonary thromboemboli,[99] and coronary artery thrombi.[83]

FIBRINOGEN UPTAKE TEST
History

Hobbs and Davies[49] in 1960 first demonstrated that an experimentally induced venous thrombus could be localized with an external radiation detector after the administration of labeled fibrinogen. Hobbs[48] subsequently found no difference in labeled fibrinogen accumulation in experimentally induced thrombo-

313

phlebitis and phlebothrombosis and was able to localize thrombi when the labeled fibrinogen was administered 48 hours after thrombosis.

Palko, Nanson, and Fedoruk[89] demonstrated that ^{131}I-fibrinogen is accumulated in forming thrombi in dogs and these thrombi can be detected by external monitoring. They also studied patients and found the test useful in detecting active venous thrombosis. They suggested that the ^{131}I-fibrinogen test could be used during surgery to follow patients who are prone to thrombosis or who have signs or symptoms suggesting deep venous thrombosis.

Atkins and Hawkins[2] in 1965 used ^{125}I-fibrinogen for detecting venous thrombi in patients. The ^{125}I-fibrinogen requires less collimation than does the ^{131}I-fibrinogen, since the energy of radiation of ^{125}I is lower than that of [131]I. Since less collimation is needed, the counting apparatus can be more portable, and the equipment can be transported to the bedside. An additional advantage in using ^{125}I instead of ^{131}I includes the longer half-life of ^{125}I, which gives the radiopharmaceutical a longer shelf life and permits the test to be followed for a longer time after injection. The disadvantages of using ^{125}I instead of ^{131}I are the greater tissue adsorption with ^{125}I and the inability to image the radiation of [125]I.

Iodination of fibrinogen

Since the results from the fibrinogen uptake test depend on the preparation of the iodinated fibrinogen, the iodination of fibrinogen will be discussed in detail. In labeling fibrinogen, two aspects need to be considered—the separation of the fibrinogen from other blood products and the iodination of the separated fibrinogen. The earliest methods for the precipitation of fibrinogen used salts and buffers, but organic solvents such as ethanol and ether were also found useful. Since fibrinogen differs from most other plasma proteins in its low solubility at low temperatures, Ware, Guest, and Seegers[119] were able to develop a simple separation based on freezing (−30° C) and slowly thawing plasma. More recent methods have employed several readily soluble amino acids such as glycine[8, 84] and β-alanine.[113] Blombäck and Blombäck[8] found that fibrinogen prepared by salt precipitation, by freezing out, or by alcohol fractionation was not sufficiently purified from prothrombin or plasminogen to be stable. Perhaps theirs is the most commonly used fibrinogen separation procedure, which will be discussed in some detail.

The Blombäck method uses glycine and alcohol fractionation to separate several fibrinogen fractions. Blood is collected in sterile vials with acid citrate dextrose (ACD) as the anticoagulant. The cells are separated by centrifugation at 1000 g and +10° C for 60 minutes. The first precipitation[14] is Cohn fraction I and is from an ethanol-sodium acetate buffer centrifuged at −3° C. The wet yield is 2.5 to 3 gm/100 ml of human plasma, and the protein is 40% to 50% coagulable with thrombin. This precipitate is extracted using citrate buffer (pH 6.0) with 6.5% ethanol and 1M glycine—ionic strength 0.3. The Cohn fraction I precipitate is suspended and stirred for an hour at −3° C followed by centrifugation at 2000 g for 12 minutes. This extraction is done twice, and the final precipitate is denoted Blombäck fraction I-0. It can be stored safely at –20° C and contains 85% to 89% coagulable protein. The conditions for the remaining Blombäck separations use ethanol-glycine solutions at low temperatures followed by centrifugation. All these preparations are from pH 6.35 ± 0.05 citrate buffer. Precipitates I-1 and I-3 are cold insoluble globulins containing 20% and 10%, respectively, of true fibrinogen. Precipitates I-2 and I-4 are good fibrinogen preparations with yields of about 175 and 100 mg/100 ml of starting plasma.

Although other fibrinogen separations have been developed,[62, 63, 84, 113] they tend to be based on the Blombäck procedure, which is the most commonly used. Because of the risk of hepatitis in using fibrinogen obtained from pooled plasma, there has been great interest in obtaining preparations of autologous fibrinogen for iodination. Bettingole et al.[7] reported a preparation requiring 3 to 5 hours to obtain low yields of labeled fibrinogen. Roberts, Sonnentag, and Frisbie[101] adapted the technique of Ingraham, Silberstein, Kereiakes, and Wellman[53] to prepare labeled autologous fibrinogen in 2 hours. In the Roberts procedure two ammonium sulfate precipitations are performed; in the Ingraham preparation a single glycine precipitation is performed. The problems with rapid preparations of autologous fibrinogen are fourfold: (1) the process will not remove cold insoluble material that clears rapidly from the blood; (2) radiopharmaceutical quality controls need to be performed on each preparation for each patient; (3) a 2-hour preparation and the time required for quality control increases the cost of the study to the patient; and (4) these fast methods of separation do not completely remove contaminants.

The contaminants most damaging to a fibrinogen preparation are plasminogen and prothrombin. Prothrombin has been effectively removed by adsorption on $BaSO_4$ (100 mg/ml of plasma),[113] and charcoal has been used for adsorption of plasminogen.[76] Plasminogen can also be inactivated by addition of ε-aminocaproic acid.[1] None of the fractionation procedures presented results in complete removal of these two contaminants. Plasminogen is the most troublesome. The use of n-octanol as an antifoaming agent during stirring of fibrinogen precipitates has been found useful and shows no negative effects.[113] Once the fibrinogen has been separated, there are several methods available for the iodination of the protein. Since fibrinogen is easily denatured, a labeling method must be examined closely to see if the preparation is a satisfactory one.

ICl iodination. In our laboratory, labeling with iodine monochloride is carried out by the Samoles and Williams[103] modification of the MacFarlane[73] procedure and also by the Helmkamp[45] modification. For the former procedure a few microliters of [125]I (or ^{131}I) are equilibrated with a small amount of ICl in 0.4 ml of 2M NaCl at pH 4.0. The amount of iodine monochloride is adjusted to give the desired number of iodine atoms per molecule of protein. This solution is added to an equal volume of borate buffer (pH 7.9, 0.4M, 0.11M NaCl). Borate buffer is then added to the fibrinogen stock solution to give a volume equal to that of the ICl solution. After mixing these two solutions, the reaction mixture is agitated for 15 minutes before removal of free I⁻, usually by Sephadex chromatography.

In the Helmkamp procedure ICl is produced by mixing 0.34 ml of KI solution (0.067 μmol), a tracer solution of Na*I, and 0.5 ml of saturated NaCl. This is diluted with water to give a total volume of 3 ml after addition of 0.15 ml of 0.5M HCl and KIO_3. Enough KIO_3 is added to give a 2:5 molar ratio of KIO_3 to I⁻. After 5 minutes an aliquot of this solution is added to the fibrinogen in 2 ml of borate buffer to which 0.25 ml of 0.5M NaOH has just been added.

Chloramine-T method. The chloramine-T method developed by Hunter and Greenwood[50, 51] has been modified by Krohn, Sherman, and Welch[68] to study the effect of the chloramine-T to protein ratio on the properties of the fibrinogen. In this procedure from 5 to 200 mg of fibrinogen was added to 50 ml of phosphate buffer (pH 7.8, 0.05M) and carrier-free Na*I followed by 25 ml of freshly prepared chloramine-T (sodium N-monochloro-p-toluene-sulfonamide) in phosphate buffer. In some cases sodium metabisulfite was added to quench the reaction mixture. Other workers have used the Bocci[9] modification of the chloramine-T method to label fibrinogen. In this method a high (250:1) ratio of chloramine-T to protein is used and the mixture is agitated for 30 minutes before addition of the sodium metabisulfite.

Electrolytic iodination. Several groups[68, 102, 117] have investigated the electrolytic method of iodinating fibrinogen. Rosa et al.[102] use a three-electrode cell made from a glass beaker with a cylindrical platinum sheet as anode, a platinum wire as cathode (surrounded by a dialysis membrane), with a reference calomel electrode in the anodic compartment. They operated the cell at constant current ($\sim$ 300 μamps) with 100 mg of fibrinogen in 0.9% NaCl and 2.5×10^{-4} mm of KI containing the radioiodine making up the electrolyte. Teulings and Biggs[117] operated at 4.5 volts (approximately 300 μamps current) in a similar cell containing only two electrodes. They iodinated using a similar solution, carrying out the iodination for 18 minutes. Krohn, Sherman, and Welch[68] followed the procedure of Katz and Bonorris[61] in which electrolysis was carried out in a 15 ml platinum crucible, which served as the anode. The crucible contained 7 ml of 0.05M phosphate buffer (pH 7.8) to which was added fibrinogen (1 to 5 mg) and Na*I; this solution is made 0.1M in sodium chloride. The cathode was a platinum wire, and various voltages and currents were studied.

Enzymatic iodination. Enzymatic labeling of fibrinogen using peroxidase, which has been used for labeling other proteins,[74, 82] has been reported.[69] This method requires the reaction of lactoperoxidase, carrier-free radioiodine, and the compound to be labeled with nanomolar quantities of H_2O_2. With the following procedure, yields as high as 75% ± 10% labeling have been observed.[69] To 100 μl of buffer (pH 8.0), 250 μg of protein, 5 μg of a crude enzyme preparation, and the desired amount of carrier-free radioiodine are added. The reactants should be equilibrated at 37° C before 10 nanomoles of H_2O_2 are added. The reaction mixture must be incubated with shaking for 30 minutes to give a maximum yield.

Properties of labeled preparations

The rate of catabolism of fibrinogen has been shown[73] to be increased by iodination at a level of 0.5 atom of iodine per fibrinogen molecule, whereas clottability measurements are not affected by large amounts of iodination.[95] Laki and Steiner[71] and Yalow and Berson[123] have studied iodinated fibrinogen with up to 90 gram atoms per 10^5 grams of native protein and found that this material still clotted with thrombin. Simply measuring the clottability does not appear to be a valid method of determining the biologic effectiveness of iodinated fibrinogen, since highly iodinated fibrinogen still clots but is cleared much more rapidly than preparations iodinated at lower levels.

Krohn, Sherman, and Welch[68] demonstrated similar findings using gel permeation chromatography on a Sepharose 4B column to evaluate the molecular weight profile of fibrinogen labeled by various methods. They found that under certain circumstances the labeling procedure tended to aggregate the fibrinogen, and, indeed, a large fraction of the fibrinogen did not even penetrate the column. When fibrinogen is radioiodinated by the chloramine-T method using the amount of reactant recommended by Hunter,[50] a product in which only 10% corresponds in molecular weight to authentic fibrinogen is obtained. Most of the remaining activity (80% ± 5%) is left on top of the column and is apparently aggregated to form a material that is physically too large to penetrate the gel. These aggregates have been separated from the gel by back flushing and have been shown to accumulate mainly in the liver.[78] The amount forming aggregates can be reduced by altering the original Hunter and Greenwood[50, 51] chloramine-T to protein ratio. As the amount of protein is increased, the amount of aggregation decreases. When using the electrolytic method under conditions of varying times, voltage, and current, approximately 47% of the fibrinogen was always found in the form of aggregates, whereas the ICl and enzymatic preparations chromatographed with little aggregation. Krohn, Sherman, and Welch[68, 69] also studied the in vitro hydrolysis of the various products and showed that in saline the iodine monochloride and enzymatic preparations were considerably more stable than the other two.

These physicochemical studies on the fibrinogen preparations have been shown[15, 77] to be in agreement with the biologic behavior of the products. Metzger et al.[77] fitted the blood clearance curves of the various labeled products to the sum of three exponential processes—the one with the longest half-life representing the catabolism of fibrinogen. The methods of preparation in order of greatest yield of fibrinogen clearing with a half-life corresponding to the catabolism of fibrinogen were iodine monochloride, enzymatic, electrolytic, and chloramine-T. The first two had considerably (two times) greater activity clearing with the correct half-life than the latter two, whereas even the chloramine-T prepared under conditions of high protein ratio behaved poorly. Coleman et al.[15] studied the thrombus to blood ratios in experimental thrombi induced in dogs. They found a similar trend with iodination method, observing that the ratios of activity in the thrombus to that in the blood were approximately 9, 6, 2.5, and 1.5

in the iodine monochloride, lactoperoxidase, chloramine-T, and electrolytic methods, respectively. It appears therefore that the physicochemical studies do give more information as to the expected biologic behavior of fibrinogen preparations and that the iodine monochloride and enzymatic methods of labeling are superior to the other two methods discussed. Since all the preparations discussed here were clottable with thrombin, it is obvious that clottability alone is no measure of the biologic effectiveness of a labeled fibrinogen preparation.

Procedure

Before the intravenous administration of ^{125}I-fibrinogen the patient is given an oral iodide solution to block thyroidal uptake of the radioactive iodine. If the labeled fibrinogen is to be injected before the oral iodide solution would be absorbed, sodium iodide (100 mg) may be administered intravenously. Oral iodide solution is continued once daily for 3 weeks. The first counts are obtained approximately 2 hours after injection. Prior to counting, the legs are elevated on a portable stand to decrease blood pooling in the legs. The legs are marked at six or seven positions on the thigh following a line from the femoral vein at the inguinal ligament to the adductor tubercle. Six or seven positions on the calf are marked from the middle of the popliteal fossa to the calcaneus. Two extra counts are obtained over each mid-calf region.

An isotope localization monitor (ratemeter), which is portable, simple, and fast is used for the study. The detector is initially placed on a previously marked location over the precordial area and the monitor adjusted to a reading of 100%. The subsequent counts are read from the monitor as a percentage of the precordial counts. Before counting the other leg, the detector is again placed over the marked precordial area to correct for any changes in the monitor.

In surgical patients, preoperative, postoperative, and alternate-day counts are obtained unless an abnormality is detected, and then counting is performed daily. In nonsurgical patients, counts are obtained 2 and 24 hours after injection and on alternate days thereafter. If any equivocal or abnormal areas are detected, counts are obtained daily.

Various criteria have been used to suggest thrombus formation in the legs. Thrombosis can be confidently diagnosed when a 20% or greater difference is noted between adjacent points on the same limb, a corresponding point on the opposite limb, or the same point from the previous day's count. The count should be elevated for at least 24 hours. Other criteria have been tried but are less accurate.

Clinical results

After the initial reports suggesting the labeled fibrinogen test to be reliable, several large studies were performed in Great Britain. Comparing the fibrinogen uptake test with phlebography, Kakkar[59] found that the two tests agreed in 82 of 88 (92%) patients. The false positive (5%) and false negative (2%) results were thought to be related to soleal vein thrombi missed by venography and old thrombi not actively forming, respectively. Browse[11] analyzed 102 patients with suspected deep venous thrombosis and found an 80% correlation with phlebography. However, several of these patients had thrombosis for more than 5 days. In a smaller group of patients, Milne et al.[81] found that all those with a positive venogram had abnormal fibrinogen uptake tests and all those with normal fibrinogen uptake tests had negative venograms. However, they did have a few patients with abnormal fibrinogen uptake tests and normal venograms.

Since the fibrinogen uptake test is reliable in detecting deep venous thrombosis and is simple to perform, it has been used to determine the incidence of venous thrombosis in various groups of patients by Kakkar and others.* Kakkar[59] found that in patients over 40 years of age undergoing elective surgery, 28% developed deep vein thombosis. Milne et al.[81] found similar results. Patients over age 50 had a greater than 50% incidence of venous thrombosis. Approximately 50% of the thrombi formed during the surgery or within 24 hours after surgery. The other thrombi occurred 3 to 7 days after surgery. In patients undergoing internal fixation for femoral neck fractures, 54% developed deep vein thrombosis. The incidence of venous thrombosis in patients undergoing retropubic prostatectomy was 50%, whereas in those having transurethral resection of the prostate the incidence was much lower (4%). The occurrence of deep vein thrombosis in obstetric patients was low (4%) but higher in gynecologic patients (18%). Gynecologic patients undergoing an abdominal operation had a greater incidence (24%) of venous thrombosis than those having a vaginal operation (9%). Of patients with acute myocardial infarction 19% developed deep vein thrombosis, and those with complications from their infarction had a greater incidence of deep vein thrombosis than those without complications.[85] The incidence of venous thrombosis following cerebrovascular accidents was 60% in a study by Warlow, Ogston, and Douglas.[120]

Some studies have not found a good correlation between the fibrinogen uptake test and venography. Mavor et al.[75] found that in 40 patients with pulmonary embolism and abnormal ileofemoral phlebography, only 2 had an abnormal fibrinogen uptake test. In 50 patients presenting with phlebographically proved occlusive ileofemoral thrombosis, only 15 had an abnormal fibrinogen test. A more recent study by Harris et al.[37] found that only 50% of fresh thrombi demonstrated by phlebography were detected by the fibrinogen uptake test. In neither of these two studies showing a poor correlation between venography and the fibrinogen uptake test is their method of labeling fibrinogen discussed or any data given concerning the labeled fibrinogen used. The fibrinogen used for evaluation can have a marked effect on the results obtained, as noted in the discussion on iodination of fibrinogen.

Limitations

Since the fibrinogen uptake test uses ^{125}I-fibrinogen with its low-energy photon, it cannot accurately detect thrombi above the middle of the thigh be-

---

*References 26-28, 30, 44, 55, 56, 58, 85, 86.

cause there is a large blood pool in this area and scattered radiation from ^{125}I in the bladder.[59] Fibrinogen labeled with radioisotopes suitable for imaging has been used to detect thrombi in the pelvis and upper thigh.[12, 19] Charkes et al.[12] using ^{131}I-fibrinogen and DeNardo et al.[19] using ^{123}I-fibrinogen have demonstrated that these radiopharmaceuticals can be used to localize thrombi in the areas in which the fibrinogen uptake test is unreliable.

Since the labeled fibrinogen must be incorporated into the thrombus so that it can be differentiated from background vascular activity, the fibrinogen uptake test will not be abnormal until 5 hours or more after injection, depending on the size and stage of the thrombus.[60] To be an accurate indicator of deep vein thrombosis, the count should be elevated for at least 24 hours. Thus the test cannot be performed as an emergency examination, and if immediate evaluation of the venous system is needed, a venogram is required.

Patients with various abnormalities of the legs may have false positive results. Experimental studies by Hobbs[48] and Hladovec, Prerovsky, and Roztocil[47] have shown that inflammation results in accumulation of fibrinogen. This is probably related to vascular permeability and not hyperemia, since labeled albumin accumulates to approximately the same amount as labeled fibrinogen but labeled red cells do not accumulate in the area. Thus cellulitis can be associated with an abnormal fibrinogen uptake test. Since ^{125}I-fibrinogen is accumulated during wound healing, the fibrinogen uptake test may be abnormal without venous thrombosis in patients with leg ulcers, wounds, or hematomas. Other conditions that can produce an abnormal fibrinogen uptake test include arthritis and superficial thrombophlebitis. The fibrinogen uptake test is useful in such conditions only if abnormal accumulation is detected in areas other than the clinically abnormal ones. These limitations of the fibrinogen uptake test may be partially overcome by using fibrinogen labeled with radioisotopes suitable for imaging, since the abnormality in the images could be compared to the clinical examination.

Another theoretical limitation of the fibrinogen uptake test is the risk of transmitting hepatitis. [59] This hazard is the main reason the radiopharmaceutical has not been approved for general use in the United States. Several large studies have been done outside the United States and have shown the test to be safe. Hicks and Hazell[46] studied 354 patients who had the fibrinogen uptake test and compared them to 354 matched control patients. The patients had careful clinical examinations, laboratory evaluations, and follow-up examinations, and there was no increase in the frequency of hepatitis in those receiving fibrinogen. The authors note that a large commercial supplier of ^{125}I-fibrinogen had received no reports of serum hepatitis from over 50,000 injections. If the fibrinogen used is from carefully selected donors screened by the latest techniques for detecting carriers of hepatitis and who have donated blood several times without the recipients' developing hepatitis, the risk of transmitting hepatitis is very low. As discussed in the section on iodination of fibrinogen, some work has been done to label autologous fibrinogen to avoid the danger of transmitting hepatitis.[93, 101]

OTHER AGENTS

Although the ^{125}I-fibrinogen uptake test is an accurate and sensitive technique for detecting deep vein thrombosis, its use is limited to monitoring the course of development of thrombi in the lower extremities over a period of several days in certain groups of high-risk patients. The nature of the test requires that the labeled fibrinogen remain in circulation for 4 or 5 days and that the radioisotope have a long physical half-life and decay characteristics suitable for detection with a simple probe-type detector. The ^{125}I-fibrinogen cannot be used in situations in which it would be desirable to image actively forming or preexisting thrombi in the deep venous system of the calf, thigh, or pelvis. Radioisotopic thrombus detection under such circumstances would require a radiopharmaceutical with properties quite different from those of ^{125}I-fibrinogen. An agent for imaging a thrombus should incorporate readily into the thrombus and clear rapidly from the circulation to produce sufficient differentiation between activity in the thrombus and the surrounding blood pool. The radionuclide should have a short physical half-life and photon decay characteristics compatible with a scintillation camera. Ideally the agent should allow imaging to be performed within a few hours following injection. This particular criterion limits the use of such agents as ^{123}I-fibrinogen[19] and ^{131}I-fibrinogen.[12] Although these preparations have been reported to be useful for visualizing thrombi, the accompanying blood background activity would be too high to permit imaging for at least 24 hours after injection. Several promising new agents for radioisotopic detection of deep vein thrombosis have been developed recently. This section considers these new agents and their potential for future clinical significance in nuclear medicine.

Fibrinogen and derivatives

Human fibrinogen labeled with ^{125}I by the mild iodine monochloride (ICl) technique has a half-life of 4 or 5 days.[17, 36] Fibrinogen and derivatives with an increased clearance rate but little change in biologic activity can be prepared and labeled with radioisotopes of short half-life and high photon yield. The rapid clearance properties can be produced by specific structural changes in the fibrinogen molecule or by the nature of the binding between the fibrinogen and the radionuclide. A key consideration is that the alterations must not denature the fibrinogen by inducing effects such as aggregation, which may result in a decrease in biologic activity.[15, 78]

Highly iodinated fibrinogen. Canine and human fibrinogen can be iodinated with as many as 4.5 iodine atoms per molecule and rabbit fibrinogen can be iodinated with as many as 3.5 without alteration of molecular size or biologic clearance behavior.[41] Introduction of additional iodine atoms, however, can produce significant changes. Fibrinogen can be iodinated with up to 100 iodine atoms per molecule by a controlled-potential electrochemical technique and with up to 25 iodine atoms per molecule by the ICl method.[38] These fibrinogen preparations all exhibit isotopic clottability of 60% to 70%, whereas the degree of aggregation and rate of blood clearance in dogs increase with extent of iodination. When the preparations are injected into dogs 4 hours after induction of femoral vein thrombosis, the thrombus-blood activity ratios 24 hours later depend on the number of iodine atoms per molecule in the order 25>50>100. The preparation with 25 iodine atoms per molecule clears from the blood with a half-life of 37 hours and gives a thrombus-blood ratio twice as high as that obtained with conventional radioiodinated fibrinogen (0.5 iodine atom per molecule) injected simultaneously.[38]

Since highly iodinated fibrinogen preparations have shorter biologic half-lives compared to conventional radioiodinated fibrinogen, ^{123}I, a short-lived (half-life of 13.3 hrs) isotope, would be more appropriate as a label than ^{131}I or [125]I. With ^{123}I as the label the agent would deliver a smaller radiation dose and could be imaged with a scintillation camera (159 keV photon emission). Highly iodinated fibrinogen containing 25 iodine atoms per molecule and labeled with ^{123}I has been prepared and evaluated as a thrombus-imaging agent.[40] Femoral vein thrombi up to 7 hours old can be well visualized in dogs 4 hours after injection.[40]

Soluble fibrin. The action of thrombin on fibrinogen produces fibrin that polymerizes through electrostatic interaction.[33] Intermolecular covalent cross-linking of the polymerized fibrin is then induced by activated factor XIII to stabilize the thrombus.[21, 72] If a clot is formed in vitro from radiolabeled fibrinogen in the presence of a factor XIII inhibitor, it can be redissolved under specific conditions of pH and ionic strength to give a radiolabeled soluble fibrin preparation that probably consists of oligomers of fibrin monomer.[16, 107] This agent may be ideally suited to incorporate into a developing thrombus. The isotopic clottability of radioiodinated soluble fibrin is greater than 80%. Its blood clearance is extremely fast, with a half-life in dogs of 5 hours. When injected into dogs 4 to 24 hours after induction of femoral vein thrombosis, radioiodinated soluble fibrin gives higher thrombus-blood ratios 24 hours later than those obtained with conventional radioiodinated fibrinogen injected at the same time.[16] This agent may be particulary suitable for imaging thrombi in regions of large blood pool soon after injection.

For routine patient use a simplification of the procedure for soluble fibrin preparation may be desirable. Such a simplification could be effected by cleaving the fibrinopeptides from radiolabeled fibrinogen to form soluble fibrin without the necessity of going through the process of clot formation and dissolution. This can be accomplished by the action of highly purified thrombin on a fibrinogen solution sufficiently dilute to prevent even electrostatic polymerization.[43] In addition, the preparation must contain no residual thrombin. This requirement can be met by adding the thrombin in a solid-phase form, which can be readily removed following incubation.[52, 88]

Like highly iodinated fibrinogen, soluble fibrin would be more appropriately labeled with ^{123}I than with ^{131}I or [125]I. Fibrinogen can be labeled with ^{123}I by the ICl or lactoperoxidase methods for use in preparing ^{123}I-soluble fibrin.[39] In dogs this agent will readily visualize femoral vein thrombi up to 6 hours old 3 hours after injection.[39]

[99m]*Tc-fibrinogen.* The ready availability, low radiation dose, and ideal com-

patibility with a scintillation camera make ^{99m}Tc very desirable as a fibrinogen label. Although the exact mechanism by which ^{99m}Tc labels proteins is unclear, ^{99m}Tc-protein binding presumably involves coordination complex formation typical of transition metals.[4, 100] The ^{99m}Tc is probably complexed by such electron-rich groups of the protein as amino, hydroxyl, and sulfhydryl.[100] This is in contrast to the labeling of proteins with iodine, which involves covalent bond formation, largely with the aromatic ring of the tyrosine residues.[96] The different nature of binding in a ^{99m}Tc-fibrinogen preparation compared to a radioiodinated fibrinogen preparation may in itself impart altered clearance behavior. Other ^{99m}Tc-labeled proteins have been found to exhibit more rapid clearance than their radioiodinated analogs.[65, 99]

The preparation of ^{99m}Tc-fibrinogen has been previously described,[6, 122] but the conditions employed involved low pH, which would denature fibrinogen and lead to loss of biologic activity.[79] Fibrinogen can be labeled with ^{99m}Tc by a simple, mild electrolytic reaction at nearly neutral pH to give a product with isotopic clottability of 60% and a rapid blood clearance (half-life in dogs of 25 hours).[42] When prepared in this way, ^{99m}Tc-fibrinogen injected into dogs 4 hours after induction of femoral vein thrombosis gives slightly higher thrombus-blood ratios 24 hours later than does conventional radioiodinated fibrinogen injected simultaneously.[42] These ^{99m}Tc-fibrinogen preparations provide clearly delineated images of 4-hour-old femoral vein thrombi in dogs 2 hours after injection.[42]

^{77}Br-fibrinogen. Fibrinogen can be labeled with bromine by an indirect mechanism involving coupling under mild conditions with a previously brominated acylating agent N-succinimidyl-3-(4-hydroxyphenyl) propionate (SHPP).[10] In this method the fibrinogen is not subjected to the oxidizing conditions inherent in direct halogenation. Fibrinogen labeled with ^{77}Br by this reaction may have two advantages for in vivo studies over conventional radioiodinated fibrinogen: the carbon-bromine bond is stronger than the carbon-iodine bond, and ^{77}Br (half-life of 56 hours) delivers a lower radiation dose than ^{131}I or ^{125}I. Fibrinogen labeled by the ^{77}Br-SHPP method has been found to exhibit biologic clearance properties and thrombus incorporation similar to conventional radioiodinated fibrinogen prepared by the ICl method.[66]

Chelates. Indirect labeling of fibrinogen with metallic radioisotopes may be possible with intermediate chelating agents. A bifunctional chelating agent, *p*-benzenediazoniumethylenediaminetetracetic acid, has been developed, which appears to be suitable for this purpose.[114, 115] In this manner fibrinogen has been labeled with ^{111}In.[35] This same chelating agent or similar ones may be useful for labeling fibrinogen with other metals. Of particular significance in this respect is ^{68}Ga, a positron-emitting isotope of short half-life (68 minutes) that may allow the imaging of thrombi by means of positron emission transaxial tomography.[92]

Fibrinolytic enzyme system

Plasminogen and plasmin. Plasminogen is the precursor of plasmin, the enzyme that catalyzes fibrinolysis and is responsible for thrombus degradation.

Plasminogen is thought to be trapped in a developing thrombus and converted to plasmin by an activating enzyme that adsorbs onto and diffuses into the thrombus; then the plasmin acts on the thrombus in situ.[108] Thus radiolabeled plasminogen and radiolabeled plasmin may be suitable for thrombus localization. A few studies of this kind have been reported. The in vivo clearance and thrombus uptake of labeled plasminogen, plasmin, and other fibrinolytic enzymes have been investigated.[3] A rapid blood clearance of only a few minutes was observed for all the agents, with labeled plasmin showing the best thrombus uptake. In a subsequent study ^{131}I-plasmin was found to localize in venous thrombi, although the blood clearance was found to be slower, with a half-life of about 2 hours.[87] The rather low purity of the enzymes used in these studies requires a reevaluation with current techniques. A more recent study with purified ^{125}I-plasmin has indicated a biologic half-life of 14.2 hours.[116]

Urokinase and streptokinase. Urokinase and streptokinase are activators of plasminogen. Urokinase is a protein that occurs naturally in man and is isolated from urine. This enzyme adsorbs onto and diffuses into an established thrombus to convert the plasminogen trapped therein to plasmin.[108] For this reason, radiolabeled urokinase may be an ideal agent for detecting older, preformed thrombi. Similarly, the enzyme streptokinase isolated from hemolytic strepto-cocci converts the plasminogen in a thrombus to plasmin.[108] Radiolabeled strepto-kinase may thus also localize in preformed thrombi, although as a foreign protein it may be less desirable than urokinase. Several groups have investigated the labeling of urokinase and streptokinase with ^{131}I and ^{99m}Tc and the use of these agents for detecting venous thrombi and thromboemboli. The results have been highly variable, especially in the case of the ^{99m}Tc-labeled agents. Some of the earlier studies[23, 98, 109] were encouraging and indicated that ^{131}I-streptokinase could be used to localize thromboemboli in experimental animals. However, in some later studies[22, 34, 99] satisfactory imaging of emboli was not achieved. Recent studies have reported successful imaging of thrombi in the deep venous system of the lower extremities with ^{99m}Tc-urokinase[80] and ^{99m}Tc-streptokinase.[64, 91] Further investigation of these agents is necessary.

OTHER COAGULATION MOIETIES

Factor XIII. The activated form of factor XIII, factor XIIIa, participates in the last stage of thrombus development by inducing covalent cross-linking of the polymerized fibrin.[21, 72] Radiolabeled factor XIII may thus have potential as a thrombus-localizing agent. Factor XIII exists in both plasma and platelets and can be isolated and purified from both sources.[104, 105] Factor XIII is activated by trace amounts of thrombin,[67] and the action of Factor XIIIa on the cross-linking of fibrin requires calcium ion.[20] Although no previous reports on radio-labeling of factor XIII or factor XIIIa have appeared, radiolabeling may be pos-sible by a mild method that will preserve the biologic activity of the enzyme.

Antifibrinogen. Immunochemical techniques have been employed in the development of new thrombus-localizing agents. Rabbit antifibrinogen antibody labeled with ^{125}I was used successfully to detect thrombi in humans.[110, 111] However, two problems with this approach have limited its use: the long half-life of the antibody (5 to 7 days) and potential adverse immunologic reactions. One proposed solution is to administer a second antibody, goat antirabbit IgG, following injection of the radiolabeled antifibrinogen.[97] This technique results in more rapid blood clearance of the antifibrinogen and reduces the likelihood of its antigenic action. Another possibility is the use of the Fab fragment of antifibrinogen rather than the intact protein. The Fab fragment appears to have a decreased antigenicity and increased blood clearance, with a half-life of 0.3 day.[32] The Fab fragment can be prepared by known technique.[18, 24] It must then be radiolabeled by a mild technique that will preserve the immunologic activity.

Platelets and leukocytes. Labeled platelets and leukocytes can be incorporated into thrombi and have been investigated as agents for thrombus detection.[22] Platelets labeled with ^{75}Se-selenite or ^{75}Se-methionine were found to localize in forming thrombi, but in insufficient amounts to be detected scintigraphically.[13] However, ^{99m}Tc–labeled leukocytes do localize sufficiently in forming thrombi to be detected by photoscanning.[13] Leukocytes labeled with ^{51}Cr have been used to detect venous thrombi by external probe monitoring.[70]

SUMMARY

Deep venous thrombosis is a common complication in hospitalized patients and is often difficult to detect clinically. The ^{125}I-fibrinogen uptake test has been used to screen large groups of patients and determine the incidence of venous thrombosis in a variety of conditions. Since there are limitations of the fibrinogen uptake test in detecting venous thrombosis, several new agents are presently being evaluated as thrombus-imaging agents.

References

1. Alkjaersig, N., Fletcher, A., and Sherry, S.: ϵ-amino-caproic acid: an inhibitor of plasminogen activation, J. Biol. Chem. **234**:832, 1959.
2. Atkins, P., and Hawkins, L. A.: The diagnosis of deep vein thrombosis in legs using ^{125}I-fibrinogen, Lancet **2**:1217, 1965.
3. Back, N., Ambrus, J. L., and Mink, I. B.: Distribution and fate of I-131 labeled components of the fibrinolysin system, Circ. Res. **9**:1208, 1961.
4. Basolo, F., and Johnson, R. C.: Coordination chemistry, New York, 1964, W. A. Benjamin, Inc.
5. Belt, T. H.: Thrombosis and pulmonary embolism, Am. J. Pathol. **10**:129, 1934.
6. Benjamin, P. B.: Aseptically sealed electrolytic cell for ^{99m}Tc-albumin micro- and macro-aggregation, J. Nucl. Med. **13**:172, 1972.
7. Bettingole, R. E., et al.: Autologous ^{131}I-fibrinogen survival: a useful technique, J. Nucl. Med. **10**:322, 1969.
8. Blombäck, B., and Blombäck, M.: Purification of human and bovine fibrinogen, Arkiv. Kemi. **10**:415, 1956.
9. Bocci, V.: Efficient labeling of serum proteins with ^{131}I using chloramine-T, Int. J. Appl. Radiat. Isot. **15**:449, 1964.
10. Bolton, A. E., and Hunter, W. M.: The labeling of proteins to high specific radioactivities by conjugation to a ^{125}I-containing acylating agent, Biochem. J. **133**:529, 1973.
11. Browse, N. L.: The ^{125}I-fibrinogen uptake test, Arch. Surg. **104**:160, 1972.
12. Charkes, N. D., et al.: Scintigraphic detection of deep vein thrombosis with ^{131}I-fibrinogen, J. Nucl. Med. **15**:1163, 1974.
13. Charkes, N. D., Malmud, L. S., and

Stern, H. S.: Comparative evaluation of current scanning agents for thrombus detection. In Subramanian, G., Rhodes, B. A., Cooper, J. F., and Sodd, V. J., editors: Radiopharmaceuticals, New York, 1975, The Society of Nuclear Medicine, Inc.

14. Cohn, E. J., et al.: Preparation and properties of serum and plasma proteins. IV. A system to the separation into fractions of the protein and lipoprotein components of biological tissues and fluids, J. Am. Chem. Soc. **68**:459, 1946.

15. Coleman, R. E., et al.: An in vivo evaluation of °I-fibrinogen labeled by four different methods, J. Lab. Clin. Med. **83**:977, 1974.

16. Coleman, R. E., et al.: Radioiodinated soluble fibrin: preparation and evaluation as a thrombus-localizing agent, Circ. Res. **37**:35, 1975.

17. Collen, D., et al.: Metabolism and distribution of fibrinogen. I. Fibrinogen turnover in physiological conditions in humans, Br. J. Haematol. **22**:681, 1972.

18. Connell, G. E., and Painter, R. H.: Fragmentation of immunoglobulin during storage, Can. J. Biochem. **44**:371, 1965.

19. DeNardo, S. J., et al.: ^{123}I-fibrinogen imaging of thrombi in dogs (Abstract), J. Nucl. Med. **15**:487, 1974.

20. DeNardo, S. J., et al.: Clinical usefulness of I-125-fibrinogen for detection of thrombophlebitis (Abstract), J. Nucl. Med. **16**:524, 1975.

21. Doolittle, R. F., et al.: Correlation of the mode of fibrin polymerization with the pattern of crosslinking. In Laki, K., editor: The biological role of the clot-stabilizing enzymes: transglutaminase and factor XIII, New York, 1972, New York Academy of Sciences.

22. Dugan, M. A., et al.: New radiopharmaceuticals for thrombus localization (Abstract), J. Nucl. Med. **13**:782, 1972.

23. Dugan, M. A., et al.: Localization of deep vein thrombosis using radioactive streptokinase, J. Nucl. Med. **14**:233, 1973.

24. Edelman, G. M., and Marchalonis, J. J.: Methods used in studies of the structure of immunoglobulins. Methods Immunol. Immunochem. **1**:405, 1967.

25. Evans, O. S., and Cockett, F. B.: Diagnosis of deep vein thrombosis with an ultra-sonic Doppler technique, Br. Med. J. **2**:802, 1968.

26. Field, E. S., et al.: Deep vein thrombosis in patients with fractures of the femoral neck, Br. J. Surg. **59**:377, 1972.

27. Flanc, C., Kakkar, V. V., and Clarke, M. B.: The detection of venous thrombosis of the legs using 125-I-labelled fibrinogen, Br. J. Surg. **55**:742, 1968.

28. Friend, J. R., and Kakkar, V. V.: The diagnosis of deep vein thrombosis in puerperium, J. Obstet. Gynecol. Br. Comm. **77**:820, 1970.

29. Frykholm, R.: The pathogenesis and mechanical prophylaxis of venous thrombosis, Surg. Gynecol. Obstet. **71**:307, 1940.

30. Gallus, A. S., et al.: Small subcutaneous doses of heparin in prevention of venous thrombosis, N. Engl. J. Med. **288**:545, 1973.

31. Gibbs, N. M.: Venous thrombosis of the lower limbs with particular reference to bed-rest, Br. J. Surg. **45**:209, 1957.

32. Gitlin, D., et al.: The selectivity of the human placenta in the transfer of plasma proteins from mother to fetus, J. Clin. Invest. **43**:1938, 1964.

33. Gladner, J. A.: The action of thrombin on fibrinogen. In Laki, K., editor: Fibrinogen, New York, 1968, Marcel Dekker, Inc.

34. Goodman, L. R., et al.: Failure to visualize experimental pulmonary emboli and clots using ^{131}I-streptokinase (Abstract), Invest. Radiol. **8**:255, 1973.

35. Goodwin, D. A., et al.: [111]Indium—labeled radiopharmaceuticals and their clinical use. In Subramanian, G., Rhodes, B. A., Cooper, J. F., and Sodd, V. J., editors: Radiopharmaceuticals, New York, 1975, The Society of Nuclear Medicine, Inc.

36. Hammond, J. D. S., and Verel, D.: Observations on the distribution and biological half-life of human fibrinogen, Br. J. Haematol. **5**:431, 1959.

37. Harris, W. H., et al.: Comparison of ^{125}I-fibrinogen count scanning with phlebography for detection of venous thrombi after elective hip surgery, N. Engl. J. Med. **292**:665, 1975.

38. Harwig, J. F., et al.: Highly iodinated fibrinogen: a new thrombus-localizing agent, J. Nucl. Med. **16**:756, 1975.

39. Harwig, J. F., and Harwig, S. S. L.: Unpublished data.

40. Harwig, J. F., Welch, M. J., Coleman, R. E.: ^{123}I-labeled highly iodinated fibrinogen: preparation and use for imaging deep vein thrombi, J. Nucl. Med. **17**:397, 1976.

41. Harwig, S. S. L., et al.: Effect of iodination level on the properties of radioiodinated fibrinogen, Throm. Res. **6**:375, 1975.

42. Harwig, S. S. L., et al.: The in vivo behavior of ^{99m}Tc-fibrinogen and its potential as a thrombus-imaging agent, J. Nucl. Med. **17**:40, 1976.

43. Harwig, S. S. L., and Sherman, L. A.: Unpublished data.

44. Heine, M., et al.: ^{125}I-fibrinogen in the prevention of venous thrombosis, Arch. Surg. **107**:803, 1973.

45. Helmkamp, R. W., Contreras, M. A., and Izzo, M. J.: I[131] labeling of proteins at high activity level with [131]ICl produced by oxidation of total iodine in Na[131]I preparations, Int. J. Appl. Radiat. Isot. **18**:474, 1967.

46. Hicks, B. H., and Hazell, J.: Safe use of ^{125}I-fibrinogen, Lancet **2**:931, 1973.

47. Hladovec, J., Prerovsky, I., Roztocil, K.: The influence of inflammation on the ^{125}I-fibrinogen uptake test in experimental thrombosis, Angiologica **10**:93, 1973.

48. Hobbs, J. T.: External measurement of fibrinogen uptake in experimental venous thrombosis and other local pathological states, Br. J. Exp. Pathol. **43**:48, 1962.

49. Hobbs, J. T., and Davies, J. W.: Detection of venous thrombosis with 131-I-labelled fibrinogen in the rabbit, Lancet **2**:134, 1960.

50. Hunter, W. M.: Iodination of protein compounds. In Andrews, G. A., Kniseley, R. N., and Wagner, H. N., Jr., editors: Radioactive pharmaceuticals, Springfield, Va., 1965, U.S. Atomic Energy Commission.

51. Hunter, W. M., and Greenwood, F. C.: Preparation of iodine-131-labelled human growth hormone of high specific activity, Nature **194**:495, 1962.

52. Hussain, Q. Z., and Newcomb, T. F.: Preparation of water insoluble thrombin, Proc. Soc. Exp. Biol. Med. **115**:301, 1964.

53. Ingraham, S. C., III, Silberstein, E. B.,

Kereiakes, J. G., and Wellman, H. N.: Preparation and tagging of autologous fibrinogen at ambient temperatures, J. Nucl. Med. **10**:410, 1969.

54. Johnston, K. W., et al.: A simple method for detecting deep vein thrombosis. An improved electrical impedance technique. Am. J. Surg. **127**:349, 1974.

55. Kakkar, V. V., et al.: Natural history of post-operative deep vein thrombosis, Lancet **2**:230, 1969.

56. Kakkar, V. V., et al.: Treatment of deep-vein thrombosis: a trial of heparin, streptokinase, and arvin, Br. Med. J. **1**:806, 1969.

57. Kakkar, V. V.: The diagnosis of deep vein thrombosis using the ^{125}I-fibrinogen test, Arch. Surg. **104**:152, 1972.

58. Kakkar, V. V.: The ^{125}I-labeled fibrinogen test and phlebography in the diagnosis of deep vein thrombosis, Millbank Mem Fund Q. **50**:206, 1972.

59. Kakkar, V. V.: Current status of the radioactive labeled fibrinogen method in the detection of venous thrombosis. In Moser, K. M., and Stern, M., editors: Pulmonary thromboembolism, Chicago, 1973, Year Book Medical Publishers, Inc.

60. Kakkar, V. V.: Deep vein thrombosis: detection and prevention, Circulation **51**:8, 1975.

61. Katz, J., and Bonorris, G.: Electrolytic iodination of proteins with I-125 and I-131, J. Lab. Clin. Med. **72**:966, 1968.

62. Kazal, L. A., Amsel, S., Miller, Q. P., and Tocantins, L. M.: The preparation and some properties of fibrinogen precipitated from human plasma by glycine, Proc. Soc. Exp. Biol. Med. **113**:989, 1963.

63. Kekwick, R. A., MacKay, M., Nance, M., and Record, B.: The purification of human fibrinogen, Biochem. J. **60**:671, 1955.

64. Kempi, V., Van der Linden, W., and von Scheele, C.: Diagnosis of deep vein thrombosis with ^{99m}Tc-streptokinase; a clinical comparison with venography, Br. Med. J. **5947**:748, 1974.

65. Kitani, K., and Taplin, G. V.: Rapid hepatic turnover of radioactive human serum albumin in sensitized dogs, J. Nucl. Med. **15**:938, 1974.

66. Knight, L. C., Harwig, S. S. L., and Welch, M. J.: Halogen-SHPP labeling

of fibrinogen: a comparison of the I-131 and Br-77 radiopharmaceuticals with I-125 fibrinogen prepared by the iodine monochloride method, J. Nucl. Med. **16:**542, 1975.

67. Konishi, K., and Lorand, L.: Separation of activated fibrin stabilizing factor from thrombin, Biochim. Biophys. Acta **121:**177, 1966.

68. Krohn, K. A., Sherman, L., and Welch, M. J.: Studies of radioiodinated fibrinogen. I. Physicochemical properties of the ICl, chloramine-T and electrolytic reaction products, Biochim. Biophys. Acta **285:**404, 1972.

69. Krohn, K. A., and Welch, M. J.: Studies of radioiodinated fibrinogen. II. Lactoperoxidase iodination of fibrinogen and model compound. Int. J. Appl. Radiat. Isot. **25:**315, 1974.

70. Kwan, H. C., and Grumet, G.: The use of ⁵¹Cr-labeled leukocytes in the detection of venous thrombosis, Clin. Res. **20:**788, 1972.

71. Laki, K., and Steiner, R.: Polymerization of iodinated fibrinogen, J. Polymer. Sci. **8:**457, 1952.

72. Lorand, L.: Fibrinoligase: the fibrin stabilizing factor system of blood plasma. In Laki, K., editor: The biological role of the clot stabilizing enzymes: transflutaminase and factor XII, New York, 1972, New York Academy of Sciences.

73. MacFarlane, A. S.: In vivo behavior of ¹³¹I-fibrinogen, J. Clin. Invest. **42:**345, 1963.

74. Marchalonis, J. J.: An enzymatic method for the trace iodination of immunoglobulins and other proteins, Biochem. J. **113:**299, 1969.

75. Mavor, G. E., et al.: Peripheral venous scanning with 125I-tagged fibrinogen, Lancet **1:**551, 1972.

76. Maxwell, R. E., Nickel, V. S., and Lewandowski, V.: Preparation of plasminogen-deficient fibrinogen and thrombin, Biochem. Biophys. Res. Commun. **7:**50, 1962.

77. Metzger, J. M., et al.: Biological clearance and distribution studies of *I-fibrinogen labeled by four methods of iodination (Abstract), J. Nucl. Med. **14:**429, 1973.

78. Metzger, J. M., et al.: Unsatisfactory biologic behavior of I-fibrinogen labeled with chloramine-T method, J. Lab. Clin. Med. **82:**267, 1973.

79. Mihalyi, E.: Structural aspects of fibrinogen. In Laki, K., editor: Fibrinogen, New York, 1968, Marcel Dekker, Inc.

80. Millar, W. T., and Smith, J. F. B.: Localization of deep venous thrombosis using technetium-99m labeled urokinase, Lancet **2:**695, 1974.

81. Milne, R. M., et al.: Postoperative deep vein thrombosis. A comparison of diagnostic techniques, Lancet **2:**445, 1971.

82. Morrison, M., and Bayse, G.: Catalysis of iodination by lactoperoxidase, Biochemistry **9:**2995, 1970.

83. Moschos, B. C., et al.: Incorporation of ¹³¹I-fibrinogen in a coronary artery thrombus, detected in vivo with a scintillation camera, Cardiovasc. Res. **8:**715, 1974.

84. Mosesson, M. W., and Sherry, S.: The preparation and properties of human fibrinogen of relatively high solubility, Biochemistry **5:**2829, 1966.

85. Murray, T. S., et al.: Leg vein thrombosis following myocardial infarction, Lancet **2:**792, 1970.

86. O'Brien, J. R.: Detection of thrombosis with iodine-125 fibrinogen: data reassessed, Lancet **2:**396, 1970.

87. Ouchi, H., and Warren, R.: Detection of intravascular thrombi by means of ¹³¹I–labeled plasmin, Surgery **51:**42, 1962.

88. Owen, W. G., and Wagner, R. H.: Preparation and properties of water insoluble thrombin, Am. J. Physiol. **220:**1941, 1971.

89. Palko, P. D., Nanson, E. M., and Fedoruk, S. O.: The early detection of deep venous thrombosis using I131-tagged human fibrinogen, Can. J. Surg. **7:**215, 1964.

90. Paterson, J. C., and McLachlin, J.: Precipitating factors in venous thrombosis, Surg. Gynecol. Obstet. **98:**96, 1954.

91. Persson, B. R. R., and Kempi, V.: Labeling and testing of ⁹⁹ᵐTc-streptokinase for the diagnosis of deep vein thrombosis, J. Nucl. Med. **16:**474, 1975.

92. Phelps, M. E., et al.: Application of annihilation coincidence detection to transaxial reconstruction tomography, J. Nucl. Med. **16:**210, 1975.

93. Pollak, E. W., et al.: Autologous ^{125}I-fibrinogen uptake test in the detection and management of venous thrombosis, Arch. Surg. **109**:48, 1974.

94. Rabinoi, K., and Paulin, S.: Roentgen diagnosis of venous thrombosis in the leg, Arch. Surg. **104**:134, 1972.

95. Regoeczi, E.: The clottability of iodinated fibrinogen, J. Nucl. Biol. Med. **15**:37, 1971.

96. Regoeczi, E., and Walton, P. L.: Effects of clotting on the label in iodinated fibrinogen in different species, Thromb. Diath. Haemorrh. **17**:237, 1967.

97. Reich, T., et al.: Detection of venous thrombosis in the human by means of radioiodinated antifibrin-fibrinogen antibody, Surgery **50**:1211, 1966.

98. Rhodes, B. A., et al.: Radioactive urokinase for blood clot scanning, J. Nucl. Med. **13**:646, 1972.

99. Rhodes, B. A., et al.: Labeling and testing of urokinase and streptokinase: new tracers for the detection of thromboemboli. In Pharmaceuticals and labeled compounds, vol. II, Vienna, 1973, International Atomic Energy Agency.

100. Richards, P., and Steigman, J.: Chemistry of technetium as applied to radiopharmaceuticals. In Subramanian, G., Rhodes, B. A., Cooper, J. F., and Sodd, V. J., editors: Radiopharmaceuticals, New York, 1975, The Society of Nuclear Medicine, Inc.

101. Roberts, R. C., Sonnentag, C. O., and Frisbie, J. H.: Rapid preparation of autologous radioiodinated fibrinogen, J. Nucl. Med. **13**:843, 1972.

102. Rosa, U., et al.: Labeling of human fibrinogen with ^{131}I by electrolytic iodination, Biochim. Biophys. Acta **86**:519, 1964.

103. Samoles, E., and Williams, H. S.: Trace labeling of insulin with iodine, Nature **190**:1211, 1961.

104. Schwartz, M. L., et al.: The subunit structures of human plasma and platelet factor XIII (fibrin stabilizing factor), J. Biol. Chem. **246**:4851, 1971.

105. Schwartz, M. L., et al.: Human factor XIII from plasma and platelets, J. Biol. Chem. **248**:1395, 1973.

106. Sevitt, S.: Venous thrombosis and pulmonary embolism: their prevention by oral anticoagulants, Am. J. Med. **33**:703, 1962.

107. Sherman, L. A., Harwig, S., and Lee, J.: In vitro formation and in vivo clearance of fibrinogen-fibrin complexes, J. Lab. Clin. Med. **86**:100, 1975.

108. Sherry, S., Fletcher, A. P., and Alkjaersig, N.: Fibrinolysis and fibrinolytic activity in man, Physiol. Rev. **39**:343, 1959.

109. Siegel, M. E., et al.: Scanning of thromboemboli with ^{131}I-streptokinase, Radiology **103**:695, 1972.

110. Spar, I. L., et al.: Isotopic detection of thrombi, Arch. Surg. **92**:752, 1966.

111. Spar, I. L., et al.: Detection of left atrial thrombi. Scintillation scanning after administration of ^{131}I rabbit antibodies to human fibrinogen, Am. Heart J. **78**:731, 1969.

112. Strandness, D. E., et al.: Ultrasound flow detection. A useful technique in the evaluation of peripheral vascular disease, Am. J. Surg. **113**:311, 1967.

113. Straughn, W., Wagner, R. H.: A simple method for preparing fibrinogen, Thromb. Diath. Haemorrh. **15**:198, 1966.

114. Sundberg, M. W., et al.: Chelating agents for the binding of metal ions to macromolecules, Nature **250**:287, 1974.

115. Sundberg, M. W., et al.: Selective binding of metal ions to macromolecules using bifunctional analogs of EDTA, J. Med. Chem. **17**:1304, 1974.

116. Takeda, Y., and Nakabayashi, M.: Physicochemical and biological properties of human and canine plasmins, J. Clin. Invest. **53**:154, 1974.

117. Teulings, F. A. G., and Biggs, G. J.: Study of electrolytic labeling of fibrinogen with iodine-131 by Sephadex G-10 gel filtration, Clin. Chim. Acta **27**:57, 1970.

118. Thomas, M. L.: Phlebography, Arch. Surg. **104**:145, 1972.

119. Ware, A. G., Guest, M. M., and Seegers, W. H.: Fibrinogen: with special reference to its preparation and certain properties of the product, Arch. Biochem. Biophys. **13**:231, 1974.

120. Warlow, C., Ogston, D., and Douglas, A. S.: Venous thrombosis following strokes, Lancet **1**:1305, 1972.

121. Wheeler, H. B., and Mullick, S. C.: Detection of venous obstruction in the leg by measurement of electrical impedance, Ann. N.Y. Acad. Sci. **170:** 804, 1970.

122. Wong, D. W., and Mishkin, F. S.: Tech-netium-99m human fibrinogen, J. Nucl. Med. **15:**343, 1975.

123. Yalow, R. S., and Berson, S. A.: Immunoassay of endogenous plasma insulin in man, J. Clin. Invest. **39:**1157, 1960.

14 Electrocoagulation of small lung tumors

Björn E. W. Nordenström

Transthoracic needle biopsy during roentgen television control[4] has been practiced since 1960. Follow-up studies[13] on our findings have proved the usefulness of the technique and the low incidence of complications. Thus early diagnosis of secondary or primary malignant tumors (2 cm or less in diameter) provides a 42% 5-year survival rate after operative removal of the tumor. In a consecutive series of small pulmonary nodules, however, two thirds were caused by granulomas or benign tumors. Of the one third that were malignant, most small primary, squamous cell carcinomas would be suitable for operation. A 5-year survival rate of 70% to 80% could be expected, but final figures for these tumors are not yet available. Among the primary lung tumors certain adenocarcinomas and oat-cell carcinomas have a poor prognosis, even at early diagnosis and surgery.[12-14] This well-recognized fact makes the value of surgical removal of these types doubtful, and some surgeons therefore refuse to operate.

In the case of tumor metastases in the lung, some solitary tumors can be removed and the patient cured. The indications for such operations are that only one metastasis exists and that the tumor is of a cell type having a relatively good prognosis.[16] A large number of different kinds of solitary metastatic tumors in the lung, however, are not appropriate for operation. Among the suitable types of lung metastases a considerable decrease in surgical cure is to be expected when two or more lesions are present in a lung. The presence of one small lesion in either lung is considered an operative contraindication by most surgeons. This is because of the small chance that the number of metastases is limited to the visible ones when there are two or more. Also the operative trauma and its effect on the patient's resistance to the disease as well as the patient's age and general condition are often contraindications to operation.[1, 2, 14]

Patients with primary or metastatic lung tumors who are not accepted for operation may be candidates for local radiotherapy. The most striking positive effect is obtained in poorly differentiated tumors, which may decrease in size considerably within a relatively short time period. This effect is augmented by increasing the oxygen tension in the blood, which can be done in several ways.[11] In spite of this, recurrence of the irradiated tumor is more or less the rule. This may partly be due to an insufficient effect of the radiation in the central part of the tumor, where a state of hypoxia is usually present. The supplementary use of

331

currently available chemotherapy and other techniques does not seem to offer a sufficient solution to this problem.

It is obvious that local treatment of malignant tumors in the lung is presently hampered by many limitations and moments of uncertainty. Thus it is worthwhile to consider the possible use of additional techniques of local treatment, which could serve as complements or alternatives to operation and radiation treatment.

This need for other methods was the reason for a preliminary study of the local application of cytostatics to lung and mediastinal tumors, which subsequently led to the development of a technique for selective catheterization of the bronchial arteries in humans.[6-9] Since the available chemotherapy is still far from ideal, these pilot studies of local treatment were abandoned temporarily.

Another possible means of local treatment of lung tumors, which I have previously written about, is electrocoagulation. This technique was the result of the following circumstances.

At the beginning of the development of diagnostic needle biopsy under television screening, objections were raised against the technique, which was considered dangerous because of the risk of local and general seeding of tumor cells. The procedure was then supplemented with local electrosterilization of the instrument tip in situ. This method is described elsewhere[4, 6] and was used in about thirty needle biopsies. The incidence of pneumothorax may have been slightly increased in these cases in comparison with needle biopsy without thermosterilization of the instrument. Otherwise, no other complications such as bleeding, etc. occurred.

The electrosterilization of the instrument could be made with local anesthesia in the chest wall and pleura. Usually the patients did not complain about any pain, but they often reported a sensation of heat "somewhere" inside the thorax. In follow-up studies of these patients it was found that very small tumors stopped growing after the biopsy with local sterilization of the instrument tip. This could be checked by a comparison between the size of the biopsied tumor and other nearby tumors or subsequently developing metastases.[2]

Later it was considered unnecessary to perform a local sterilization of the instrument in situ, and this part of the technique was given up.* In one patient[1] the surgical removal of every small nodule that was encountered resulted in the same 5-year survival rate for the malignant tumors as for the small tumors that we diagnosed by needle biopsy prior to operation.[12]

There has been considerable experience with electrocoagulation of tumors in organs other than the lung. In electrocoagulation of cancer of the vulva, a large

---

*A local tumor implant in a lung is of academic interest only. In the case of cell implantation in the vicinity of a tumor, the tumor and the implant will be removed at operation. Implantation into the pleura and chest wall can be avoided if a direction of the needle is chosen that gives a minimum distance of 4 cm between the tumor surface and the pleura.

piece of the involved tissue can be locally removed without bleeding. There have been hundreds of cases of percutaneous electrocoagulation in the brain without bleeding.[5] In addition to local tissue destruction, a certain amount of edema usually occurs.

With this background some preliminary attempts have been made to sterilize small verified malignant lesions in the lung by means of electrocoagulation.

SELECTION OF PATIENTS

The ideal patient for this procedure must be young and in good condition with one or two small, easily accessible metastases for which surgery or radiation treatment is considered questionable. Clinical colleagues were informed about these preliminary indications, and with these restrictions the number of suitable cases has been very limited. Twenty-five cases have therefore been collected over a 10-year period, during which time it has become obvious that the electrode technique and the control of sufficient heat transmission in the tissue are the critical points of the procedure.

TECHNICAL CONSIDERATIONS

Sufficient experience now exists for percutaneous needle biopsy of lung lesions as small as 5 mm by means of biplane roentgen television screening. With sufficient experience in diagnostic needle biopsy, one should be able to insert electrodes in small lesions for electrocoagulation. The lungs are, from a technical point of view, probably more suitable for local electrocoagulation than the brain because by means of fluoroscopy it is possible to have continuous control of the position of the electrodes, the local effect on the tissue, etc. Thermoelectric elements can be positioned on the tissue for the control of heat transmission. Even though bleeding is not considered to occur in intracerebral electrocoagulations, the possibility of the development of a hematoma in the brain could be disastrous. Such a complication in the lung is likely to be detected immediately and could be treated before the development of serious effects. The possible risks of bleeding in the lung seem, however, to be minimal or absent, as in the experience with intracranial electrocoagulations. The reason for the lack of bleeding is the heat application in this technique, which differs from that in surgical diathermy.

In surgical diathermy the "electric knife" is moved through the tissue, producing a continuous new wet tissue contact that keeps the circuit open, even with the application of a large electric effect on the knife edge. In electrocoagulation a relatively low electric effect is applied on the instrument to coagulate the surrounding tissue over a relatively long period of time. The transmission of heat is therefore largely dependent on the conductivity of the surrounding tissue, and this can be influenced in several ways.

The effect distribution is obtained from the following

$$P = \int \cdot i^2$$

where

$$P = \text{effect per volume unit (watt/m}^3)$$
$$\int = \text{resistivity ohmmeter}$$
$$i = \text{current density ampere/m}^2$$

The current density (i) at a distance (r) from a thin long thread conductor (of the length 1) gives

$$2 \pi r \cdot 1 \cdot i = I_1 = \text{total current from electrode}$$

which means:

$$i = \frac{I_1}{1 \cdot 2 \pi r} \sim \frac{I_1}{1 \cdot r}$$

This gives:

$$P \sim \int \cdot \left(\frac{I_1}{1 \cdot r}\right)^2$$

The effect per volume unit is consequently four times as great at the surface of the thread with the radius (r_t) as the effect at a distance equal to twice the length of the radius from the center of the thread (Fig. 14-1).

The current density (i) at a distance (r) from a spherical conductor (Fig. 14-2) gives

$$4 \pi r^2 \cdot i = I = \text{total current}$$

which means:

$$i = \frac{I}{4 \pi r^2} \sim \frac{I}{r^2}$$

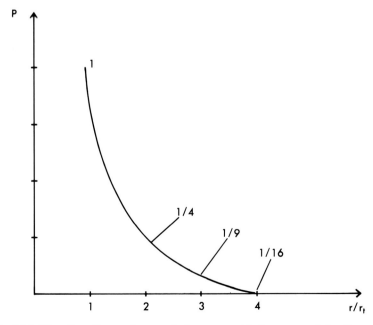

Fig. 14-1. The effect *P* per volume unit decreases with the square of the distance.

This gives:

$$P \sim \int \cdot \frac{I^2}{r^4}$$

The effect per volume unit is consequently sixteen times as great at the surface of the sphere as at a distance 2r from the center of the sphere (Fig. 14-3).

The current density between two very large parallel plates is of equal magnitude everywhere between the plates in the case of constant resistivity. In

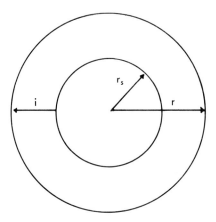

Fig. 14-2. *i*, Current density; r_s, radius of spherical electrode; *r*, arbitrary radius of medium surrounding electrode.

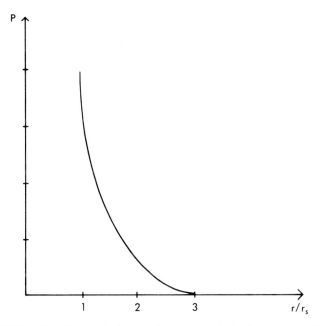

Fig. 14-3. The effect *P* per volume unit decreases with the fourth power distance.

reality, when the plates are relatively small, the current and effect density is greater close to edges, as compared with the density in a plane between the plates.

METHODS

Current generator. The current generator used is a standard diathermy apparatus (Erbotom). Separate settings for electrocoagulation and the use of cutting instruments are available as well as adjustment of current-voltage levels. As a rule, the application of heat should be made slowly at low settings of the apparatus. As resistivity increases, higher output has to be applied. No specific level can be predicted or recommended because factors such as elective distance (when two active electrodes are used) and tissue resistance vary in different types of tissue and during the course of heating.

Biopsy. Teflon catheters 16 cm long and 1.3 mm thick are threaded on 1 mm thick needles and introduced under local anesthesia to the surface of the tumor. Biplane television fluoroscopy is then used. Cell material is removed by means of aspiration biopsy or the use of a needle screw. A cytologist immediately examines the cell material, and if a malignancy is present, is usually able to confirm the diagnosis within a few minutes. In the meantime, steps are taken to introduce one or several electrodes and one electrothermometer for each through a separate Teflon catheter.

Electrodes. Because electrodes are applied percutaneously, their size and construction must meet certain specifications.

In the first 18 cases one metal string was inserted into the tumor through an insulating Teflon catheter and used together with a large indifferent grounded surface electrode under the patient.

In 8 cases two to five electrodes were inserted through teflon catheters into the tumor. Varying pairs of electrodes were connected to the terminals of the current generator. This method produces a simultaneous heat generation at two places at a time, which is more efficient than heat generation at only one electrode. The electrodes used for the purpose were stainless steel threads 22 cm long and 0.55 mm thick with a 15 mm long tapered tip shaped like a screw. This instrument, originally constructed for improvement of the sampling of cell material at needle biopsy,[10] is provided with a 0.1 mm thick Teflon layer over the metal. Only the spiral tip of the screw was allowed to make contact with the tissue. When one or several pairs of active electrodes are used in a tumor, the current generator as well as the patient should be insulated from ground.

Temperature measurements. The amount of heat supplied to a tumor should be controlled by means of a thermoelement. A 1.0 mm thick string-shaped thermoelement was used in 5 patients. The instrument is inserted through a Teflon catheter of the same type as that used for insertion of the electrodes. The thermosensitive tip of the instrument is then placed in the tissue close to the tumor surface and preferably at the most distant position in relation to the electrodes.

The outgoing signal from the instrument is written on a recording chart, which makes it possible to obtain the time-temperature integral (Fig. 14-13).

To prevent the thermoelement from acting as an accessory diathermy electrode, it should have a high impedance against the electrocoagulation circuit. This is obtained by providing the thermoelement probe with an electrically insulating material such as a thin Teflon coat. The probe may also produce a high impedance to ground at high frequencies by means of a drossel interconnected at the supplying cables.

RESULTS
Electrocoagulation with one active electrode

Electrocoagulation with only one active electrode was performed in 18 cases. Of these, at least 2 patients have shown a convincing cure, and several others have shown a possible temporary arrest in their growth. In a number of the cases the tumor has shown continued growth.

The 3 tumors in which good effect was observed were the smallest in this group. In one patient a melanosarcoma metastasis 10 by 13 mm in size was electrocoagulated for 4 minutes. It did not show any further growth within an observation period of 13 months. During the same time other metastases

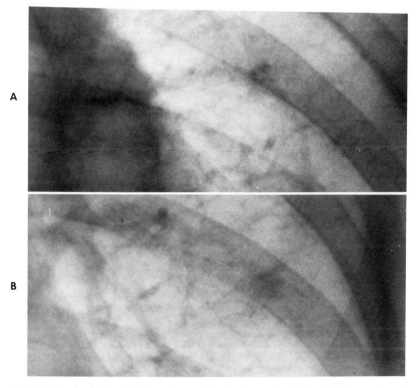

Fig. 14-4. **A,** Poorly differentiated embryonic testicular metastasis with 5 mm diameter in the lingula lobe (1969). **B,** In 1971, diameter of tumor is 10 mm.

appeared in the lungs showing a rapid growth. This case is reported in detail elsewhere.[4]

The second patient, a 25-year-old man, presented with a 10 by 10 mm solitary metastasis containing a poorly differentiated embryonic testicular tumor in the left lung. He had earlier been operated on for this tumor. He received postoperative radiation treatment and was maintained on chemotherapy. Needle biopsy revealed numerous very large atypical cells from an undifferentiated tumor. The cytologic material corresponded well with material obtained earlier from the testicular tumor. Fig. 14-4, A, shows the tumor as it appeared in 1969. By 1971 the tumor increased in size (Fig. 14-4, B) in spite of treatment with chemotherapy.

Before diagnostic needle biopsy the tumor was the size shown in Fig. 14-5, A. A small hematoma occurred in connection with needle biopsy (Fig. 14-5, B). Following electrocoagulation for 3 minutes a local reaction occurred around the tumor (Fig. 14-5, C). The reaction in the surrounding lung had partly disappeared a week later, but the tumor appeared denser than before (Fig. 14-5, D). Six months later the tumor had reduced in size, but some scar tissue was seen in the surrounding lung parenchyma (Fig. 14-5, E). In 1975, four years after the treatment, the tumor is not visible. Only some scar formation is seen (Fig. 14-5, F).

The patient is still taking chemotherapy 10 years after the operation of the primary tumor but is in good condition. No further metastases have been found in his lungs or elsewhere.

The patient illustrated in Fig. 14-6 is a 59-year-old man who had undergone nephrectomy for hypernephroma and then a leg amputation for a hypernephroma metastasis. Shortly after the amputation a solitary tumor was observed below the hilum of the right lung. When diagnostic needle biopsy was performed, the tumor measured 15 mm in diameter. Cytologic material verified the presence of a hypernephroma. Electrocoagulation was made with one active electrode for 10 minutes with a temperature of up to 60° C at the tumor surface. Minimal thermic reaction occurred. A 4 cm pneumothorax disappeared spontaneously within 2 days. The tumor did not show any change in size after the electro-coagulation. In Fig. 14-6, A, the tumor is seen immediately before the electro-coagulation. Fig. 14-6, B, shows the same size of the tumor 16 months later at the latest control examination. At that time, however, new large tumor masses had appeared in the left lung.

This is the only case in the group of 18 patients in which temperature control was applied. No complications occurred other than a small or medium-sized pneumothorax, which is common in ordinary diagnostic needle biopsy.

The radiologic appearance of local bleeding inside and outside a tumor is characterized by rather dense irregular infiltrations and is very well known from diagnostic needle biopsies. The local edema around a tumor due to a thermic reaction is a valuable sign of efficient heat transmission and is characterized by a rather light, diffuse density without sharp, irregular borderlines. This is

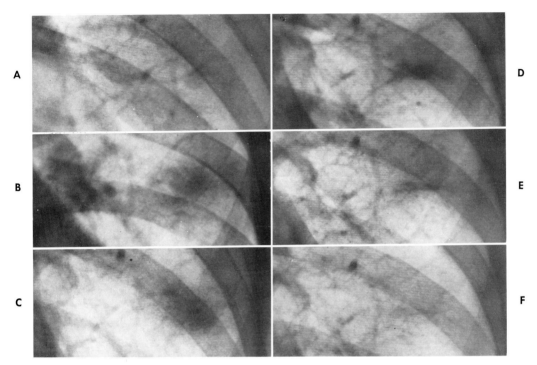

Fig. 14-5. Same case as Fig. 14-4. **A,** Tumor immediately before needle biopsy. **B,** After needle biopsy, local bleeding has occurred inside and around tumor. **C,** Local edema around tumor after electrocoagulation. **D,** Two months after electrocoagulation, increased density is seen in tumor along with scar formation in surrounding parenchyma. **E,** Six months later, tumor has decreased considerably in size. **F,** Four years after electrocoagulation, only minor scars are visible at tumor site.

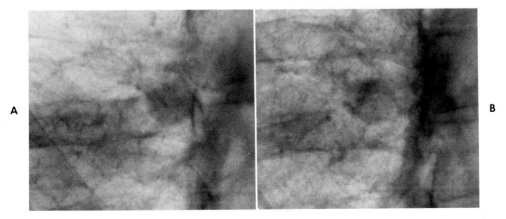

Fig. 14-6. **A,** Hypernephroma metastasis in apical segment of right lower lobe immediately before electrocoagulation. **B,** Sixteen months after treatment, tumor shows no sign of further growth.

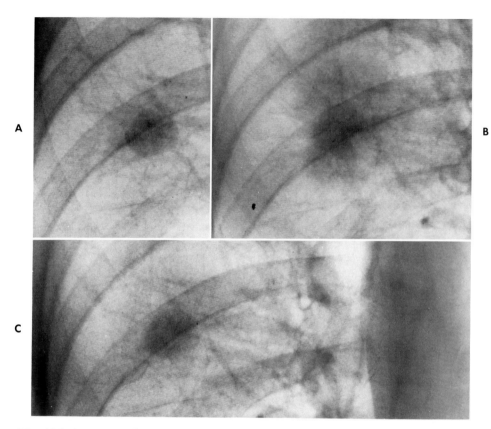

Fig. 14-7. **A,** Hypernephroma of right upper lobe before electrocoagulation. **B,** Heat production causes edema in lung, characterized by a rather homogeneous light density. **C,** The following day edema has almost disappeared.

illustrated in Fig. 14-7, which shows a hypernephroma immediately before (Fig. 14-7, *A*) and immediately after (Fig. 14-7, *B*) electrocoagulation. The next day almost all the edema had disappeared (Fig. 14-7, *C*).

Electrocoagulation with two or more active electrodes

This type of electrocoagulation was performed in only 7 cases. Fig. 14-8, *A,* shows a melanosarcoma metastasis 12 mm in diameter in the right lower lobe of a 44-year-old woman. She had been operated on for a melanosarcoma in the skin in 1965 and for a regional metastasis of the same tumor in 1970. A new metastasis in the lung was found in 1974. It grew rapidly and measured 20 by 25 mm 2 months later (Fig. 14-8, *B*). Electrocoagulation was then performed with three stainless steel electrodes with screw tips, which were anchored at the periphery of the tumor. The position of the electrodes in an AP and lateral view is seen in Fig. 14-8, *C* and *D*. Electrocoagulation was performed with 3 × one pair electrodes during a total coagulation time of about 4 minutes. After coagulation the tumor diminished rapidly in size (Fig. 14-8, *E*) and 16 months later

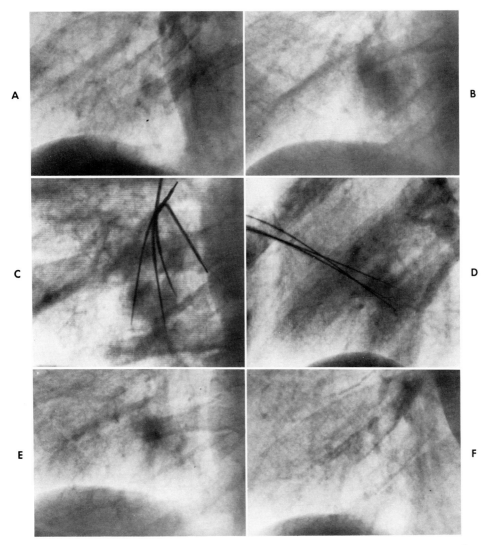

Fig. 14-8. A, Melanosarcoma metastasis in right lower lobe. **B,** Two months later, tumor has rapidly increased in size. **C** and **D,** AP and lateral views of tumor after positioning of three electrodes prior to electrocoagulation. **E,** At control examinations after electrocoagulation, tumor showed decreasing size. **F,** Sixteen months after electrocoagulation no obvious tumor residual is seen.

measured only 5 by 6 mm (Fig. 14-8, *F*). The patient was in good condition without any signs of new metastases. She died from brain metastases 2 years 5 months later. At autopsy no tumor residual was found in the lungs.

A metastatic mammary carcinoma diagnosed at needle biopsy is illustrated in Fig. 14-9, *A* and *B*. Because of the general condition of the patient, surgical removal was not performed. After irradiation with 4000 rads, the tumor diminished in size (Fig. 14-9, *C* and *D*). In the period shortly after the irradiation the patient developed a pulmonary embolus in the right lung. Fig. 14-10, *A*,

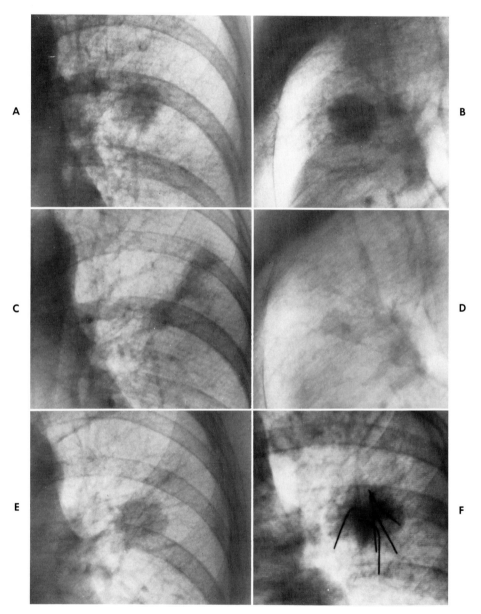

Fig. 14-9. **A** and **B**, AP and lateral views of a metastasis from a mammary carcinoma in anterior segment of left upper lobe. **C** and **D**, Tumor decreased in size rapidly after irradiation with 4000 rads. **E**, Eight months later, tumor has grown to size it had before irradiation. **F**, Implantation of five electrodes in tumor before electrocoagulation.

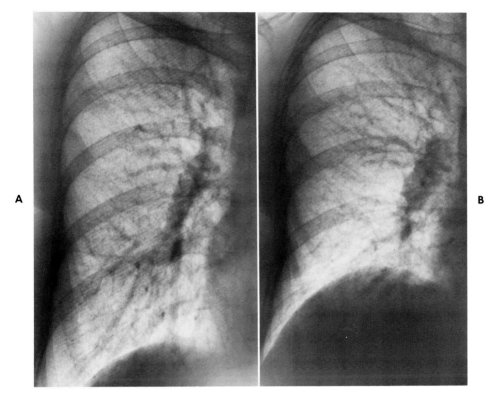

Fig. 14-10. Same patient as in Fig. 14-9. **A,** Right lung before development of pulmonary embolism in right lower lobe. **B,** Pulmonary embolism in right lower lobe, which occurred shortly after irradiation of left-sided lung tumor.

shows the normal lung vessels shortly before the irradiation and Fig. 14-10, *B,* the blocking of the right lower lobe artery by the embolus.

Eight months after the irradiation the tumor had grown to the same size as before the irradiation (Fig. 14-9, *E*). Since surgery as well as further irradiation was not considered suitable, attempts were made to electrocoagulate the tumor. Because of the size of the tumor, five electrodes were introduced (Fig. 14-9, *F*). Current was applied between different pairs of electrodes, which produced a temperature rise of 50° to 60° C, at least in one measuring place at the tumor surface. A small amount of local edema occurred around the tumor as well as a 4 cm pneumothorax, which disappeared spontaneously after 2 days. On the fifth day, however, the patient suddenly died from a new pulmonary embolus.

In patients with less tendency to develop pulmonary embolism, electrocoagulation of residual tumor after irradiation may be considered in the future. Technically it should have been relatively easy to destroy the residual of the tumor when it had diminished to the size seen in Fig. 14-9, *C* and *D*.

No bleedings have occurred during electrocoagulations with multiple active

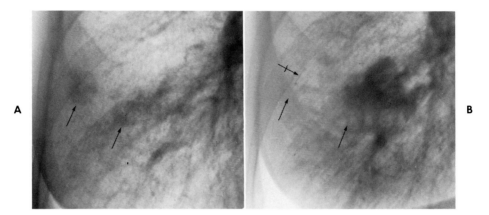

Fig. 14-11. A, Two hypernephroma metastases in right lung (arrows). **B,** About a year later electrocoagulated tumor (left arrow) is considerably reduced in size. Uncoagulated tumor has grown (right arrow). Note position of lost electrode tip (⇥).

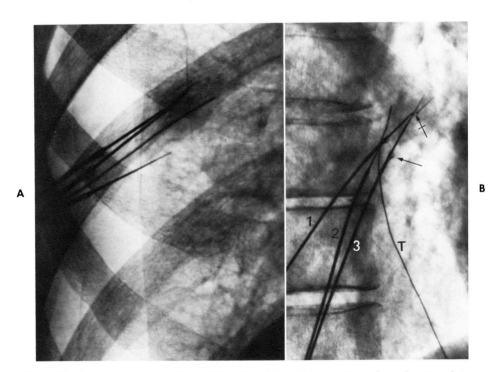

Fig. 14-12. Same patient as in Fig. 14-11. AP and lateral views. Two electrodes (*1* and *3*) are inserted in tumor. Third electrode (*2*) was displaced out of tumor at development of a pneumothorax. Thermoelement (*T*) is positioned close to posterior surface of tumor. Note funnel-shaped widening of Teflon tubings (←) due to heat production and too-close position of electrodes *1* and *3*, which caused a welding effect that cut the tip of electrode *1* (⇤).

electrodes. A pneumothorax of 2 to 6 cm in width has been produced in every case, but they have all resorbed spontaneously.

An unexpected complication occcurred in one patient in this series. A 62-year-old woman was treated with chemotherapy after operative removal of a hypernephroma. Later she developed several pulmonary lesions, one about 15 mm in diameter (Fig. 14-11, *A*). Needle biopsy of one of them yielded cell material showing hypernephroma. In connection with the sampling of cell material, a sterilization of the needle track and the punctured tumor was performed.

Three radiopaque Teflon tubes threaded on 1 mm wide needles were introduced percutaneously to the tumor surface after local anesthesia of the skin and pleura. Cell material was taken out through two of the needles by means of 0.55 mm wide stainless steel strings with tapered screw ends. After the cytologic diagnosis had been made, the needles were replaced by new stainless steel string electrodes covered with insulating surfaces, except on the 15 mm long screw ends. A thermoelement string was then introduced and positioned close to the back surface of the tumor (Fig. 14-12). Current was applied between two of the electrodes positioned inside the tumor. The temperature at the tumor surface rose to more than 60° C for different time intervals (Fig. 14-13). During the manipulation with the electrodes a pneumothorax of about

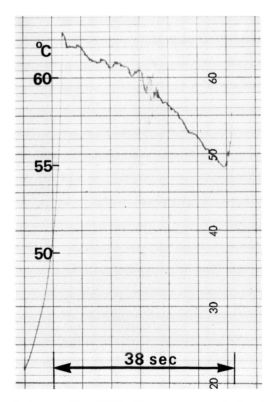

Fig. 14-13. Same patient as in Fig. 14-11. Temperature registration from posterior part of tumor shows a temperature rise over 60° C.

5 cm in depth developed, which resulted in the displacement of one of the three electrodes (3) to a position below the tumor. The two other electrodes (1 and 2) were displaced within the tumor and thus were positioned very close to each other at one point. This resulted in a heat strong enough to melt the stainless steel, so that 10 mm of the tip of one of the electrodes became dislodged. The electrodes and the thermoelement were then removed as well as the third electrode, which never was used. The patient had noticed only the usual vague sensation of heat. The pneumothorax resorbed spontaneously after 2 days.

A control film of the lungs a year later showed that the metal tip of the electrode was positioned in the lung above the electrocoagulated tumor (Fig. 14-11, *B*), which had diminished considerably in size. A second metastasis that had been observed close to the electrocoagulated one had grown in spite of treatment with chemotherapy to such a size that electrocoagulation was impossible. Further new metastases were developing in other parts of the lungs.

CONCLUSIONS

Experience has shown that local electrocoagulation of lung tumors in situ can be done relatively easily under local anesthesia with good local effect on the tumor and no important effects on the surrounding lung or on the patient in general. It should be possible to utilize the technique on multiple occasions in the same patient and as a supplementary method to reduce the patient's total tumor burden. Local radical surgery of a single primary tumor or metastasis should always be considered as the first therapy, but often a patient's condition or various circumstances (e.g., bilateral single small tumors, a poor prognostic type of tumor, or other general or local contraindications) make surgery questionable. In cases in which lesions are small or there is residual tumor after radiation treatment, local electrocoagulation should be considered. Yet it must be emphasized that experience with the method is not sufficiently large for a final evaluation of its usefulness. On the other hand, further improvements in this technique are being developed.

References

1. Birath, G.: Bronchialcancerns diagnostik och behandling, Sven. Läkartidningen 63:937, 1966.
2. Björk, V. O.: Bronchiogenic carcinoma, Acta Chir. Scand. (supp. 123) 95:1, 1947.
3. Churchill, E. D., Sweet, R. H., Scanell, J. G., and Wilkins, E. W.: Further studies in the surgical management of carcinoma of the lung, J. Thorac. Surg. 36:301, 1958.
4. Dahlgren, S., and Nordenström, B.: Transthoracic needle biopsy, Almqvist & Wiksell, Publishers, 1966.
5. Leksell, L.: Personal communication, 1975.
6. Nordenström, B.: Therapeutic roentgenology, Acta Radiol. [Diagn.] 3:115, 1965.
7. Nordenström, B.: Selective catheterization with Tifocyl injection of bronchomediastinal arteries in bronchial carcinoma, Acta Radiol. [Ther.] 4:298, 1966.
8. Nordenström, B.: Selective catheterization and angiography of bronchial and mediastinal arteries in man, Acta Radiol. [Diag.] 6:14, 1967.

9. Nordenström, B.: Bronchial arteriography, Bronches **19**:368, 1969.
10. Nordenström, B.: New instruments for biopsy, Radiology **17**:474, 1975.
11. Nordenström, B., Nordén, I., and Norhagen, Å.: Oxygen tension distally to a temporary occlusion of the pulmonary artery during oxygen breathing, Acta Radiol. [Ther.] **4**:385, 1966.
12. Overholt, R. H.: Curability of primary cancer of the lung. Early recognition and management, Surg. Gynecol. Obstet. **68**:435, 1939.
13. Paulson, D. L.: Survival rates following treatment for bronchogenic carcinoma, Ann. Surg. **146**:997, 1957.
14. Shaw, R. R., and Paulson, D. L.: The treatment of bronchial neoplasms, Springfield, Ill., 1959, Charles C Thomas, Publisher.
15. Sinner, W. N.: Transthoracic needle biopsy of small peripheral malignant lung lesions, Invest. Radiol. **8**:305, 1973.
16. Tala, P., and Virkkula, L.: The malignant solitary pulmonary lesion, Thorax **15**:252, 1960.

15 Some basic considerations of cerebrospinal fluid physiology as reflected by CSF imaging studies

A. Everette James, Jr., and Hugh Davson

with the collaboration of Ernst-Peter Strecker,* William Flor,** Barry Burns,‡ and Melvin Epstein§

In this chapter we shall relate some of the radiographic observations encountered in patients with communicating hydrocephalus and altered cerebrospinal fluid (CSF) physiology. We will present a review of studies by ourselves and others of normals and animals after development of communicating hydrocephalus. The anatomic changes we depict with imaging studies are reflections of abnormal function that have existed for sufficient periods of time to result in structural derangements. Serial analysis of the development of some of these changes will aid in basic understanding of why and when they occur and allow us to interpret in a meaningful fashion the resulting diagnostic radiographic images.

DEVELOPMENT OF COMMUNICATING HYDROCEPHALUS

The underlying mechanism in the development of communicating hydrocephalus is an imbalance of cerebrospinal fluid production and absorption or drainage.[28, 37, 50] In hydrocephalus, CSF–containing spaces within the brain (i.e., the ventricles) enlarge at the expense of neural tissue. Experimental evidence shows that initially there is diminished absorption either due to a dysfunction at the arachnoidal villi-venous sinus interface or to obstruction in or obliteration of the communicating pathways that allow movement of CSF to absorptive sites. Under these conditions, normal CSF production may eventually

---

*Fellow, Laboratory for Radiological Research, The Johns Hopkins Medical Institutions, Baltimore, Md.; Institute of Radiology, Freiburg, West Germany.
**Department of Experimental Pathology, Armed Forces Radiobiological Research Institute, Bethesda, Md.
‡Department of Environmental Medicine, The Johns Hopkins School of Hygiene and Public Health, Baltimore, Md.
§Department of Neurosurgery, The Johns Hopkins Medical Institutions, Baltimore, Md.

result in a volume of fluid greater than the existent space. Thus, as the spaces containing the relatively increased amount of cerebrospinal fluid enlarge, alterations in CSF production, movement, and absorption occur. These pathophysiologic changes appear to represent attempts to resist the derangements caused by diminished absorption and are grouped together as "compensatory" mechanisms, about which limited data are presently available. The most likely mechanisms for compensation appear to be the following:

1. Decrease in CSF production commensurate with diminished absorptive ability
2. Production of secondary or alternative pathways of CSF drainage to provide an adequate method of CSF removal
3. Enlargement of CSF-containing spaces to aid in absorption

Only fragmentary data can be gathered from our clinical experience regarding the changes associated with the development of communicating hydrocephalus. Neurologic, radiographic, and laboratory studies have inferred that certain sequential events may occur. Following an insult to the drainage structures from subarachnoid hemorrhage[43, 60] or infection,[33, 57] absorption is impaired; exactly what structures do not function properly is not entirely clear. In both human and nonhuman primate the areas of greatest CSF drainage appear to be the arachnoid villi located in the parasagittal region, although some absorption may occur through similar structures in the spinal region. In other species there are normal absorptive pathways that may or may not be present in humans. These areas may become available during the development of hydrocephalus in humans and provide alternative pathways that assist in compensation. Certain studies designed to evaluate these routes will be discussed.

Another theory of compensation in the development of hydrocephalus is that production of CSF diminishes commensurate with the defect in the drainage mechanism to reestablish harmony between production and absorption. However, CSF production (choroidal and extrachoroidal) does not appear to diminish in animals with communicating hydrocephalus.[31, 37] Cerebrospinal fluid is formed mainly by the choroid plexus in the cerebral ventricles, although data have been presented to suggest production in other sites such as the ventricular ependyma and even outside the ventricular region. Examination of this fluid leads to the conclusion that CSF is not an ultrafiltrate of plasma but is formed by an active process. The relative concentrations of various ions and molecules in CSF and comparisons with blood made by Davson[12] and others have confirmed this belief. The metabolism of the choroid plexus has not been studied in detail. It is known that certain substances such as carbonic anhydrase inhibitors at least temporarily diminish CSF production,[15] but no effective treatment method has been developed. We have attempted to examine the respiration of the choroid plexus cells in vitro in animals with hydrocephalus and compare the data to those from normal animals. The experimental method and preliminary results will be presented in this chapter.

The response of CSF pressure to changes in absorption is not well documented.

Some data suggest that CSF pressure is transiently normal, but as the absorptive rate becomes slower, CSF pressure rises, and sustained increased pressures are recorded. The cerebrospinal fluid pressure continues to increase, and the cerebral ventricles, which are initially of normal size, soon begin to enlarge.[28, 49, 51] As CSF pressure increases and the ventricles enlarge, it is unclear whether CSF volume studies show normal or decreased production,[31, 45] nor is it certain whether cerebral blood volume is normal or diminished.[27] Data from our laboratory will be discussed and compared with the findings of others.

Several investigators believe that as CSF pressure increases, the outward vector force at the ependymal surface is transmitted through the brain substance to the rigid bony calvarium.[28, 29] This outward force acting along the surface of the ventricle is opposed not only by the peripheral subarachnoid space, but also by the rigid calvarium and the interposed brain. Since the brain is a viscoelastic substance with the small, thin-walled cerebral vessels being the most compliant structures, the effect of this force may first cause changes of these vessels. Fluid and lipids are initially lost from the brain due to the outward forces acting on the ependymal surface, and the small vessels in the periventricular area probably collapse.[28, 55] These changes seem to occur first in the immediate subependymal white matter, especially at the superior ventricular angles (junction between the corpus callosum and the caudate nucleus). The location of these initial changes has been explained by the fact that the outward force of the CSF against the ependymal surface in this area is effective in two directions. Thus a separation force at the angle is more effective than one acting at right angles to the ventricular lining.

DETECTION AND STUDY OF COMMUNICATING HYDROCEPHALUS
CSF-imaging studies

With continued CSF production at a normal or near-normal rate and impaired absorption, the ventricles progressively enlarge initially at the expense of the white matter.[35] This is probably due to the compressive effect on the cerebral veins in this area. Computerized transaxial tomograms, cerebral angiograms, and pneumoencephalographic studies have been used to document this enlargement of the internal CSF-containing spaces. At carotid angiography the sweep of the callosal vessels in the arterial phase and measurements of distance from the thalamostriate to the internal cerebral vein are rather insensitive secondary signs of ventricular enlargement. Pneumoencephalography will demonstrate "rounding" of the ventricular angle even before the measurements exceed normal limits.[3] Pneumoencephalography is an accurate diagnostic procedure, but with inherent morbidity. The use of reconstructed images from the differential absorption of radiation appears to be an extremely promising method of detecting hydrocephalus. For these determinations this imaging technique will probably replace other diagnostic studies.

CSF imaging (cisternography) allows not only detection of hydrocephalus, but recording of abnormal CSF movement as well. In communicating hydrocephalus, radioactively labeled macromolecules injected in the lumbar sub-arachnoid space or the cisterna magna show abnormal movement into the ventricular system.[3, 19, 33] This entry of radiopharmaceutical does not normally occur, presumably due to the fact that the major portion of CSF is produced intraventricularly and is absorbed in the area of the arachnoid villi, resulting in a net current of flow outward.[34] Although this explanation for the normal movement of labeled macromolecules seems reasonable, the pathophysiology is probably much more complex. The cerebral blood flow, volume, CSF pressure, and other important physiologic parameters are rapidly changing, and structural alterations occur in response. These interrelationships and the time course of changes are not well documented.

As hydrocephalus progresses, the ventricles continue to enlarge, and move-ment of macromolecules in the CSF appears even more abnormal. If a labeled macromolecule is now injected into the lumbar subarachnoid space or the cis-terna magna, almost immediate movement into the ventricle (suggesting an ac-tive process) is seen.[19, 33, 65] Once in the ventricles, these labeled substances re-main there for protracted time periods.[46] This "stasis" is accompanied by enlarge-ment of the apparent ventricular size on delayed images, as noted by James et al. and Milhorat.[36, 49, 50] A number of explanations have been offered for this sequence of ventricular entry, stasis, and ventricular "enlargement," including changes in the radiopharmaceutical, separation of the radioactive label and recirculation, increased background in the periventricular area, and transependy-mal migration of the labeled macromolecule (usually ^{131}I human serum albumin). At present, data tend to support the explanation of transependymal movement of the radiopharmaceutical.[30, 34, 53, 61]

Serial neurologic studies of patients with developing communicating hydro-cephalus show a progression of neurologic problems initially affecting the lower extremities and later involving the upper.[77] These phenomena have been related to the relative anatomic location of long tract fibers and the surfaces of the lat-eral ventricles.[77] The fibers responsible for motor activity in the hands and upper extremities originate near the level of the superior surface of the lateral ventricle. As a consequence, these fibers course in such a direction that they are parallel to the ventricular surface for only a short distance. The motor fibers for the lower extremities and feet arise near the superior surface of the cere-bral cortex and course in such a direction that the fibers are parallel to the sur-face of the lateral ventricle for a much greater distance. Thus a force acting at right angles to the ependymal surface in a lateral direction would stretch and compress the fibers to the lower extremities much more than those to the upper extremities. We shall attempt to correlate these ideas with the serial neurologic findings in a model that produces communicating hydrocephalus over a time period that is long enough to allow sequential observation.

No serial pathologic studies on a large series of patients with acute, subacute, or chronic communicating hydrocephalus are available.[10, 17, 18, 72] Several small series suggest that obliteration of the subarachnoid space over the cerebral convexities, obstruction of the communicating pathways such as the basal or ambient cisterns, obstruction around the cerebellar tentorium, or fibrosis in the parasagittal arachnoid villi are the most common findings. These data support the theory that CSF cannot reach the area of greatest absorption, causing an eventual hydrocephalus. Serial studies in animals show that initially there is a loss of the cilia of the ependymal cells lining the lateral ventricles. These ependymal cells also change from their normal cuboidal shape and become flattened.[39, 51] They then become separated and denuded, and the lining (which appears normally to effect a partial barrier to large molecules) is lost. Enlargement of the extracellular space in the white matter surrounding the brain is present, and a paucity of the small cerebral vessels is seen.[10, 30, 31, 37] Specific in-depth analysis of the gray matter and cord, which would allow definitive statements about the presence of chronic nonspecific degenerative changes, is not available.[22, 39] From the neurologic symptoms encountered clinically and in the laboratory, one would predict that studies of chronic hydrocephalus would demonstrate abnormalities in these areas.

The CSF-brain-blood barrier has not been adequately investigated using histochemical or radioactive markers. Transfer of labeled molecules from the subarachnoid space into the intravascular compartment has been utilized both in clinical practice and in the laboratory to separate humans and animals with communicating hydrocephalus from normals.[1, 69] In humans with communicating hydrocephalus there is a delay in transfer of ^{125}I human serum albumin from the CSF space into the blood. This was also found to be true in animals with developing or well-developed communicating hydrocephalus (Fig. 15-1). However, because of the wide range of values in the hydrocephalic group,

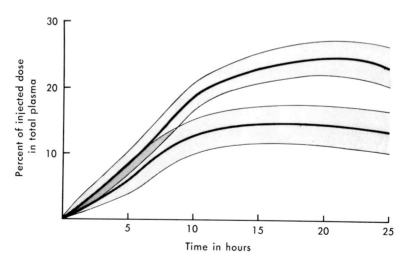

Fig. 15-1. Graph comparing transfer of radiopharmaceutical from the subarachnoid space into blood in normal animals (upper band) and in animals after development of hydrocephalus (lower band). Shaded area represents the standard deviation. Transfer of labeled molecule from CSF space into blood is both delayed and diminished following induction of chronic communicating hydrocephalus. (Modified from James, A. E., et al.: J. Neurosurg. **41:**32, 1974.)

humans with hydrocephalus due to an absorptive abnormality cannot be separated from those with hydrocephalus due to generalized atrophy. In the animal groups, those animals with ventricular entry and movement of the radiopharmaceutical out of the ventricles by the 24-hour cisternographic view cannot be separated from those with ventricular penetration and stasis. For these reasons, blood sampling to measure transfer has been abandoned as a primary procedure for diagnosis in most clinical laboratories. In general, pattern interpretation is utilized to diagnose hydrocephalus and to select patients that might benefit from a CSF diversionary shunt.

Following subarachnoid injection of any appropriate radiopharmaceutical a predictable sequence of images is seen, depending on the anatomy and physiology of the CSF spaces and the relation of CSF production and absorption. In normals, following lumbar radiopharmaceutical injection, radioactivity appears in the area of the basal cisterns within 1 or 2 hours (Fig. 15-2, A).

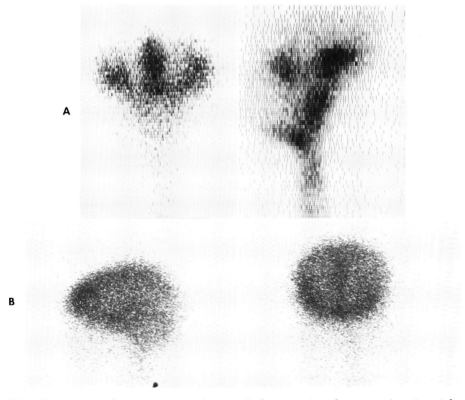

Fig. 15-2. A, Normal cisternogram in human. Early views (rectilinear scan) at 1 to 2 hours show movement of radiopharmaceutical (1 mCi of ^{111}In DTPA) from site of injection (lumbar subarachnoid space) to basal cisterns and cisterna magna. No ventricular radioactivity is visible. B, Delayed cisternographic views (camera) at 24 to 48 hours show generalized distribution of radiopharmaceutical in subarachnoid space over cerebral cortex. Concentration in area of arachnoid villi is also seen normally, especially with labeled albumin in adults imaged with a rectilinear scanner.

The communicating pathways are seen in 4 to 6 hours, and radioactivity is present over the cerebral cortex. No ventricular radiopharmaceutical entry is seen. After 6 to 12 hours the radioactivity moves over the cerebral cortex and collects in the parasagittal region in 24 hours. In adults the basal cisterns begin to clear of radioactivity at 24 hours, and concentration in the area of the arachnoid villi is seen (Fig. 15-2, *B*). This concentration may become more dramatic on the 48- to 72-hour views and is better defined with the labeled albumin (mol wt 69,000) than with the chelates (mol wt 600 to 800). The chelates show prolonged basilar retention. The "capping" over the cranial vault is more distinct on images made with the rectilinear scanner than with the scintillation camera. This is probably due to differences in the inherent planes of optimum resolution with the two types of collimators employed.

Identification of detailed structural anatomy present on cisternograms will become of secondary importance in the future because of more widespread use of computerized axial tomographic devices. These machines elegantly resolve small changes in anatomic configuration and size and adequately document the presence or absence of ventricular enlargement as well as changes of the cerebral sulci (Fig. 15-3). It may be predicted that soon radionuclide studies of CSF will be used to answer queries regarding abnormal function, not changes of structural anatomy. The general directions of CSF movement, however, are of significant importance, and serial studies such as CSF images and CAT with water-soluble contrast media will provide useful information.

Diversionary shunts

Treatment of certain patients with chronic communicating hydrocephalus by CSF diversionary shunts has been associated with dramatic improvement.[3, 46, 62] However, as further experience has been acquired, complications and failures have been emphasized.[47] More specific preoperative selection of patients is recommended, not only to avoid a number of the complications due to the surgery, but also to improve overall results. Several modifications in shunt design have diminished complications, but, at the very least, surgical revision at certain time intervals is predictable. Surgical establishment of an alternative drainage pathway is a traumatic procedure and is to be undertaken only in those patients likely to benefit. Alternative methods of treatment have been attempted, but, to date, no other effective form of therapy is available. It would appear that with data regarding the basic mechanisms associated with the development of communicating hydrocephalus and with more fundamental understanding of CSF production and absorption more appropriate methods of treatment will be developed.

Production of communicating hydrocephalus in animal models

Current investigations of the pathophysiologic mechanisms involved in communicating hydrocephalus have been limited by the lack of a satisfactory animal model. A great number of methods to produce communicating hydrocephalus

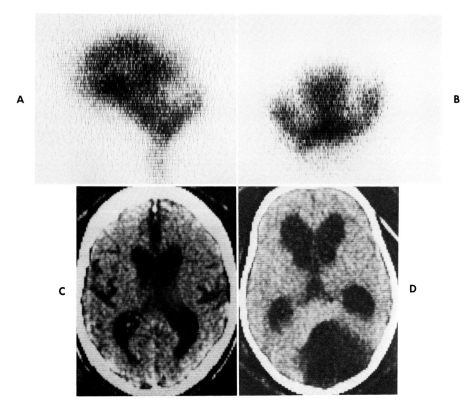

Fig. 15-3. A and **B**, CSF-imaging study (cisternogram) in patient with chronic communicating hydrocephalus. Early views at 1 to 2 hours show radiopharmaceutical (1 mCi of [169]Yb DTPA) in lateral ventricles. This localization of radioactivity persists for protracted time periods in patients with chronic communicating hydrocephalus and normal CSF pressures. **B,** Clearing of ventricles on delayed views is usually seen in patients with communicating hydrocephalus due to atrophy. **C,** Transaxial computerized tomographic view through lateral ventricles showing enlargement. In addition, there is dilation of subarachnoid space over cerebral cortex, characteristic of generalized cerebral atrophy. **D,** EMI scan (transaxial computerized tomogram) of child with hydrocephalus and a large Dandy-Walker–type cyst. Cortical sulci are not seen, since this does not represent a primary atrophic process. (Courtesy Fred J. Hodges, M.D., and A. L. Bahr, M.D., Johns Hopkins Hospital.)

have been reported.[40, 76] Beginning with the concept that hydrocephalus results from an imbalance of production and absorption, these techniques diminish CSF absorption by a variety of means. Some are too traumatic to the animal to be utilized in a chronic time frame; others produce inflammation and closure of the outlets of the fourth ventricle and cause noncommunicating hydrocephalus. The most commonly used method has been injection of a noxious substance into the subarachnoid space. Studies by Strecker, James, Konigsmark, and Merz[67] have shown that this provokes a generalized inflammatory response resulting in histologic changes with healing, altering the normal movement of CSF and probably changing the dynamics of the CSF-brain-blood interfaces. This method often results in profound symptoms, death of a large percentage of animals, and closure

of the aqueduct of Sylvius or ventricular outlets, resulting in obstructive hydrocephalus. Some animals will develop communicating hydrocephalus, but the
yield in primates is low.

Early in this century, Dandy and his colleagues described a surgical procedure involving wrapping of the brain stem to cause hydrocephalus.[40] Since that
time, injection of agents such as lampblack and kaolin has been recommended.
Because subarachnoid hemorrhage from any cause may produce hydrocephalus
clinically, injection of blood into the subarachnoid space has been attempted by
us and others. Radiographic contrast media of the type that causes a localized
inflammatory reaction and subsequent granuloma formation has been used to
produce communicating hydrocephalus, as has the surgical obliteration of venous
return. Temporary obstruction of the CSF pathways by balloons or cotton plugs
has also been advocated. As stated, we attempted these methods, and they failed
to produce the type of hydrocephalus we wished to study, were inappropriate for
investigations involving a chronic time frame, or failed to produce hydrocephalus
at all.

A very promising method was described in which subarachnoid infusion of
silicone oil produced hydrocephalus in young animals.[75, 76] This technique appeared suitable for a chronic model because no marked meningeal inflammation
occurred. It was only limited by the inability to control the location of the
silicone oil once it was injected into the subarachnoid space. A simple, successful,
and relatively atraumatic technique has subsequently been developed to produce
chronic communicating hydrocephalus.[35, 40] This method allows differentiation
of the various phases of development of hydrocephalus in a manner similar to that
employed in patient evaluation. With this technique 1 to 2 ml of a Silastic-type
material is injected through a catheter into the basal subarachnoid space. The
mixture contains 3 ml of polysiloxane polymer, 3.5 ml of dimethylpolysiloxane,
and 2 drops of the catalyst stannous octoate.* One milliliter of powdered tantalum
can be added for radiographic localization (Fig. 15-4). The advantages of Silastic
(room temperature–curing silicone rubber) are that it enters the subarachnoid
space as a fluid and then hardens to effect an obstruction in a predictable manner and location. Additionally, it does not cause significant meningeal inflammation. In the proportions described, this mixture requires 20 to 40 minutes to
harden in CSF. For this reason the animal is placed on the side during the
cisterna magna puncture, catheter manipulation to the basal cisterns, and injection. The animal is then positioned supine with the head hanging to facilitate flow toward the dependent cerebral cortex. This mixture was chosen
because the combination of polysloxane polymer and dimethylpolysiloxane has
been used as an injectable prosthesis for soft tissue augmentation and appears
physiologically and chemically inert in other spaces; thus we felt it would act
similarly in the subarachnoid space. Histologic studies supported this concept—
there was no inflammatory reaction in the meninges unless we added radio-

---

*Dow Corning Corp., Midland, Mich.

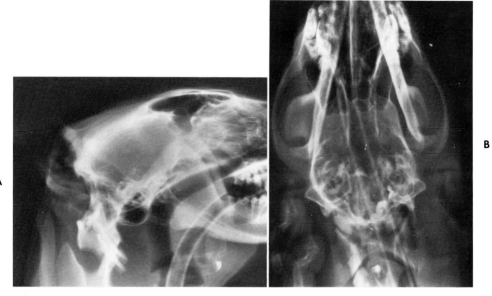

Fig. 15-4. **A,** Lateral and, **B,** dorsoventral skull radiographs of dog following injection of Silastic (rendered radiopaque by mixing powdered tantalum at time of injection) into basal cistern through an intracatheter. In this animal, Silastic localized anterior to pons but superior to outlets of fourth ventricle. Localization in area of arachnoid villi also occurred with this animal model.

graphic contrast media, which provoked an inflammatory response. However, the subarachnoid space is obliterated by this semisolid substance in many areas, especially the parasagittal region in dogs, the basal regions in puppies, and the tentorial region and communicating pathways in primates.

In summary, this method produces a communicating hydrocephalus that develops over a period of weeks or months, not unlike that seen clinically in both adults and children, and reconstruction of the clinical circumstances of chronic communicating hydrocephalus is obviously important in any related experimental study. In the small number of patients with chronic communicating hydrocephalus not due to generalized atrophy, the most common pathologic findings have been obliteration of the subarachnoid space in the basal cisterns, in the communicating CSF pathways (such as the ambient cisterns), in the tentorial region, or over the cerebral convexities and around the arachnoid villi. As stated earlier, no large necropsy series of patients is available, but it may be presumed that these findings represent the chronic stage of a process that began as cranial vault trauma, subarachnoid hemorrhage, or meningitis. These pathologic findings correlate well with reported pneumoencephalographic manifestations and appearance on CSF images (cisternograms) in patients with chronic communicating hydrocephalus. If removal of certain substances from the cerebrospinal fluid is impaired by any of these insults, alterations in CSF composition and/or volume may occur. It does not appear that the composition of CSF is greatly changed in hydrocephalus, but the volume relative to the available CSF space may be.

Comparison of CSF pressures in normal and hydrocephalic subjects

Correlation of cisternograms, radioactive transfer from the subarachnoid space into the blood, and CSF pressure measurements allowed us to separate the animals into two distinct groups, normals and hydrocephalics. In normal animals the CSF pressure measurements were in the range of 8 to 20 cm of water despite serial cisterna magna punctures (Fig. 15-5, A). Recordings were made with the animal intubated and lying on the left side, anesthetized with pentobarbital sodium (30 mg/kg intravenous), and following administration of intramuscular atropine (0.02 mg/kg). The cisterna magna was punctured using the external occipital protuberance and the lateral masses of the atlas as landmarks. Correct placement of the needle within the cisterna magna was assured by the presence of clear CSF, radiographic monitoring, and pressure tracings. Without loss of CSF, the needle was connected to a Sanborn model 267A pressure transducer coupled to a Sanborn 350-1100C carrier preamplifier and a Sanborn 7700 series recorder. Anatomic localization of the needle was confirmed radiographically. The pressure transducer was positioned at the level of the cranial midline during the measurement of ventricular pressure. Calibration was performed with a fluid manometer in centimeters of water. A second recording was obtained 1 or 2 minutes after the removal of 2 ml of CSF. In those animals with communicating hydrocephalus, the two pressure readings were nearly identical due to increased volume of the CSF compartment.

Validity of CSF pressure measurements was confirmed by the characteristic "arterial-like" waveforms induced by the pulsations of the choroid plexus and cerebral vessels. If these waveforms were absent, it was assumed that the needle was not within the subarachnoid space of the cisterna magna. The cisternograms in these animals (Fig. 15-5, B) showed distribution of the radioactivity in the basal cisterns on the early views at 30 minutes and 4 hours, with movement over the cerebral cortex by 24 hours. In the animals in which noncommunicating hydrocephalus developed, the CSF pressure was elevated within days after Silastic injection and continued to increase until the time of death. The cisternographic pattern did not differ from that seen in the control animals.[65] In the animals in which communicating hydrocephalus was induced, elevated CSF pressures were observed initially. Later the CSF pressure measurements decreased and eventually fell into the normal range.[41] The cisternograms were normal before Silastic injection but showed ventricular radiopharmaceutical entry in all animals as pressures began to decline in 20 to 45 days after injection (Fig. 15-5, A). Radiopharmaceutical was well delineated in the lateral ventricles on the 30-minute and 4-hour views (Fig. 15-5, C). By the 24-hour view, movement over the cortex was present, although some ventricular radioactivity remained. Subsequent cisternograms showed prompt ventricular entry without later cortical activity but persistent radioactivity in the ventricles. A comparison of cisterno-

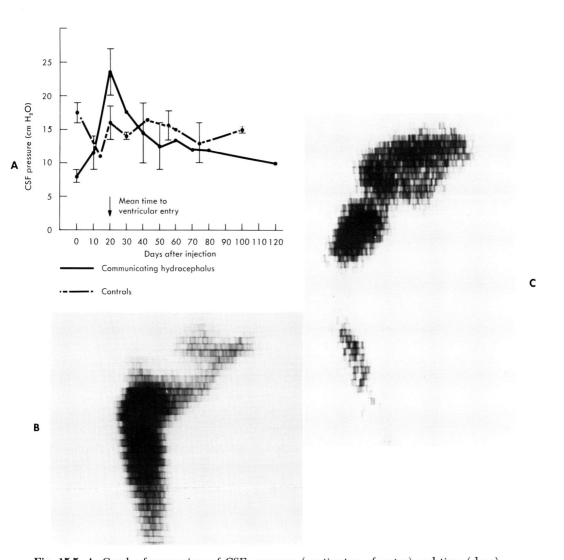

Fig. 15-5. **A,** Graph of comparison of CSF pressures (centimeters of water) and time (days) in normal animals and animals following subarachnoid Silastic injection. CSF pressure increases for some time following Silastic injection, but after approximately 15 to 30 days, CSF pressure decreases and again returns to normal range. **B,** Right lateral view of a cisternogram in a normal dog taken approximately 30 minutes after injection of 500 μCi ^{111}In DTPA. Radioactivity is concentrated in cisterna magna area as well as upper cervical spine. Anterior extension of radioactivity is in basal cisterns and communicating pathways. No ventricular radioactivity is seen. **C,** Right lateral view of a cisternogram in an animal 30 days after Silastic injection. Radiopharmaceutical (500 μCi of ^{111}In DTPA) was placed in cisterna magna and this right lateral view obtained with a rectilinear scanner 30 minutes after injection. Radioactivity is concentrated at injection site, but superiorly a large area of radioactivity representing lateral ventricles, which are enlarged, is noted. This pattern is characteristic of that seen in both animals and humans with communicating hydrocephalus. (**A** modified from James, A. E., Strecker, E. P., Novak, G. R., and Burns, B.: Neurology 23:1226, 1973; **B** from James, A. E., et al.: J. Neurol. Sci. 24:151, 1975.)

grams with pressure measurements in animals with communicating hydrocephalus showed that the pressure began to increase before ventricular radiopharmaceutical entry was detected on the cisternograms and continued to increase during the phase of ventricular entry and "clearing." Pressures were significantly elevated (p<0.05) before and during ventricular entry of radiopharmaceutical.[41] CSF pressure began to decrease about the time that ventricular entry and "stasis" appeared on the cisternograms and eventually reached normal range. The decline of CSF pressure could be correlated with the increased localization of radiopharmaceutical entry in the ventricle and the increasing length of time it remained there. From these studies using multiple punctures and finite sampling periods, we have extended our observations by the use of improved methods of CSF pressure measurement. By using indwelling ventricular catheters and subdural pressure transducers to monitor CSF pressure both intraventricularly and over the cerebral cortex, the same general findings were obtained. These studies are to be continued not only to more accurately document CSF pressure changes but also to characterize by continuous monitoring the pressure waveform and to determine whether "spikes" of intermittent increased pressure occur. The significance of transient increases in CSF pressure is not known, but their presence has been related to improvement by CSF diversionary shunting.

A number of theories and elegant mathematical expressions have attempted to explain the concomitant findings of normal CSF pressure measurements and large ventricles. Some investigators believe that although the CSF pressures are in the normal range, their effective force on the brain is greater than the same pressure with ventricles of normal size.[28] They reason that the forces are acting on the ependymal surface of the ventricles in a lateral or outward direction. Since the area (ventricular surface) is markedly enlarged in hydrocephalus, the pressure is distributed over a larger surface and the outward thrust is increased. While these forces may be reflected by an increase in CSF pressure around the periphery of the cerebral cortex, there is a transient imbalance when the internal CSF pressure exceeds that in the peripheral subarachnoid space and the outward force is opposed by the rigid bony calvarium, as occurs at this time. During these periods of imbalance, which may be initiated by a reduced drainage capacity, the internal spaces enlarge, despite a normal production of CSF. This enlargement would produce an increase in cranial vault size if the sutures have not fused, as in children. If the cranial vault is rigid and resists expansion of intracranial contents, the more complaint brain is compressed between the outward force of the CSF in the ventricles and the inner table of the bony calvarium. During this period the CSF pressure is elevated, and if cisternograms are obtained (which we do not advocate), no ventricular entry is seen. At some point the ventricles enlarge enough so that radiopharmaceutical injected in the subarachnoid space in the spine or cisterna magna enters the ventricles and is delineated there (Fig. 15-5, *C*). However, CSF pressure abnormalities are accompanied by related anatomic and physiologic alterations, which will be presented later. It is difficult to accept the fact that the transient pressure differences between the ventricles and the subarachnoid space over the cerebral hemispheres would be sustained for a sufficient period of time to allow such profound internal changes. Since the outlet foramina of the fourth ventricle are patent and probably enlarged, the pressure differences must be very transient.

During the phase of increased pressure on the ventricles from the outward force of the CSF, one form of compensation would be an adjustment of CSF production to the diminished absorptive capacity. Several studies to measure CSF production in animals and humans with hydrocephalus have produced conflicting results. In general, during periods of marked increased intracranial pressure, CSF production is diminished.[11] It is not known if the pressure elevation must be intermittent or continuous to decrease CSF production. Moderate increases of CSF pressure do not appear to diminish CSF production, and studies have found animals and humans with chronic hydrocephalus and apparently normal CSF volume production. We wanted to examine these phenomena from two aspects: (1) the volume of CSF production and (2) the metabolism of the choroid plexus cells during and after development of communicating hydrocephalus.

Volume of CSF production

Employing the ventriculocisternal perfusion techniques of Pappenheimer, Heisey, Jordan, and Downer[54] modified by Rall, Oppelt, and Patlak,[58] and Fenstermacher et al.,[25] [3]H polyethylene glycol and ^{14}C inulin were utilized to determine the dilution of the radioactive marker by the production of CSF during the testing period. Perfusion was begun after immobilization of the animal, ventricular cannulation by stereotactic techniques, and placement of a cannula in the cisterna magna (Fig. 15-6). Since radioactive markers were used for the perfusion studies, at the conclusion of the procedure, the brain was fixed for subsequent pathologic and morphologic studies.

Using this method, in the absence of CSF production, the outflow radioactivity (C_o) will equal the inflow radioactivity (C_i), since the molecules utilized are too large (under normal circumstances) to enter the blood or to leave the CSF compartment in a significant amount during this time period. Some movement into the periventricular cerebral tissues occurs initially, but stops within 25 minutes after the perfusion begins. With production of CSF, the radioactive marker is diluted as it passes through the system, and by measuring the extent of this dilution, the CSF production rate can be determined. This relationship is expressed mathematically

$$Q_i C_i = Q_o C_o$$

where Q_i = flow in and Q_o = flow out.

However, the term for outflow (Q_o) is composed of the inflow plus the flow due to CSF production. This means that $Q_o = Q_i + Q_{CSF}$. Thus the first equation can be modified to:

$$Q_{CSF} = \frac{C_i - C_o}{C_o} \cdot Q_i$$

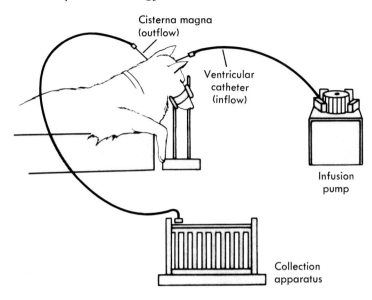

Fig. 15-6. Placement of ventricular and cisternal cannulae for ventriculocisternal perfusion studies. (Modified from James, A. E., Novak, G., and Burns, B.: Exp. Brain Res. **27:**1977.)

In this calculation the volume of CSF production per minute is determined and can then be related to body or brain weight. Normal animals tolerate the procedure well, and the only difficulty is insertion of the ventricular cannula into the small, normal-sized ventricles. In animals studied during the phase of elevated pressure, it is sometimes difficult to regulate the other physiologic parameters. This disadvantage is offset somewhat by the ease with which free flow of CSF from the cisterna magna catheter is established. After development of communicating hydrocephalus, animals require smaller amounts of anesthesia, and failure to adjust the anesthetic levels will result in profound respiratory depression. The enlarged lateral ventricles are quite easy to cannulate, and once the preparation is initiated, there are fewer technical difficulties in studying hydrocephalic animals than normals.

The data regarding CSF production are combined because not enough studies have been performed to date to separate clearly each hydrocephalic group. However, enough data were accumulated for the combined groups of animals with hydrocephalus to compare with the measurement of CSF production in normals. The volume of CSF production was expressed as $\mu l/min/kg$. In six normal animals, the range was 2.01 to 5.10 $\mu l/min/kg$, the average being 3.73 ± 0.49 SE $\mu l/min/kg$. Animals with communicating hydrocephalus had a range of 1.20-4.64 $\mu l/min/kg$. The average CSF production in these animals was 2.46 ± 0.61 SE $\mu l/min/kg$. No statistically significant difference between the two groups was observed, but the trend was for lower rates of CSF production in the hydrocephalic animals. These studies were with small numbers of dogs, and only two animals in the group were studied at times less than 2 weeks following subarachnoid Silastic injection (subacute). If one examines the findings in this group separately, the average volume of CSF production was 1.45 μl/min/kg. Because the CSF production seemed reduced in animals during the phase of increased CSF pressure, this group of dogs was subsequently studied and the findings of diminished CSF production were confirmed. Since there were elevated CSF pressures during this stage, a study of nonhuman primates during this period would be of particular importance.

Ventriculocisternal perfusion measurements of CSF production and simultaneous CSF pressure recordings demonstrate that the rate of production is not directly pressure dependent over a wide pressure range, although our studies and those of others suggest that in a semiquantitative manner there is some relation.[11, 31, 45] The rates of CSF formation vary for different species,[12, 13, 38] but if expressed as a fraction of the total volume of CSF, the rate is reasonably consistent and found to be approximately 0.5% per minute. In humans the rate of CSF formation is approximately 0.37 ± 0.1 SD ml/min. Since the total CSF volume is approximately 140 ml, the CSF is renewed in 6 to 8 hours. As previously discussed, the rate of CSF formation is reasonably pressure independent for a range of –10 to 240 mm of H_2O.[45, 48, 49] In the initial development of hydrocephalus, before significant ventricular enlargement has occurred, the CSF pressures may exceed this upper limit and cause diminished CSF production. Recently, Lorenzo, Page, and Watters[45] have shown a response to pressure in CSF production.

CSF formation rate can be temporarily modified by acetazolamide and methazolamide, recognized inhibitors of carbonic anhydrase.[15] In rabbits a 50% reduction of CSF formation can be produced by intravenous and intracisternal injection of these substances. In humans the effect of these drugs is reached in approximately 90 minutes and lasts for less than an hour. Since the site of action of these carbonic anhydrase inhibitors is the cells of the choroid plexus, a study of the metabolism of these cells in normal and hydrocephalic animals seemed appropriate. A reduction in absorption, CSF volume production, and choroid plexus metabolism would explain the loss of the net flow of CSF from the ventricles to the peripheral space. This would be reflected on cisternograms by "reversal" of radiopharmaceutical movement and entry into the enlarged ventricles, as occurs with communicating hydrocephalus.[19, 36]

Choroid plexus cell metabolism

We stated earlier that CSF is mainly produced in the choroid plexus of the cerebral ventricles, although some ependymal and extraventricular production may occur. It has been suggested that in the early development of hydrocephalus a reduction of choroid plexus metabolic activity (as reflected by cellular respiration) might provide a potential compensatory mechanism to lessen the effects of diminished absorption and to minimize the progression of ventricular enlargement. CSF volume production represented one method to study this possibility; another would be an in vivo or in vitro investigation of the respiration of choroid plexus cells.

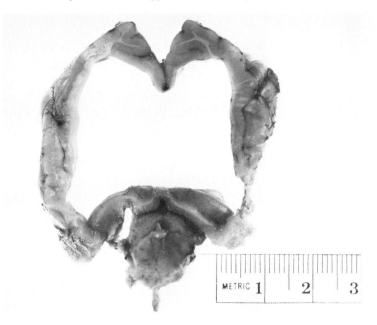

Fig. 15-7. Coronal section of a 7-week-old puppy 10 days after injection of Silastic into basal subarachnoid space. Communicating hydrocephalus, which was confirmed by cisternography, is profound. This specimen was fixed by immersion in formalin. Perfusion with either formalin or a glutaraldehyde mixture was precluded by studies that were performed on the choroid plexus respiration. However, enlargement of lateral ventricles is striking.

The most sensitive means available for measuring gaseous exchange in biologic material is the ampulla-diver respirometer developed by Zajicek and Zeuthen[78] as a modification of the Cartesian diver described by Linderstrom-Lang.[23, 24, 44] We used this instrument to measure the respiration (oxygen consumption) of choroid plexus cells during the development of communicating hydrocephalus in puppies.[38] Puppies were chosen as the experimental model for several reasons: littermates could be used as controls, the development of hydrocephalus was rapid (7 to 10 days after injection) and profound (Fig. 15-7), and the required large numbers of animals were readily available.

Immediately after induction of sufficient anesthesia, the choroid plexus was removed and placed in a substrate buffer. Microdissection of the choroid plexus from the supporting structures was performed. Groups of isolated choroid plexus cells along with substrate buffer were placed in a series of small ampulla divers. These divers were individually suspended vertically in flotation chambers, which were placed in a large water bath (Fig. 15-8, *A*). Temperature and pressure were rigidly controlled.[23, 24] The height of the meniscus between the liquid (substrate buffer and cells) and the gas phase in the ampulla diver was adjusted to a mark under direct visualization through a single-aperture microscope. The change in position of this meniscus for some period of time was recorded by manually increasing the pressure in a vernier buret to adjust the meniscus to its former level (Fig. 15-8, *B*). This change reflected the decrease in partial pressure of oxygen

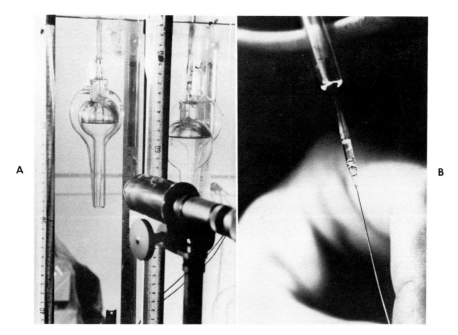

Fig. 15-8. A, Single-aperture microscope and small (5 cm) ampulla diver contained in flotation chamber suspended in water bath. Scales for measurement of pressure adjustment are seen vertically on each side of flotation chambers. There are several flotation chambers in the water bath so that samples from choroid plexus in hydrocephalic puppies can be measured simultaneously against those from their littermate normal controls. **B,** Detailed view of small ampulla diver being held above by pipetting device and secured between thumb and index finger of laboratory technologist. In expanded portion of diver are choroid plexus cells and substrate buffer. Meniscus between air-containing portion of diver and substrate buffer is aligned to cross members of single-aperture microscope at end of each measuring period.

due to metabolism of the glucose in the buffered substrate by the choroid plexus cells. In this manner one can accurately calculate the choroid plexus cell respiration.[23, 24, 78, 80]

The gas exchange per unit time is calculated by the formula

$$\frac{\Delta O_2}{\Delta t} = \frac{x \cdot v \cdot g \cdot f \cdot (B + h - e) \, .273}{(V + v) \cdot 10,300 \, (273 + t°)}$$

where V = gas volume in amplifier chamber; x = change in the position of the diver per unit time (adjustment in the vernier buret at the end of each hour); v = volume of the vernier buret in microliters; g = dry weight of the diver (usually 30 to 50 mg); f = buoyancy factor or tendency of the glass to float in water; B = barometric pressure in millimeters of water; h = initial equilibrium pressure of the diver measured in millimeters of water; e = vapor tension of 0.1 NaOH at 30° C in millimeters of water; and t = temperature in the system, which is maintained at 30° C.

Following the above calculation, which yields a result of $\Delta O_2/\Delta t$ in each ampulla diver, division by the dry weight of the choroid cells will measure the oxygen consumption for each microgram per hour. These determinations for each of the divers are averaged and compared with those of the control animals. Measurement of the oxygen consumption of the choroid plexus cells per unit weight are shown in Table 15-1. Samples of choroid plexus (4 to 8) were placed in the flotation chamber at the same time as the litter matched controls. Four hydrocephalic animals and their controls were analyzed on separate days. From these data the ΔO_2 in $\mu l/\mu g/hr$ for the normals averaged 3.70×10^{-4} and 3.91×10^{-4} for the hydrocephalic puppies. These differences, according to the student T test, are not statistically significant, nor did there appear to be changes in the early phases of the development of hydrocephalus when correlated with gross pathologic findings.

To study the effect of increased pressure in three animals (two hydrocephalics, one control), the adjustment (h) was moved so that the microdiver would be below that of the initial equilibration. The distance chosen in millimeters on the vertical scale corresponded to 300 to 400 mm of water in vivo. In the normal, increased pressure resulted in an oxygen consumption of 3.70×10^{-4} $\mu l/\mu g/hr$, and in the two hydrocephalic animals it was 4.63×10^{-4} and 5.38×10^{-4} $\mu l/\mu g/hr$, respectively (Table 15-2). Again, the difference between the consumption in the hydrocephalic animals and the normal animal seemed large, but, after analysis, did not appear to be statistically significant.

These results, which show no change in oxygen consumption by choroid plexus cells, may not reflect the in vivo circumstance for the following reasons. The overall oxidation of glucose, a process involving many enzyme pathways, may not prove the most sensitive measure of the metabolic activity of the cho-

Table 15-1. Effect of hydrocephalus on choroid plexus cell respiration*

Animals	O_2 consumption ($\mu l/\mu g/hr$)
Normal	4.22×10^{-4}
Normal	3.27×10^{-4}
Normal	4.52×10^{-4}
Normal	2.77×10^{-4}
Communicating hydrocephalus	5.28×10^{-4}
Communicating hydrocephalus	3.24×10^{-4}
Communicating hydrocephalus	4.57×10^{-4}
Communicating hydrocephalus	2.56×10^{-4}

*Modified from James, A. E., Epstein, M. H., and Smith, T. C.: Invest. Radiol. **10**:366, 1975.

Table 15-2. Effect of increased pressure on choroid plexus cell respiration*

Animals	O_2 consumption ($\mu l/\mu g/hr$)
Normal	3.70×10^{-4}
Communicating hydrocephalus	4.63×10^{-4}
Communicating hydrocephalus	5.38×10^{-4}

*Modified from James, A. E., Epstein, M. H., and Smith, T. C.: Invest. Radiol. **10**:366, 1975.

roid plexus cells. By using specific substrate systems, we may also be able to more accurately understand choroid plexus metabolism and, hence, CSF production. By the same token, various substances to inhibit choroid plexus cell metabolism may be evaluated. In the intact animal, control of regional blood flow to the vessels supplying the choroid plexus cells may provide an in vivo mechanism to alter metabolic activity that could not be measured by this in vitro method. Although a decline in CSF production by decreased choroid plexus cell metabolism would tend to diminish the net current of CSF from the ventricles, the appearance of radioactivity in the ventricles soon after a lumbar injection suggests a more rapid process.[36]

CSF drainage and absorption

Alteration of metabolism of the cells that produce CSF and changes in the volume of CSF production during and after development of hydrocephalus are but two of the mechanisms by which compensation might be produced. Another very important mechanism may well be alteration of the pathways or site(s) of mechanism of CSF drainage or absorption. Several alternative pathways of drainage have been proposed, including increased movement down the central canal and the subarachnoid space of the spinal cord and absorption in the arachnoid granulations there[22] and transependymal movement of CSF into the periventricular space and eventual removal from that site.[37, 50, 61] Neither of these mechanisms has been established as the proper explanation, and other possibilities certainly exist.

Using the radiopharmaceuticals injected for CSF-imaging studies, we correlated autoradiographic findings (gross, histologic, and semiquantitative) with the histologic and ultrastructural appearance.[30, 37, 61] Investigations using normal animals or animals with noncommunicating hydrocephalus have demonstrated transependymal movement of large molecular weight substances consistent with diffusion through the periventricular extracellular space of the brain.[25, 30, 37, 58, 61] However, transependymal bulk flow of these large molecules has not been demonstrated in normals as in animals with chronic communicating hydrocephalus. Autoradiography was employed to trace pathways of altered CSF movement and to compare them with normal pathways.[6] Iodine 131 serum albumin (150 to 300 μCi) was initially used for the autoradiographic studies. Before intracisternal or intraventricular injection the unbound ^{131}I was determined by paper electrophoresis. Radiopharmaceutical preparations with more than 2% "free" iodine were excluded because the movement pattern reflected by autoradiographs might be altered by the small molecules of ^{131}I not bound to the albumin.[67] Both general- and specific-area analysis of proposed sites of CSF absorption were studied for the distribution and gradients of radioactivity. The areas were selected from the distribution of radioactivity on gross autoradiographs. At necropsy the size of the ventricular system in the normal and hydrocephalic animals was noted as well as the location of the Silastic. Histologic slides were obtained from all animals, particularly from the ependyma, periventricular white matter, and meninges. All animals with ventricular radio-pharmaceutical entry following cisterna magna injection had obvious hydro-cephalus grossly at necropsy (Fig. 15-9). Animals with ventricular "stasis" of the radiopharmaceutical during cisternography had more severe hydrocephalus than those with transient ventricular entry of the labeled albumin that cleared on later studies. The most prominent dilation of the ventricles occurred in the midportion, body, and inferior horn of the lateral ventricles, with associated loss of the periventricular white matter in these areas. The third and fourth ventricles and the aqueduct of Sylvius were enlarged, but not as significantly as the lateral ventricles.

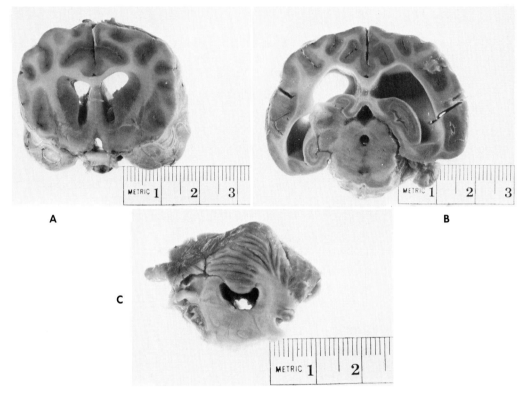

Fig. 15-9. Gross pathologic sections in animal with chronic communicating hydrocephalus produced by injection of Silastic into subarachnoid space. **A,** Coronal section through area of corpus callosum above lateral ventricle and caudate nucleus laterally. Ventricular enlargement is noted with left lateral ventricle being greater than right. Rounding of left ventricular angle is also more prominent, but both are definitely changed from normal acute angle present in animal sacrified prior to Silastic injection. **B,** Coronal section at level of the midportion to posterior portion of the midline ventricle showing extensive nature of ventricular enlargement. **C,** Coronal section through cerebellum demonstrating enlargement of fourth ventricle. At gross pathologic examination, orifices of fourth ventricle are examined for patency. These were found to be dilated and open. This had been confirmed earlier by cisternography, since radiopharmaceutical entered from injection in the cisterna magna into the ventricular system and was present on images taken as early as 10 minutes after injection. Thus this appearance certainly represents communicating hydrocephalus.

In the area of the dorsolateral ventricular angles, severe flattening of the ependyma could be detected microscopically. There was degeneration of the underlying periventricular tissue with apparent enlargement of the extracellular space consistent with a localized edema. This was manifested histologically by areas devoid of cells, which appeared as fluid-filled "lakes" (Fig. 15-10). The choroid plexus was normal in histologic appearance. The ependyma of the third ventricle, cerebral aqueduct, and fourth ventricle was not significantly altered. Control dogs were examined in the same manner and showed no abnormal changes. In dogs with severe communicating hydrocephalus, following intra-cisternal injection of the radiopharmaceutical, silver grains representing the labeled albumin were found adjacent to the free border of the ventricular ependymal wall, between ependymal cells, on the surface of the choroid plexus, and in the interstitial tissue of that structure (Fig. 15-11, A). Labeled albumin was detected in the walls of the veins and intraluminally in vascular structures of the choroid plexus. Increased radioactivity was present in the periventricular

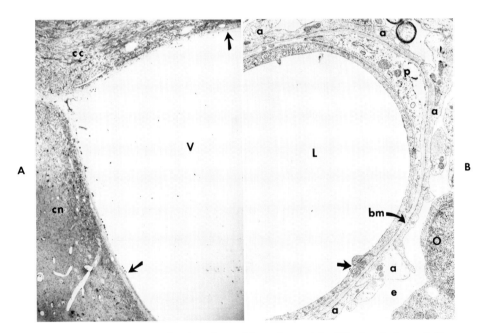

Fig. 15-10. A, Light micrograph of surface of lateral ventricle (*V*) of a hydrocephalic monkey (83 days after injection of Silastic) at angle formed by corpus callosum (*cc*) and caudate nucleus (*cn*). Between arrows, ependymal cells have become stretched and flattened or have rounded up, and ependymal lining has lost its integrity. Note parenchymal edema in subependymal tissue, especially nearest to angle. **B,** Electron micrograph of a small vessel (*L*, lumen) in periventricular region of corpus callosum of a hydrocephalic monkey (113 days after injection of Silastic). Perivascular ring of astrocyte end feet (*a*) is still intact, although glial processes contain increased numbers of reactive glial filaments. Note parenchymal edema (*e*) beneath this ring of end feet. Endothelial cell junction (arrow) remains intact. An oligodendrocyte (*O*) is present as well as pericyte cytoplasm (*p*) within basement membrane (*bm*) of vessel. (**A,** Epon, 1 *μ*, methylene blue and azure II; ×150; **B,** uranyl acetate and lead citrate; ×11,600.)

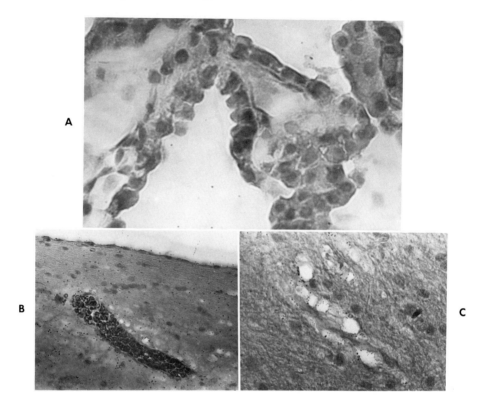

Fig. 15-11. A, Histologic section of autoradiograph of choroid plexus area. Grains of silver representing position of radiopharmaceutical in ventricular space and adjacent to choroid plexus cells are visible. It is not certain whether this represented accumulation of radiopharmaceutical within the choroid plexus because this study provides rather nonspecific anatomic information. **B,** Histologic section of ventricular ependyma and periventricular region in a dog with chronic communicating hydrocephalus. This autoradiograph was obtained 45 days after Silastic injection, and the animal was sacrificed at approximately 30 minutes after intraventricular injection by slow infusion of 100 μCi of ^{131}I-labeled albumin. The brain was fixed by formalin immersion. Multiple grains of silver are visible in area of flattened ventricular ependyma and in periventricular region. There are a number of acellular areas, representing an incease in extracellular space, probably due to edema. Finely packed cellular layer just below ependymal surface is lost. **C,** Histologic section of periventricular region of a dog with chronic communicating hydrocephalus. This autoradiograph was obtained 1 hour after perfusion of the cisterna magna with 100 μCi of ^{131}I albumin. Silver grains appeared to be oriented around small cerebral vessels. Whether there is radioactivity within the vessels cannot be determined by this particular study.

brain tissue in the white as well as the gray matter (nuclei). The greatest concentration was in the first 2 to 3 mm below the ventricular ependymal surface, and there was a definite gradient from the ependyma to the cerebral cortex (Fig. 15-11, *B*). This observation will be considered in detail later. Radioactivity appeared to localize around the walls of capillaries and venules (Fig. 15-11, *C*), especially in the subependymal veins.

There was no significant difference in the distribution of the grains in the animals with communicating hydrocephalus that received the intraventricular infusion of radiopharmaceutical and those that received an intracisternal injection. Labeled albumin was observed in the periventricular structures of those hydrocephalic animals having radiopharmaceutical entry and "clearing" in cisternograms. Radioactivity was found in the same distribution as in the animals with ventricular radiopharmaceutical entry and "stasis." In addition, silver grains were detected in (1) the arachnoid and pia matter over the cerebral convexities, (2) the arachnoid vessels and the subpial area, especially around the subpial capillaries, and (3) the first 2 mm of cerebral cortex below the pia.

In control dogs with cisterna magna injection of radiopharmaceutical, distribution of radioactivity was as follows: (1) no labeled albumin was present in the ventricular system or adjacent tissue, and (2) most of the labeled albumin was in the subarachnoid space surrounding the cervical spine, the basal cisterns, the CSF space over the cerebral hemispheres, and in the area of the arachnoid villi. In control dogs, following ventricular infusion of the labeled albumin, penetration of the labeled albumin into the periventricular tissue and choroid plexus was noted. The most significant penetration appeared to be in the lateral ventricles in the angles between the corpus callosum and caudate nucleus. Less penetration was observed through other ventricular borders. The number of silver granules was much less when compared with the number in the hydrocephalic animals (even with intracisternal injection), especially at distances greater than 2 mm from the ventricular ependyma. The more distant from the ependymal surface toward the cerebral cortex, the greater the difference between hydrocephalic and normal animals became.

In general, gross autoradiographs confirmed the findings on the microscopic slides. In the control animals with intracisternal injection, no radioactivity could be detected within the ventricular system. In animals with communicating hydrocephalus, the greatest amount of radioactivity was in the ventricles, with little in the subarachnoid space over the cerebral hemispheres (Fig. 15-12). After intraventricular injection, radioactivity was present in the periventricular tissue in both the control and the hydrocephalic animals. However, the density of radioactivity was much greater in the hydrocephalic animals, and the penetration into the periventricular tissue was to a much greater distance from the ependyma.

We have performed only a few autoradiographic studies in primates, but the findings have correlated well with those noted in dogs. At cisternography no ventricular entry is seen, but there is generalized distribution of the radioactivity over the cerebral cortex on delayed views in normals (Fig. 15-13, A). Following development of communicating hydrocephalus, entry of the radiopharmaceutical from a cisterna magna injection in the ventricles occurs (Fig. 15-13, B). Autoradiographs of hydrocephalic primates show movement of labeled albumin from the ventricle into the neurophil and orientation around the cerebral veins (Fig. 15-13, C).

Although the distribution of the radiopharmaceutical in normals and animals with hydrocephalus was different, the dynamics of movement in the sub-

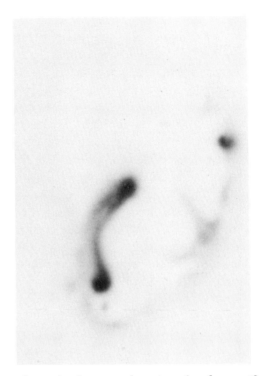

Fig. 15-12. Gross autoradiograph of a coronal section of a dog sacrificed 30 minutes after slow infusion of 100 μCi of serum albumin into cisterna magna. Radioactivity (^{131}I) appears in ventricle and along ventricular ependyma. Concentrations of radioactivity are visible at angles of lateral ventricles. Little radioactivity is present over cerebral cortex in this coronal section of a single hemisphere. This distribution of radioactivity appears to be the same as that noted on the cisternograms.

ependymal area were of particular interest. To determine the tissue concentration of the labeled albumin as a function of distance from the ventricular surface, silver grains per unit area of periventricular tissue were counted. The concentration of the radiopharmaceutical in the tissue was considered proportional to the number of silver grains present on the autoradiographs. Semiquantitative analysis was achieved by counting the number of grains per rectile visualized in a light microscope with 1000× magnification. After counting of the first rectile aligned over the surface of the ventricular ependyma, the microscopic slide was moved by one rectile length in the direction of the cerebral cortex and distal to the lateral ventricle. This method of counting was continued until the area of the cerebral surface (subarachnoid space) was reached. To obtain a large statistical population of counts per field, three separate counts through the same tissue area on the same slide were obtained. The number of grains over a distance of 1 mm were then combined and the mean ± standard deviation was determined. To facilitate comparison of the different animals, the number of grains at the ventricular ependyma was taken to represent 100%

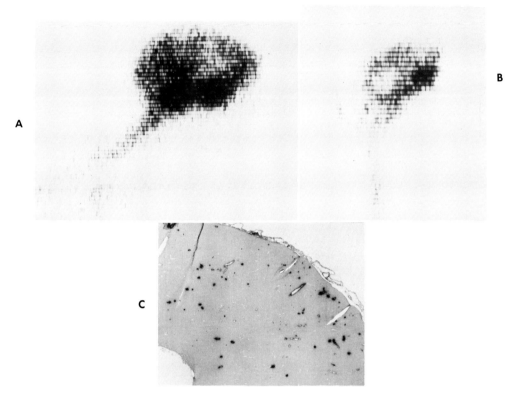

Fig. 15-13. **A,** Right lateral view of cisternogram in a normal monkey 6 hours after injection of 1 mCi of ^{111}In DTPA into cisterna magna. Generalized radioactivity is seen over cerebral cortex; no ventricular entry is noted. **B,** Right lateral view of cisternogram in a rhesus monkey 45 days after subarachnoid injection of Silastic. For this cisternogram 1 mCi of ^{111}In DTPA was injected into cisterna magna 6 hours before this view was obtained. Ventricular entry of radiopharmaceutical is seen. **C,** Autoradiograph in monkey with communicating hydrocephalus. The animal was sacrificed 2 hours after intraventricular injection of 150 μCi of ^{131}I-labeled serum albumin. In this low-power magnification study, orientation of radioactivity around small cerebral vessels is seen ($\times$45).

radiopharmaceutical concentration and served as a reference (Fig. 15-14). Concentration in tissue distal to the ependyma was expressed by the ratio between the amount of radiopharmaceutical in the brain parenchyma and that at the ependymal surface. This method was used as an alternative to that proposed by Rall, Oppelt, and Patlak,[25] and Fenstermacher et al.[58] by which the amount of radioactivity per gram of tissue is determined by sample counting and weighing.

Subsequently, using ^{14}C inulin as the radioactive marker we did make the measurements in the same manner and confirmed the distribution of radioactivity that was suggested from the histologic method. In this technique, samples of neural tissue (approximately 1 mm^3) are serially obtained beginning at the ventricular surface and proceeding out toward the cerebral cortex. They are weighed, placed in counting vials, and homogenized, and the amount of ac-

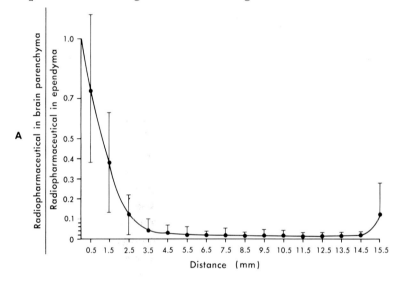

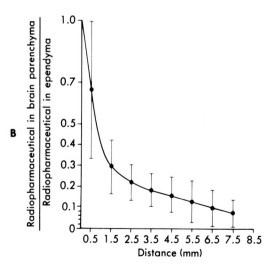

Fig. 15-14. A, Plot of amount of radioactivity within cerebral cortex compared to that on surface of ventricular ependyma in a normal dog. This graph represents distribution on arithmetic paper of the ratio of radiopharmaceutical in the brain parenchyma compared to the ependyma at each distance in millimeters from the ventricular surface. In the normal, a very rapid decrease in the amount of radioactivity is seen as one moves distal to the ventricular ependyma. **B,** This same type of plot in an animal with communicating hydrocephalus shows that there is more radioactivity in the periventricular region, which correlates well with the appearance of the histologic autoradiographs. (Modified from James, A. E., et al.: Radiology 111:341, 1974.)

tivity is determined. In general, the distribution was the same as that obtained by the histologic autoradiographic method, although the actual structural localization was not as precise.

The relative tissue concentration of radioactivity was plotted against distance from the ependyma on arithmetic paper (Fig. 15-14) as well as on arithmetic probability paper (FD Form 6-134, modified by Schantz and Lauffer[63]) (Fig. 15-15). From this data presentation, the size of the extracellular space and the diffusion coefficient for the radiopharmaceutical can be calculated utilizing Schantz's method for diffusion measurements in agar gel.[63] When the fraction C_t/C_e (tissue concentration/ependymal concentration) is plotted against distance on probability paper, the data do not extrapolate to 1.0 (where X = 0) but to a lower value. The intercept can be considered as a direct measure of percentage of extracellular space (ECS) of the brain. When the ECS is determined, it can be used to convert the values C_t/C_e to C/C_e. C represents the amount of solute radiopharmaceutical concentration per unit volume of ECS, and is obtained by using the formula:

$$C_e = C\ (1 - ECS)$$

The diffusion coefficients can be calculated by plotting the values of C/C_e against X. Using the slope Y/X of this plot, one can calculate the diffusion coefficient in the brain by the following equation:

$$D_B = \frac{1}{(Y/X^2)\ 2t}$$

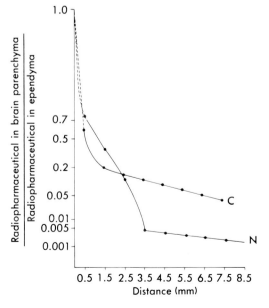

Fig. 15-15. Plot of radioactivity distribution within brain of a normal dog and one with communicating hydrocephalus. Amount of radioactivity is compared to distance from ventricular ependyma on arithmetic probability paper. The straight line portion of the graph in the normal dog (N) has the configuration seen with processes that occur by simple diffusion. The upward curvature of the plot of the distribution of radioactivity in the animal with communicating hydrocephalus (C) suggests some form of facilitated diffusion. Since the radioactive marker employed in this instance was labeled albumin, this probably represents bulk flow. (Modified from James, A. E., et al.: Radiology **111**:341, 1974.)

X = the distance in the brain in centimeters, t = time in seconds, and Y is a function of the concentration in the relationship shown:

$$C/C_e = 1 - \frac{2}{\sqrt{2}} \int_0^Y e^{-\frac{y^2}{2}} DY$$

The value of Y was obtained from calculations published by Schantz and Lauffer.[63] The value of D, the diffusion coefficient of the solute in brain tissue, is calculated by the equation:

$$D = D_B \left(1 + \frac{2\ ECS}{3}\right)$$

We determined the radiopharmaceutical concentration from the superior surface of the body of the lateral ventricle (through the corpus callosum and white matter) to the cerebral cortical surface. In the control animal, radiopharmaceutical was injected into the lateral ventricle. Labeled albumin was found 3.3 mm deep into the periventricular tissue after 4 hours. At a distance greater than 3.5 mm from the ependyma, the tissue concentration was near zero (1% to 2% of the ependymal concentration) and was not utilized in the calculations. These data of decrease of radioactivity from the ependyma outward plotted on probability paper are represented by a straight line (Fig. 15-15). Since almost all the labeled albumin remains in the extracellular space of the brain during the first 4 hours and all the molecules of the radiopharmaceutical are homogeneous, one can assume that this movement is due to diffusion. The calculated diffusion coefficient was 107×10^{-5} cm² sec⁻¹. The size of the ECS measured 5%, similar to the calculations of other investigators.[4, 25, 58]

In animals with communicating hydrocephalus, the tissue concentration versus distance function was quite different from that in normals. On arithmetic paper, the initial slope (1.5 mm distal to the ventricular surface in the periventricular tissue) is steeper for all animals with communicating hydrocephalus. The same data plotted on probability paper are biphasic and composed of two straight line regions with different slopes. The slope of the first part represents an apparent diffusion coefficient of 0.75×10^{-5} cm² sec⁻¹ which is lower than in the control animal. The second part has a significantly higher diffusion coefficient, reflecting low resistance to radiopharmaceutical movement. In dogs with communicating hydrocephalus, the calculated ECS was 8% in the periventricular tissue.

Evidence that protein and other molecules of large size migrate from the ventricular system into the brain parenchyma has been documented microscopically in normal and hydrocephalic animals.[4, 6, 37, 58, 61] Although radioactive labeled albumin appears in the circulation, the pathways from the ventricle into the brain parenchyma and from there into the circulation are still unknown. Studies using ventriculocisternal perfusion suggest that in normal animals substances that are restricted to the extracellular space of the brain parenchyma, such as inulin or sucrose, diffuse from the ventricle into the neuropil.[58] These studies seem to show that the ventricular ependyma and the periventricular area show a different response to presentation of macromolecules in hydrocephalics and in normals. In normal circumstances a passive movement by diffusion is present, whereas in communicating hydrocephalus "facilitated" diffusion is present. Since the labeled molecule is serum albumin, the term "bulk flow" might be accurately applied. These observations are supported by the images seen at cisternography. In humans with very large ventricles it is not unusual to see radioactivity move from the lumbar injection site to the cerebral ventricles within 30 minutes to 2 hours after injection—a time course suggesting a much more active process than movement by simple diffusion.[63, 66] If the labeled molecules of radiopharmaceutical then passed by bulk flow into the periventricular space, continued radioactivity would be expected in this area (ventricular stasis). Thus the initial cause of ventricular radiopharmaceutical penetration may be loss of the net current of CSF movement from the ventricles, aided by continued enlargement of the ventricular space.[19, 36] As the pathologic changes in the ventricular ependyma and periventricular region progress, radiopharmaceutical crosses what was previously a partial barrier to large molecules.[51, 68] These phenomena would explain the apparent enlargement on later views of the cisternographic study and recent reports of periventricular diminished attenuation seen on CAT scans.[19, 50]

We were interested in the movement of macromolecules from the CSF directly into the blood as well as by a more circuitous route through the extracellular space to the blood. Compartmental analysis was applied to our data to study these dynamics. Twenty-three animals (mongrel and beagle dogs) were used in this study and divided into two groups: (1) a control group of 15 animals with normal cisternograms and normal-sized ventricles at autopsy and (2) animals with communicating hydrocephalus (acute or chronic).

To assess transfer, each dog was given an intracisternal injection of 1 to 2 mCi in 1 ml of ^{99m}Tc–labeled serum albumin. Blood samples of 3 to 5 ml were taken every 30 minutes for the first 4 hours, then every 2 hours for up to 28 hours after injection.[1, 14, 69] Venous blood samples were obtained and counted in a well scintillation counter. (Counts were corrected for unbound ^{99m}Tc in the original preparation.) Standards prepared at the time of injection were used to correct for radioactive decay.

To calculate accurately the amount of radiopharmaceutical that transferred from the subarachnoid space into the blood to obtain the measured radiopharmaceutical blood concentrations, the rate of disappearance of the radioactively labeled albumin from the circulatory system into other compartments (such as liver, kidneys, lymphatic system, and extracellular space) was determined. We measured the disappearance of ^{99m}Tc–labeled albumin in four animals after intravenous injection over a time period of 26 hours. These data reflect the arithmetic mean of the concentrations after injection. The blood concentrations (which represent transfer from the CSF) were corrected at 2-hour intervals for both groups. The blood concentration 2 hours after radiopharmaceutical injection was not altered. The corrected 4-hour value consists of the sum of the

2-hour value and the amount transferred during the 2- to 4-hour interval. This value is the difference between the measured 4-hour blood concentration and that portion of the 2-hour blood concentration which remains in the circulation during this interval. After 2 hours this value represented 43% of the initial amount. Sequentially, each concentration is the sum of the corrected value at the beginning of that time interval and the amount of radiopharmaceutical that transferred from the CSF to the plasma during the interval measured. This is the difference between the measured 6-hour blood concentration and the sum of radiopharmaceutical remaining in the circulation for 2 to 6 hours and that transferred between 2 and 4 hours (34% of the 2-hour value and 43% of the amount transported in the 2- to 4-hour interval). These calculations were performed in the same manner for both animal groups from time of injection until 26 to 28 hours after injection.

The sums of the values of radiopharmaceutical that passed from the subarachnoid space into the blood from time zero (injection) until 26 to 28 hours after cisterna magna injection were plotted for all animal groups on linear and arithmetic probability paper.

The amount of radiopharmaceutical remaining in the CSF space at the conclusion of the study was considered as 100% minus the amount that had transferred into the blood. This function was used to calculate the mean transit time ($\bar{t}$) of the labeled albumin from the site of injection to the exit from the CSF system. Employing the method described by Zierler,[80] we calculated the mean transit time. While these assumptions have been proved valid for calculations in the blood circulation, we recognize that their application to CSF physiology has heretofore been largely unexplored. The mean transit time is determined by the fraction of the area under the reverse of the blood accumulation function and the zero time radioactivity in the CSF.[79]

$$t = \frac{\text{Area}}{\text{Peak (or zero line) concentration}}$$

The mean transit time through the system is the ratio of the volume in which the indicator is distributed to the flow from the system. From this value one obtains by the equation

$$\bar{t} = \frac{V}{F} \text{ or } \frac{F}{V} = \frac{1}{\bar{t}}$$

a flow-to-volume ratio of radiopharmaceutical leaving the CSF space to the volume of the radiopharmaceutical distribution space. In this circumstance of equal dispersion of labeled albumin within the CSF, these calculations would provide information regarding the relation of CSF flow entering the circulation to the CSF distribution space:

$$\frac{F}{V} = \frac{1}{\bar{t}}$$

In normal dogs the ventricular CSF volume was not included in the radiopharmaceutical space because (as demonstrated by cisternography) radiopharmaceutical entry into the ventricular system is prevented by the CSF flow leaving the ventricles and the anatomic arrangement of the fourth ventricular outlet.[19, 37] In animals with communicating hydrocephalus the ventricular volume was considered as a part of the radiopharmaceutical distribution space because the ventricles are clearly delineated on the cisternographic images.

The observed circulating blood levels of ^{99m}Tc serum albumin were plotted against sampling time for all groups and the blood levels recorded as percentage of injected activity:

$$\frac{\text{Total activity circulating in blood}}{\text{Total activity injected into CSF}} \times 100$$

Certain features of the curves indicate that animals with hydrocephalus may be distinguished from controls on the basis of their transfer kinetics. Normal animals reach maximum concentration at a different time from those with chronic communicating hydrocephalus. The apparent transfer of radiopharmaceutical, not corrected for disappearance from the circulation after intracisternal injection, can be shown by curves of the mean plasma concentration (as percentage of the injected dose) of the radiopharmaceutical plotted against elapsed time after injection (in hours).

The blood may be regarded as the end organ of CSF blood transfer of ^{99m}Tc–labeled albumin, if the measured radiopharmaceutical blood concentration is corrected for passage of the radiopharmaceutical from the circulation into other compartments.[69, 71] After this correction, one can obtain the amount of labeled albumin transferred. This can be illustrated by curves that represent accumulation of labeled albumin transferred into blood from time zero to the end of blood sample collection. The amount of radiopharmaceutical versus time interval curves (the differentials of the accumulation curve) specifies what percentage of the injected labeled albumin moved out of the subarachnoid space into the blood during a selected time interval.[69, 71] When these differential curves ascend from zero to maximum, the first part of the radiopharmaceutical accumulation curve is convex upward. As these curves reach their maximum, the radiopharmaceutical accumulation functions have a flex point. When the differential curves fall to zero, the accumulation curves are deflected in a concave fashion, approaching 100% of labeled albumin. Because it is not practical to wait until all the radiopharmaceutical has been transferred into the blood or the radiopharmaceutical accumulation curves have reached 100%, the curves were extrapolated to 100%.

In the control group the maximum rate of transfer occurred 10 hours after subarachnoid injection and was 9.7% every 2 hours. The radiopharmaceutical accumulation curve demonstrates that in the control animals 50% of the injected radiopharmaceutical has left the CSF compartment after 13.6 hours and 85% after 24 hours. In dogs with chronic communicating hydrocephalus, transfer of labeled albumin from the CSF to the blood was slower than in normals. The accumulation curve in the first 3 hours showed only a slight upward slope;

the steepest slope occurred between 4 and 8 hours. The maximum amount of radiopharmaceutical transferred in a 2-hour time interval was 6.8%, which occurred 8 hours after injection. Twenty-four hours were required for 50% of the labeled albumin injected into the CSF to be transferred into the circulation.

The mean transit time of the radiopharmaceutical through the CSF spaces and the ratios of CSF flow from CSF space to CSF distribution space showed the characteristics of transfer in these two different physiologic circumstances. The mean transit time in dogs with communicating hydrocephalus was more than twice that of controls. This determination may be interpreted to mean alternatively that radiopharmaceutical flow from the CSF space (in milliliters per hour) to intravascular space (in milliliters) is less than 50% of that in control dogs or that the volume of the CSF compartment is twice that of normals.

We regarded the radiopharmaceutical accumulation functions as cumulative relative frequently distributions. The values of these accumulation functions were plotted on standard probability graph paper. The degree to which all plotted points lie on a line on this type of graph paper determines the closeness of fit of a given distribution to a normal distribution. Plots on semilogarithmetic paper did not appear useful because derived data did not appear to reflect exponential functions.

The data of the control group form a straight, ascending line on standard probability paper during the period of 12 to 26 hours after intracisternal radiopharmaceutical injection. This period was preceded by a curve ascending in a convex fashion. In dogs with communicating hydrocephalus there was a curve of similar contour, which formed a straight line between 16 and 26 hours. A lower slope was preceded by a curved portion in the first 16 hours after radiopharmaceutical injection. Analysis of these data allowed characterization of CSF to blood transfer in normal and hydrocephalic animals.

The method to determine radiopharmaceutical blood transfer after instantaneous subarachnoid or intraventricular injection has been performed previously by other investigators.[1, 71] The method we employed has the advantage of avoiding repeated puncture of the subarachnoid space, complicated perfusion studies, or leakage around the puncture needle. The time for blood sample collection can be extended over several days because the animal does not have to be anesthetized during this period. Finally, the minimal volume and protein content of the radiopharmaceutical injected into the subarachnoid space is unlikely to disturb CSF dynamics.

Previous investigations have failed to provide accurate information about the transfer of radiopharmaceutical from the CSF into the circulation because the leakage of labeled albumin from the circulatory system into other compartments was not considered. After entry of radioactively labeled albumin into the blood, it disappears from the circulatory system, distributes in the lymph system, disintegrates in the intestinal fluid, and is metabolized by other organs. Recirculation into the central nervous system has not been measured in this investigation because the rate of recirculation was assumed.[1, 4, 14, 69] These modifications of the measured radiopharmaceutical-blood composition curves for CSF physiology enable one to utilize methods of calculation that have been found useful in blood and circulatory compartment analysis.[42, 79]

When an indicator is introduced by instantaneous injection into a system (such as the subarachnoid space) and the output can be determined at the exit from this system, the amount of radiopharmaceutical transferred versus time can be calculated.[42, 71, 79] It is to be expected that the accumulation curves that have been customarily plotted on semilogarithmic graph paper would fit a straight line (as is usual in most circulatory studies). This is considered to be a two-compartment system. According to observations of Zierler,[80] there is reason to suspect that transfer curves with a long time of transfer do not reflect exponential functions. It is suggested that these functions more closely resemble frequency distribution functions.[80] This concept has proved valid for the radiopharmaceutical accumulation functions of this study (which greatly resemble cumulative frequency distributions) and was demonstrated by the plots on probability graph paper.[58]

The degree of slope of the accumulation frequency functions, the slope of the straight lines on the probability paper, and the radiopharmaceutical transfer versus time curves in our studies demonstrated that there are individual frequency functions of transit time for each cumulative hour.

It is possible to obtain more information about the nature of the CSF compartments if two assumptions are made:

1. The rate of CSF formation is equal in both animal groups. This seems to be valid from other investigations.[11, 45] An assumption of this sort would mean that during the experimental period, the CSF volume entering the total CSF compartment is equal to CSF volume transfer into the circulatory compartment.[28]

2. The radiopharmaceutical is uniformly distributed within the CSF.

If these assumptions are correct, the data suggest that the varying flow-to-volume ratios $\frac{1}{t} = \frac{F}{V}$ are due to different radiopharmaceutical distribution spaces in normal and hydrocephalic animals—a conclusion in keeping with observations on the cisternographic images. A steep upward slope of the radiopharmaceutical accumulation curve is documented by our investigations, which utilized cisternography, autoradiography, and radiochemistry.

In hydrocephalic animals mean transit time is more than twice as long as in the control group, which means that the total radiopharmaceutical space is more than doubled. This space represents several anatomic compartments in animals with communicating hydrocephalus:

1. The extraventricular subarachnoid space of the spine and (to some extent) the space over the cerebral hemispheres

2. The enlarged ventricular space

3. An enlarged extracellular space of the brain, especially in the periventricular region[10, 17]

When the blood is regarded as the end organ of transfer, compartmental analysis of the spaces and the time-course of movement can be characterized.[71, 80] The data from these experiments suggest that it is possible to determine clearance functions, mean transit times of the radiopharmaceutical through the CSF system, and CSF absorption-to-CSF distribution space ratios in normal dogs and those with chronic communicating hydrocephalus. The data also suggest that this method may be used as an adjunct to cisternographic image interpretation in the diagnosis of communicating hydrocephalus. This type of analysis may prove sensitive in the early detection of CSF absorptive abnormalities.[1, 69] Since this method is easily performed in combination with cisternography and provides data regarding the CSF and transfer dynamics, expanded use in clinical situations seems warranted.

Various studies have resulted in disagreement about the size of the CSF drainage pathways and the method by which macromolecules are removed from the CSF space.[64, 70, 73, 74] There have been a number of qualitative studies on the behavior of materials injected intraventricularly or subarachnoidally, but few quantitative studies to determine how rapidly different substances disappear from the CSF.[14, 32, 56] Valuable information regarding the nature of the barrier between the CSF and nervous tissue (often called the CSF-brain barrier) as well as the CSF-blood barrier could be obtained from such measurements. Davson, Kleeman, and Levin[14] injected a measured volume of labeled substances in the cisterna magna of rabbits and measured their disappearance. ^{24}Na was utilized as a reference marker and the relative loss of the injected substance was expressed as a percentage of ^{24}Na loss. A rapid rate of escape was found with lipid-soluble substances. The speed of escape of inulin was the slowest measured and was believed to represent escape through the arachnoid villi exclusively. Since there is data to support the conclusion that albumin also follows this route, the speed of its disappearance from the CSF and accumulation in the intravascular compartment would be important. For this reason we have attempted to evaluate dynamics of the entry of labeled albumin into the blood from the CSF compartment by mathematical analysis.[69]

The CSF-blood barrier concept is intimately related to the idea of the blood-brain barrier (BBB). This observation was made in studies showing that certain dyes injected intravenously stain most organs but not the brain.[7, 59] These dyes are bound to plasma proteins that apparently do not cross the endothelial junctions of cerebral capillaries. Using horseradish peroxidase (43,000 mol wt) and ultrastructural analysis, Reese and Karnovsky[59] found that the passage of peroxidase was due to the existence of open channels between endothelial cells and the small number of micropinocytotic vesicles present. Vesicles in cerebral capillary endothelium are fewer in number and less active than those in muscle capillary endothelium. Thus the brain capillary system seems impermeable to large molecules such as protein.[7, 8, 59] Because the ependyma acts as only a partial barrier to movement of large molecules into the periventricular extracellular space, the changes present in hydrocephalus will only result in expansion of this compartment, since these large molecules are not removed by the small cerebral vessels when the blood-brain barrier is intact.[7, 8, 13, 73] These molecules must be removed at the site of CSF absorption, the arachnoid villi.[73, 74]

Welch and Friedman[74] have shown that the channels in an isolated arachnoid villus are approximately 12 μ in size, and they propose that large molecules travel through a series of projections acting as baffles to pass from the CSF into the intravascular compartment. Other investigators have failed to observe patent large channels in their electron microscopic studies and have believed that this represents an artifact of the preparation.[64, 70] However, large molecules such as albumin are removed from the CSF. Theories have been proposed to explain these phenomena. Brightman, Klatzo, Olsson, and Reese[8] believe that large molecules may be transported across endothelial barriers by an active mechanism of vesicle formation. The large molecules could be surrounded by an invagination or pit on the CSF side of the endothelium, which would then be incorporated, transported across the endothelium as cytoplasmic vesicles, and discharged into the blood on the opposite side. In studies of both the cerebral arachnoid villi and the drainage mechanism of the anterior chamber of the eye, Tripathi[70] has demonstrated an active formation and closure of channels through which the large molecules of the CSF can be removed into the intravascular compartment. Thus a number of studies have resulted in conflicting data regarding the mechanism by which macromolecules move from the CSF into the intravascular compartment.

We decided to study the dynamics of transfer in vivo by employing radioactive labels of molecular sizes varying from that of a small ion to a particle 15 to 30 μ in size. By this method, we hoped to establish a model by which to determine the normal initial time of transfer from the CSF, the time course of movement, and the effective size of the pathways. New Zealand white rabbits weighing 1.7 to 3.1 kg were used. They were anesthetized with pentobarbital (Nembutal). The renal artery, vein, and ureter were tied simultaneously to prevent removal of the radiopharmaceutical by this route. Potassium perchlorate (200 mg) was given intravenously and infused with artificial CSF to diminish choroid plexus and glandular uptake of technetium. Bilateral ventricular perfusion was accomplished by a modification of the method described by Pollay, Davson, and Purvis.[12, 16, 56] Separate syringes were used to infuse the artificial CSF with radioactive markers into each lateral ventricle. Using ^{99m}Tc as pertechnetate or ^{99m}Tc or ^{111}In–labeled diethylenetriamine pentaacetic acid (DTPA, 800 mol wt) as a reference marker, we measured the transfer of the following radiopharmaceuticals from the CSF space to the intravascular compartment:

1. ^{14}C dextran (16,000 or 75,000 mol wt)
2. ^{3}H dextran (16,000 or 75,000 mol wt)
3. ^{99m}Tc or ^{113}In–labeled sulfur colloid (0.01 to 1.0 μ)
4. ^{99m}Tc serum albumin "mini"-microspheres (0.1 to 1.0 μ)*
5. ^{99m}Tc–labeled rabbit red blood cells (approximately 7 μ)
6. ^{99m}Tc or ^{113m}In serum microspheres (15 to 30 μ)*

---

*Microspheres, 3M Corporation, St. Paul, Minn.

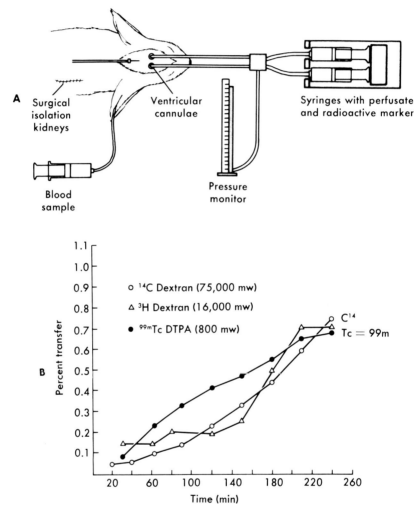

Fig. 15-16. A, Apparatus for ventricular perfusion while monitoring CSF pressure. Radioactive marker is infused through ventricular cannulae at a rate and volume that keep the rabbit's CSF pressure within normal limits. Serial blood samples are obtained by an indwelling catheter in the ear. Perchlorate is administered intravenously, and renal structures are isolated surgically to ensure that blood levels of chelated radiopharmaceuticals remain sufficiently high to statistically reflect transfer from CSF space. **B,** Graph of transfer of labeled dextran and a reference marker following intraventricular perfusion in a normal rabbit. Dextran molecule appears to transfer from CSF space into intravascular compartment in time period studied. CSF pressure is at upper limit of normal.

After insertion of the ventricular cannulae, the perfusion rate (0.013 to 0.017 ml/min) was regulated to keep the CSF pressure in a normal range (90 to 180 mm H_2O). Using the methodology previously described, the CSF pressure measurements were obtained every 5 minutes until they became stable ($\pm$ 10 mm on consecutive measurements).[15] Blood samples were obtained during perfusion beginning at 15 minutes for 1 to 4 hours (depending on the stability of the radiopharmaceutical). At the termination of the experiment, the animal was sacrificed and appropriate tissue specimens taken. To determine if each radiopharmaceutical was behaving in a predictable manner, intravenous injections were made in animals and the disappearance rate and body distribution studies performed.

Samples drawn at various time intervals and tissue samples were prepared and counted in a well scintillation counter or an AutoAnalyzer.* Using a standard prepared from a count of the radioactivity present in the CSF perfusate, the plasma samples were expressed as a percentage for each time period in which a sample was obtained.

Evaluation of the transfer of the reference radioactive marker showed that, by this system, movement from the CSF into the blood could be demonstrated. With in vivo and other testing of the radiopharmaceuticals, expected characteristics of stability and whole-body distribution were demonstrated. Those preparations in which early "leaching" or separation of the label from the large molecule had been demonstrated by previous studies were repeatedly washed of "free" radioactive label and the amount of separation determined. Microscopic studies, pore filtration, and column chromatography were used to document radiopharmaceutical size and stability. From the blood determinations, the two dextran molecules (16,000 and 75,000 mol wt) transferred across the CSF-blood barrier (Fig. 15-16). Molecules of larger size did not appear to transfer (the measurement of blood samples was confirmed by the tissue specimens) (Fig. 15-17). No significant reticuloendothelial activity was demonstrated with either the colloid or the "mini"-microspheres. The spleen did not contain significantly increased radioactivity when the red blood cells were employed nor were there increased amounts present in the capillaries of the lungs when the 15 to 30 μ sized albumin microspheres were utilized.

In the rabbit, CSF is believed to drain by nonspecific flow into the dural sinuses and transfer across the pia into the neural tissue and thence into the cerebral capillaries and those of the pia itself.[13, 21, 75] Our study was designed not to determine the sites of this transfer (although the arachnoid villi appear to be the route of egress of proteins), but to analyze the size of molecules that rapidly cross the CSF-blood barrier.

The use of particles to measure effective size of pathways, whether they are arteriovenous malformations, intercellular or intracellular channels, or clefts in the endothelial cells of membrane linings, has been well established. One objec-

---

*Hewlitt-Packard, Stanford, Calif.

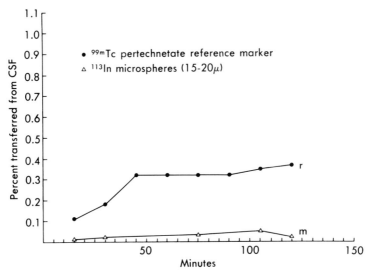

Fig. 15-17. Graph of transfer of labeled small albumin microspheres from intraventricular perfusion into blood. No significant transfer occurred despite movement of reference marker.

tion is that the particles (due to surface configuration, charge, or other properties) may not remain separate or may form larger aggregates that would change their individual effective diameters. With a number of the macromolecules we employed, many of these properties were determined. Microscopic examination of the radiopharmaceutical failed to demonstrate these aggregates. Tissue distribution studies also failed to provide evidence that this occurred. Since separation of the label from the large molecule could result in spuriously high values in the blood, studies of the radiopharmaceutical stability for these time periods were obtained.[69] In addition, the results suggested less transfer than expected, reducing the probability that this was an important factor.

The time course by which the blood was sampled was a compromise between radiopharmaceutical stability, animal survival, and expected course of movement from the entry of perfusion to the sites of drainage. It has been demonstrated that a labeled molecule intraventricularly injected as a bolus is in a matter of minutes homogeneously distributed throughout the ventricle.[12, 14] Movement from the ventricle to the remainder of the subarachnoid space also occurs rapidly.[19, 20] Since the ventricular perfusion was constant during the time period of the studies, no artifactually low values for transfer to the blood can be expected to occur because of uneven distribution or failure of the radiopharmaceutical to reach the normal drainage sites. Although certain ultrastructural studies[74] seem to show the pathways for movement of macromolecules across to be significantly greater than 1 μ in size, we were not able to confirm this. Rather, the data suggest that the effective limiting size is less than 0.1 μ—a figure considerably smaller than predicted. Since in clinical practice we use radiopharmaceuticals that are smaller than the 75,000 mol wt dextran, limitations for transfer should not affect our images. It has been noted that the retention of human serum albumin in the parasagittal region to produce "capping" is not nearly so common with the smaller chelates.[33, 36]

SUMMARY

Although considerable data regarding the physiology of CSF have been omitted from this chapter, we wished to select those studies which, in our opinion, provided data that directly or indirectly would assist in our understanding of the diagnostic radiographic images we produce in patients with communicating hydrocephalus. Ventricular enlargement, which we can readily depict, probably does not occur until the force, as a result of pressure on the ventricular surface, exceeds the resistance of the brain.[26, 28, 37] As the ventricles enlarge, the ependyma becomes flattened and stretched and loses its property as a partial barrier to the movement of large molecules from the CSF into the extracellular periventricular space.[5, 10, 18, 72] Although CSF is produced in normal or near normal quantities by the choroid plexus, the drainage or absorption is inadequate, and the net movement of CSF from the ventricles to the arachnoid villi is diminished. In the circumstance of diminished absorption, choroid plexus metabolism and CSF production are not significantly diminished.

The alterations of the ependymal surface or the CSF-brain barrier may not directly influence our pattern recognition of diagnostic studies. However, the structural alterations we see are expressions of basic pathophysiologic changes, some of which are not completely understood at this time. Original investigations concerning these pathologic changes may be stimulated and made relevant by our clinical imaging studies. Selection of more appropriate patients for CSF diversionary shunts and development of improved methods of treatment may result from the combination of refinements of our diagnostic techniques and a greater understanding of normal and abnormal CSF physiology.

Acknowledgment

We are grateful to Martin Donner for use of the facilities of the department of Radiology and Radiological Science of the Johns Hopkins Medical Institutions and to Henry Wagner's Division of Nuclear Medicine for the radiopharmaceuticals. Michael Maisey and his staff at Guy's Hospital provided the radiopharmaceuticals and tested them for the study of CSF drainage pathway size. Jillian H. Christian and J. Gordon McComb also made that study possible. Timothy Merz evaluated the autoradiographs and Ed Sperber and Don Price gave us advice with the neuropathology, as did Ramesh Tripathi. Gary Novak provided invaluable technical assistance. Joe Fenstermacher demonstrated the proper technique of ventriculocisternal perfusion, and Cliff Patlak showed us the proper manner to present the probability plot data. Giovanni DiChiro gave us emotional support and inspiration. Finally, we express our appreciation to the Royal Society of Medicine, The James Picker Foundation, and the National Foundation for financial support.

References

1. Abbot, M., and Alksne, J. F.: Transport of intrathecal I^{125} RISA to circulating plasma. A test for communicating hydrocephalus, Neurology (Minneap.) **18**:870, 1968.

2. Adams, R. D., et al.: Symptomatic oc-

cult hydrocephalus with "normal" cerebrospinal fluid pressure, New Engl. J. Med. **23**:117, 1965.

3. Benson, D. F., LeMay, M., Patten, D. H., and Rubens, A. B.: Diagnosis of normal-pressure hydrocephalus, New Engl. J. Med. **283**:609, 1970.

4. Bito, L. Z., and Davson, H.: Local variations in CSF composition and its relation to the composition of ECS of the cortex, Exp. Neurol. **14**:264, 1966.

5. Blakemore, W. F., and Jolly, R. D.: The subependymal plate and associated ependyma in the dog. An ultrastructural study, J. Neurocytol. **1**:69, 1972.

6. Bowsher, D.: Pathways of absorption of protein from the CSF: an autoradiographic study in the cat, Anat. Rec. **128**:23, 1957.

7. Brightman, M. W.: The intracerebral movement of proteins injected into blood and cerebrospinal fluid of mice, Prog. Brain Res. **29**:19, 1967.

8. Brightman, M. W., Klatzo, I., Olsson, Y., and Reese, T. S.: The blood-brain barrier to proteins under normal and pathological conditions, J. Neurol. Sci. **10**:215, 1970.

9. Brightman, M. W., and Palay, S. L.: The fine structure of ependymal in brain of the rat, J. Cell Biol. **19**:415, 1963.

10. Clark, R. G., and Milhorat, T. H.: Experimental hydrocephalus. III. Light microscopic findings in acute and subacute obstructive hydrocephalus in the monkey, J. Neurosurg. **32**:400, 1970.

11. Cutler, R. W., Page, L., Galicich, J., and Waters, G. Y.: Formation and absorption CSF in brain, Brain **91**:707, 1968.

12. Davson, H.: The physiology of CSF, London, 1967, J. & A. Churchill, Ltd.

13. Davson, H., Hollingsworth, J., and Segal, M. B.: The mechanism of drainage of CSF, Brain **93**:665, 1970.

14. Davson, H., Kleeman, C. R., and Levin, E.: Quantitative studies of the passage of different substances out of the CSF, J. Physiol. (Lond.) **161**:126, 1962.

15. Davson, H., and Luck, C. P.: The effect of acetazolamide on the chemical composition of the aqueous humour and CSF of some mammalian species and on the rate of turnover of ^{24}Na in these fluids, J. Physiol. **137**:279, 1957.

16. Davson, H., and Purvis, C.: An apparatus for controlled injection over long periods of time, J. Physiol. **149**:135, 1952.

17. De, S. N.: A study of the changes in the brain in experimental internal hydrocephalus, J. Path. Bact. **62**:197, 1950.

18. DeLand, F. H., et al.: Normal pressure hydrocephalus: a histological study, Am. J. Clin. Pathol. **58**:58, 1972.

19. DiChiro, G.: Movement of cerebrospinal fluid in human beings, Nature **204**:290, 1964.

20. DiChiro, G., et al.: Descent of CSF to spinal subarachnoid space, Acta Radiol. **14**:379, 1973.

21. Domer, F. R., Davson, H., and Hollingsworth, J. R.: Subarachnoid versus ventricular perfusion in the rabbit, Brain Res. **58**:81, 1973.

22. Eisenberg, H. M., McLennan, J. E., and Welch, K.: Ventricular perfusion in cats with kaolin-induced hydrocephalus, J. Neurosurg. **41**:20, 1974.

23. Epstein, M. H., and O'Connor, J. S.: Respiration of single cortical neurons and of surrounding neuropile, J. Neurochem. **12**:389, 1965.

24. Epstein, M. H., and Thorne, P. R.: Respiration of isolated cerebellar neurons using an automatic fiber optic Cartesian diver, Exp. Neurol. **26**:586, 1970.

25. Fenstermacher, J. D., et al.: Ventriculocisternal perfusion as a technique for analysis of brain capillary permeability and extracellular transport. In Capillary permeability, The Alfred Benzon Symposium II, Copenhagen, 1970, Munksgaard.

26. Geshwind, N.: The mechanism of normal pressure hydrocephalus, J. Neurol. Sci. **7**:481, 1968.

27. Greitz, T.: Cerebral circulation in adult hydrocephalus studied with angiography and the ^{133}Xenon method, Scand. J. Clin. Lab. Invest. **22**(supp. 102):12C, 1969.

28. Hakim, S.: Biomechanics of hydrocephalus. In Harbert, J. C., editor: Cisternography and hydrocephalus, Springfield, Ill., 1972, Charles C Thomas, Publisher.

29. Hakim, S., and Adams, R. D.: The special clinical problem of symptomatic hydrocephalus with normal cerebrospinal fluid pressure, J. Neurol. Sci. **2**:307, 1965.

30. Hochwald, G. M., Lux, W. E., Sahar, A., and Ransohoff, J.: Experimental hydrocephalus: changes in cerebrospinal fluid dynamics as a function of time, Arch. Neurol. **26**:120, 1972.

31. Hochwald, G. M., Sahar, A., Sadik, A. R., and Ransohoff, J.: Cerebrospinal fluid production and histological observations in animals with experimental obstructive hydrocephalus, Exp. Neurol. **25**:190, 1969.

32. Hochwald, G. M., and Wallenstein, M.: Exchange of albumin between blood, CSF, and brain in the cat, Am. J. Physiol. **212**:1199, 1967.

33. James, A. E., et al.: A cisternographic classification of hydrocephalus, Am. J. Roentgenol. Radium Ther. Nucl. Med. **115**:39, 1972.

34. James, A. E., et al.: An alternative pathway of cerebrospinal fluid absorption in communicating hydrocephalus, Radiology **111**:143, 1974.

35. James, A. E., et al.: An experimental model for chronic communicating hydrocephalus, J. Neurosurg. **41**:32, 1974.

36. James, A. E., et al.: A pathophysiologic mechanism for ventricular entry of radiopharmaceutical and possible relation to chronic communicating hydrocephalus, Am. J. Roentgenol. Radium Ther. Nucl. Med. **122**:38, Sept., 1974.

37. James, A. E., et al.: Pathophysiology of chronic communicating hydrocephalus in dogs (Canis familiaris): experimental studies, J. Neurol. Sci. **24**:151, 1975.

38. James, A. E., Epstein, M. H., and Smith, T. C.: In-vitro measurement of respiration of choroid plexus cells in communicating hydrocephalus, Invest. Radiol. **10**:366, 1975.

39. James, A. E., Flor, W. F., Strecker, E. P., and Bush, M.: The pathological alterations in chronic communicating hydrocephalus. Proceedings of the International Congress of Radiology, Excerpta Medica, Amsterdam, 1975.

40. James, A. E., Strecker, E. P., Bush, R. M., and Merz, T.: Use of Silastic to produce chronic communicating hydrocephalus, Invest. Radiol. **8**:105, 1973.

41. James, A. E., Strecker, E. P., Novak, G. R., and Burns, B.: Correlation of serial cisternograms and cerebrospinal fluid pressure measurements in experimental communicating hydrocephalus, Neurology **23**:1226, 1973.

42. Kety, S. S.: Measurement of regional circulation by the local clearance of radioactive sodium, Am. Heart J. **38**:321, 1949.

43. Kusske, J. A., Turner, P. T., Ojemann, G. A., and Harris, A. B.: Ventriculostomy for the treatment of acute hydrocephalus following subarachnoid hemorrhage, J. Neurosurg. **38**:591, 1973.

44. Linderstrom-Lang, K.: Principle of the cartesian diver applied to gasometric technique, Nature **140**:108, 1937.

45. Lorenzo, A. V., Page, L. K., and Watters, G. V.: Relationship between cerebrospinal fluid formation, absorption and pressure in human hydrocephalus, Brain **93**:679, 1970. (See also Arch. Neurol. **30**:387, 1974.)

46. McCullough, D. C., Harbert, J. C., DiChiro, G., and Ommaya, A. E.: Prognostic criteria for CSF shunting from cisternography in communicating hydrocephalus, Neurology **20**:594, 1970.

47. Messert, B., and Wannamaker, B. B.: Reappraisal of the adult occult hydrocephalus syndrome. Neurology **24**:224, 1974.

48. Milhorat, T. H.: Choroid plexus and cerebrospinal fluid production, Science **166**:1514, 1969.

49. Milhorat, T. H.: Hydrocephalus and the CSF, Baltimore, 1972, Williams & Wilkins Co.

50. Milhorat, T. H., and Clark, R. G.: Some observations on the circulation of PSP in the CSF: normal flow and flow in hydrocephalus, J. Neurosurg. **32**:522, 1970.

51. Milhorat, T. H., et al.: Structural, ultrastructural, and permeability changes in the ependyma and surrounding brain favoring equilibration in progressive hydrocephalus, Arch. Neurol. **22**:397, 1970.

52. Millen, J. W., Woolam, D. H. M., and Lamming, G. F.: Congenital hydrocephalus due to experimental hypovitaminosis A, Lancet **267**:679, 1954.

53. Nanagas, J. C.: Hydrocephalus, Bull. Johns Hopkins Hosp. **32**:385, 1970.

54. Pappenheimer, J. R., Heisey, S. R., Jordan, E. F., and Downer, D. E. C.: Perfusion of the cerebral ventricular system

in unanesthetized goats, Am. J. Physiol. **203**:763, 1962.

55. Penfield, W., and Elridge, A. R.: Hydrocephalus and the atrophy of cerebral compression. In Penfield, W., editor: Cytology and cellular pathology of the nervous system, New York, 1932, P. B. Hoeber, Inc.

56. Pollay, M., and Davson, H.: The passage of certain substances out of the CSF, Brain **86**:137, 1963.

57. Prockop, L. D., and Fishman, R. A.: Experimental pneumococcal meningitis, Arch. Neurol. **19**:449, 1968.

58. Rall, D. P., Oppelt, W. W., and Patlak, C. S.: Extracellular space of brain as determined by diffusion of inulin from the ventricular system, Life Sci. **2**:43, 1962.

59. Reese, T. S., and Karnovsky, M. J.: Fine structural localization of a blood-brain barrier to exogenous peroxidase, J. Cell Biol. **34**:207, 1967.

60. Rudd, T. G., and Nelp, W. B.: Cisternograms following subarachnoid hemorrhage, J. Nucl. Med. **11**:358, 1970.

61. Sahar, A., Hochwald, G. M., and Ransohoff, J.: Alternate pathway of cerebrospinal fluid absorption in animals with experimental obstructive hydrocephalus, J. Exp. Neurol. **25**:200, 1969.

62. Salmon, J. H.: Adult hydrocephalus: evaluation of shunt therapy in 80 cases, J. Neurosurg. **37**:423, 1972.

63. Schantz, E. J., and Lauffer, M. A.: Diffusion measurements in agar gel, Biochemistry **1**:658, 1962.

64. Shabo, A. L., and Maxwell, D. S.: Electron microscopic observations on the fate of particulate matter in CSF, J. Neurosurg. **29**:464, 1968.

65. Strecker, E. P., Bush, R. M., and James, A. E.: Cerebrospinal fluid imaging as a method to evaluate communicating hydrocephalus in dogs, Am. J. Vet. Res. **34**:101, 1973.

66. Strecker, E. P., James, A. E., Kelly, J., and Merz, T.: Semiquantitative studies of transependymal albumin movement in communicating hydrocephalus, Radiology **111**:341, 1974.

67. Strecker, E. P., James, A. E., Koningsmark, B., and Merz, T.: Autoradiographic observations in experimental communicating hydrocephalus, Neurology **24**:192, 1974. See also Strecker, Invest. Rad. 8: 33-42, Jan.-Feb., 1973.

68. Strecker, E. P., Kelley, J. E. T., Merz, T., and James, A. E.: Transventricular albumin absorption in communicating hydrocephalus: semiquantitative analysis of periventricular extracellular space utilizing autoradiography, Arch. Psychiatr. Nervenkr. **218**:369, 1974.

69. Strecker, E. P., Scheffel, E., Kelly, J., and James, A. E.: CSF absorption in communicating hydrocephalus: evaluation of transfer of radioactive albumin from subarachnoid space to plasma, Neurology **23**:854, 1973.

70. Tripathi, R.: Tracing of the bulk outflow route of cerebrospinal fluid by transmission and scanning electron microscopy, Brain Res. **80**:503, 1974.

71. van Wart, C. A., Dupont, J. R., and Kraintz, L.: Transfer of radioiodinated human serum albumin (RISA) from cerebrospinal fluid to plasma, Proc. Soc. Exp. Biol. Med. **103**:708, 1960.

72. Vessal, K., Sperber, E., and James, A. E.: Normal pressure hydrocephalus: a cisternographic-pathologic correlation, Ann. Radiol. **17**:785, 1974.

73. Weed, L. H.: Studies on the CSF. The pathways of escape with particular reference to the arachnoid villi, J. Med. Res. **26**:51, 1914.

74. Welch, K., and Friedman, V.: The cerebrospinal fluid valves, Brain **83**:454, 1960.

75. Weller, R. O., and Wisniewski, H.: Histological and ultrastructural changes with experimental hydrocephalus in adult rabbits, Brain **29**:819, 1969.

76. Wisniewski, H., Weller, R. O., and Terry, R. D.: Experimental hydrocephalus produced by the subarachnoid infusion of silicone oil, J. Neurosurg. **31**: 10, 1969.

77. Yakovlev, P. I.: Paraplegias of hydrocephalus, Am. J. Ment. Defic. **51**:561, 1947.

78. Zajicek, J., and Zeuthen, E.: Quantitative determination of cholinesterase activity in individual cells, Exp. Cell Res. **11**:568, 1956.

79. Zeuthen, E.: Growth as related to the cell cycle in a single-cell culture of tetrahymena performis, J. Embryol. Exp. Morphol. **1**:239, 1953.

80. Zierler, K. L.: Equations for measuring blood flow by external monitoring of radioisotopes, Circ. Res. **6**:309, 1965.

16 Radionuclide liver imaging

Tuhin K. Chaudhuri and James H. Christie

When radioisotope scanning of the liver was introduced in the early 1950s,[59] it provided the only noninvasive method of detecting mass lesions within the liver. Today, despite the inherent limitations of the scanning system in demonstrating voids in a sea of radioactivity and the introduction of other techniques such as selective angiography and sonography, its usefulness has not waned. On the contrary, with the development of new radiopharmaceuticals and improved instrumentation, including gating methods to reduce the effect of respiratory motion[17] and tomographic scanning to better detect lesions in depth, its popularity has increased. Within its limitations it provides important information regarding the anatomic and physiologic configuration of the liver not readily obtained by other methods. In those centers where it has lost credibility, the fault lies not with the technique but with those whose understanding of the technique is limited and whose expectations are unrealistic. A frequently heard criticism of liver scanning is its nonspecificity. Although this is true in the main, correlation of scan findings with the patient's clinical profile renders this complaint unfounded in the vast majority of cases.

RADIOPHARMACEUTICALS

It has been traditional to consider two groups of radiopharmaceuticals in liver scanning: those removed by the reticuloendothelial system—the radiocolloids—and those removed by the parenchymal cells—the radiolabeled dyes. Recently two additional groups have been included: blood pool and tumor-seeking radiopharmaceuticals. Of the radiocolloids, ^{99m}Tc sulfur colloid[26] and ^{198}Au colloid[59] are most commonly used although ^{131}I rose bengal[22, 62] and colloids of ^{113m}In,[25, 51] ^{131}I,[16] and others* have been used to varying extent. ^{131}I rose bengal has lately been used almost exclusively to evaluate parenchymal cell function and bile excretion; historically, ^{131}I Bromsulphalein (^{131}I BSP)[50] and ^{131}I tetraiodophenolphthalein[42] have had limited use in the past. Static blood pool scanning in the investigation of hepatic mass lesions has utilized ^{113m}In transferrin and ^{131}I and ^{99m}Tc human serum albumin, whereas dynamic vascular studies of liver blood flow usually have incorporated early ^{99m}Tc sulfur colloid distribution. Recently agents such as ^{75}Se selenomethionine, ^{67}Ga gallium citrate, ^{113m}In bleomycin, and others

---

*References 1, 2, 7, 8, 19, 58.

have been used in the differential diagnosis of hepatic tumors, utilizing their metabolic selectivity; but discussion of these is not appropriate in this chapter.

　　Radiocolloids for reticuloendothelial cell imaging. Intravenously injected colloids are selectively removed from the blood by the reticuloendothelial system. Removal is exponential, and organ concentration depends on the total number of reticuloendothelial cells within the organ and its relative blood supply. In normal individuals approximately 80% of the colloid is removed by the liver, 15% by the spleen, and the remainder by the bone marrow and (to a minimal extent) lungs. Alterations in reticuloendothelial cell distribution, (e.g., in chronic debilitating disease) or decreased organ blood supply (e.g., in cirrhosis) will significantly alter these percentages.

　　Of the several available radiocolloids, ^{198}Au colloid was initially and is still used in some areas of the world where ^{99m}Tc is not available. Its major advantage is that it is a true colloid (1.00 $\mu\mu$ to 0.1 μ in size) with a reproducible particle size of about 0.02 to 0.036 μ. Its disadvantages are its relatively long half-life and its high gamma energy and beta emission, all of which limit the injectable dose and consequently reduce available image information.

　　To overcome these disadvantages, numerous other radiocolloids have been developed from the generator-produced short-lived radioisotopes of ^{99m}Tc,[26] ^{113m}In,[25, 51] and ^{87m}Sr.[2, 8] Of these, ^{99m}Tc sulfur colloid is most widely used because of its widespread availability and its ideal properties for scanning. A disadvantage, however, is that ^{99m}Tc sulfur colloid with its average particle size of 0.5 to 1.0 μ is not a true colloid. Particles can vary even more depending on preparation. For example, the addition of more gelatin results in larger particle sizes, and reheating the sulfur colloids can change the suspension from opalescent to clear, making particles invisible under the microscope.[33] Leakage of trace amounts of aluminum in the effluent can result in the formation of macroaggregates.[15]

　　It has been demonstrated that the in vivo distribution of ^{99m}Tc sulfur colloid is at least in part dependent on the colloid particle size. When colloid particles have a diameter of 0.5 to 1.0 μ, there is a relatively equal uptake in the liver and spleen with no appreciable uptake in the bone marrow. With larger particles there is increased relative deposition in the spleen, and with smaller particles there appears to be more uptake in the bone marrow. Particles with diameters greater than 10 μ are, of course, trapped in the pulmonary capillaries. Despite these observations, the fact that chromic ^{32}P phosphate (particle size 1.0 μ) and ^{198}Au colloid (0.022 to 0.036 μ) have nearly equal distributions suggests that factors other than particle size may be involved.

　　With controlled particle size, alterations in organ distribution may give insight into the underlying pathology. Therefore it is important to standardize colloid preparation and to institute quality control techniques. In many instances 2 or more patients scanned with the same preparation act as their own controls, but the period elapsing between preparation and injection must be considered because there can be colloid deterioration with time.

^{99m}Tc sulfur colloid has more or less replaced the other radiocolloids for liver imaging, but, as previously mentioned, ^{198}Au colloid is still used in areas where ^{99m}Tc is not available. Although the liver images obtained with the two radio-colloids are similar, there are subtle differences, primarily due to the decreased information on the ^{198}Au colloid scan. In theory, the higher gamma energies of ^{198}Au and ^{113m}In should permit better delineation of deep liver lesions because

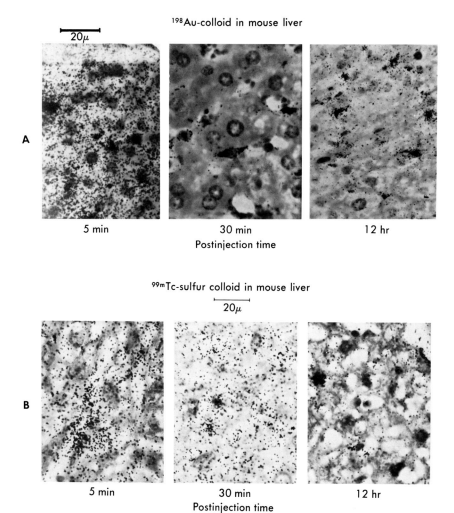

Fig. 16-1. **A,** Five-minute and 30-minute autoradiographs of mouse liver with ^{198}Au. The 12-hour picture is of conventional histologic preparation. Note concentration of silver grains in sinusoids at 5 minutes, intracellular localization of radioactivity in Kupffer's cells at 30 minutes, and aggregated metallic gold visible in plain histology 12 hours postinjection. **B,** Autoradiographs of mouse liver at different time intervals following injection of ^{99m}Tc-sulfur colloid. Note silver grains concentrated in sinusoids at 5 minutes and a generalized distri-bution of radioactivity at 30 minutes and later. Autographic grains overlie both parenchymal and reticuloendothelial cells. (From Chaudhuri, T. K., Evans, T. C., and Chaudhuri, T. K.: Radiology **109:**633, 1973.)

of decreased photon absorption with depth. However, this has not been evident clinically, probably because any minor advantage gained is overshadowed by a loss in resolution due to increased collimator septal penetration.

A recent study[12] has shown observable differences in the way in which the liver handles [198]Au colloid and ^{99m}Tc sulfur colloid. Serial autoradiographs after intravenous injection in mice have shown that [198]Au colloid passes through three distinct phases of phagocytosis by the reticuloendothelial cells; ^{99m}Tc sulfur colloid does not (Fig. 16-1).

Radiopharmaceuticals for parenchymal cell imaging. Intravenously injected ^{131}I rose bengal is loosely bound to plasma proteins, and its distribution is identical to the Evans blue space. Its rate of extraction by the polygonal cells of the liver is determined by the function of the polygonal cells and the liver blood flow, provided doses of less than 60 mg of dye are given.[56] Extrahepatic extraction of ^{131}I rose bengal is minimal and certainly less than BSP in normal individuals.[30] In its passage through the liver, conjugation or other transformation of ^{131}I rose bengal does not occur, and there is little if any enterohepatic recirculation.[49]

Since ^{131}I rose bengal does not cross the gastrointestinal epithelium, fecal measurements realistically reflect biliary excretion. These factors make ^{131}I rose bengal a useful agent for the evaluation of liver disease. However, the prolonged extraction times in patients with hepatocellular disease and delayed excretion in biliary obstruction may result in the liberation of ^{131}I iodide, which can simulate intestinal and fecal ^{131}I rose bengal excretion.

The disadvantages of ^{131}I rose bengal are similar to those of [198]Au and include a relatively long half-life and high gamma energy and beta emission. Because of these factors, the injectable dose is limited, and thus reducing available image information.

Attempts to overcome these problems with ^{123}I rose bengal have been thwarted by its limited availability and cost. New ^{99m}Tc–labeled compounds[37, 39] that have been used successfully in animals and humans without undesirable effects appear to be promising.

INSTRUMENTATION AND TECHNIQUE

Regardless of recent significant advances in instrumentation and the development of short-lived radiopharmaceuticals with ideal imaging energies, radioisotope imaging continues to be a relatively coarse imaging technique with inherent limitations. These limitations are most evident in liver scanning, which attempts to visualize voids within a comparatively large sea of radioactivity.

Liver imaging can be performed satisfactorily with both the rectilinear scanner and the gamma camera. It is interesting, however, that most individuals are strongly biased to one technique, and few are willing to routinely use both interchangeably. These biases are understandable, since the single most important factor in the accurate assessment of the liver scan is appreciation of the normal range of variation and it is difficult to transfer this appreciation from one technique to the other.

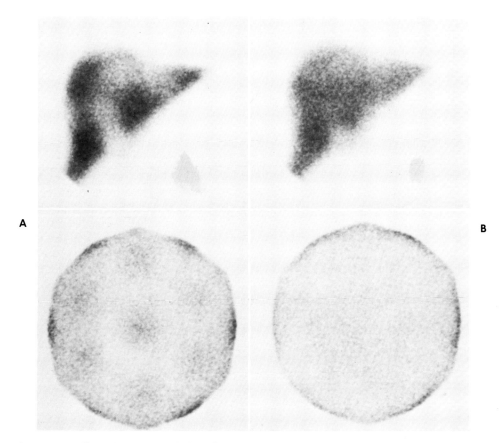

Fig. 16-2. Effect of improper (**A**) and proper (**B**) tuning of photomultiplier tubes on liver images with corresponding flood fields.

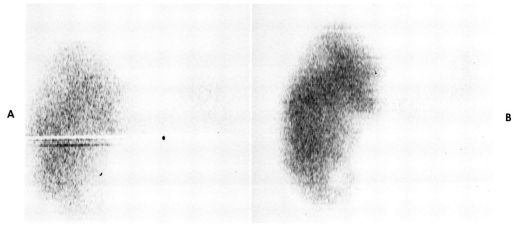

Fig. 16-3. Effect of information density on scan images. **A,** 1300 counts per square centimeter. **B,** 2600 counts per square centimeter.

To overcome the inherent limitations of the technique, investigators have attempted to manipulate the data to amplify counting rate changes, which hopefully would permit the detection of smaller lesions within the liver. In rectilinear scanning such techniques as background cutoff and data accentuation or enhancement have been employed; computer averaging and accentuation have been used with the gamma camera. Fortunately, enthusiasm for such manipulation has waned. Although these techniques have yielded desirable results in controlled laboratory settings, their clinical application has usually resulted in an unacceptable rate of false positive examinations. In the final analysis, the precise instrument or technique is not of critical importance. It is critical, however, that all parameters of a given technique be standardized and that adequate quality control techniques monitor daily equipment performance. Figs. 16-2 and 16-3 illustrate two of the virtually infinite number of variables or problems that may be encountered.

RETICULOENDOTHELIAL CELL IMAGING

Normal liver. The normal liver varies considerably in size and shape in different individuals and in the same individual under varying conditions. Many attempts have been made to classify the shape of the normal liver, primarily from the anterior scan image, resulting in thirty-nine different types in 125 patients in one series.[48] An appreciation of normal variations in shape may be useful, but an understanding of why these variations exist is more productive. The liver is a pliable organ that conforms to and is affected by the space it occupies. It is fixed to the diaphragm and to the anterior abdominal wall by the falciform ligament, which lies between the right and left lobes of the liver; posteriorly, the right triangular and coronary ligaments form attachments to the right hemidiaphragm. The superior contour of the liver is defined by the right hemidiaphragm and the rib cage; the portion below the costal margin is less confined and may vary considerably with patient positioning, especially in patients with pendulous abdomens.

The liver is divided into two major lobes, the right and left. In normal individuals the right lobe makes up about four fifths of the liver mass. Posterior and medial to the right lobe are two smaller lobes—the caudate lobe posterosuperiorly and the quadrate lobe anteroinferiorly. The left lobe is normally much smaller than the right, is anterior and flat, and typically extends 2 to 5 cm to the left of the midline. The appearance of the "normal" liver and its relationship to adjacent structures in anterior, posterior, and right and left lateral views are shown in Fig. 16-4.

The so-called Riedel's lobe, most commonly seen in women, is not a true lobe and represents a tonguelike, inferior projection of the right lobe, occasionally extending to the iliac crest. The caudate lobe, which is immediately adjacent to the superior portion of the posterior aspect of the right lobe, is almost enveloped by the right lobe and cannot be identified on scans as separate from the right lobe, even when enlarged. The quadrate lobe, also adjacent to the posterior

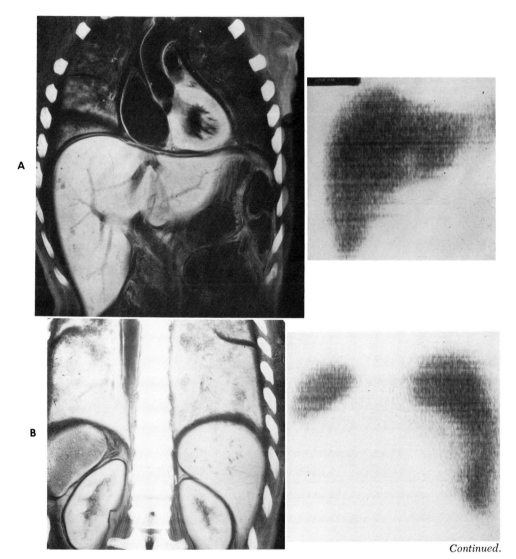

Continued.

Fig. 16-4. Relationship of liver-spleen scan images with other intra-abdominal structures. **A,** Anterior view. **B,** Posterior view. **C,** Right lateral view. **D,** Left lateral view.

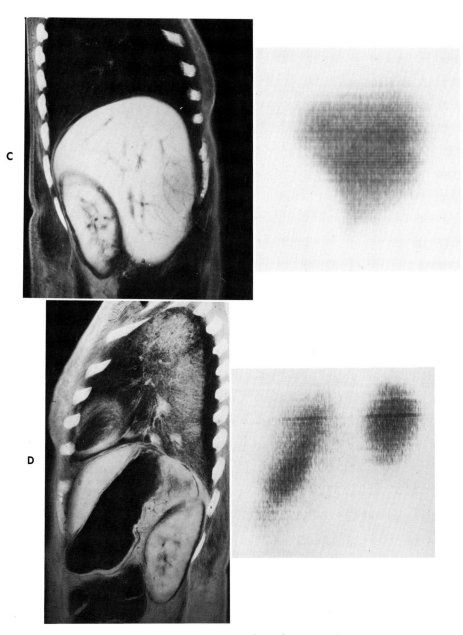

Fig. 16-4, cont'd. For legend see p. 397.

aspect of the right lobe, is inferior and, when enlarged, projects caudad between the right and left lobes, resulting in a "cloverleaf" appearance of the liver on the anterior scan image (Fig. 16-5).

In the interpretation of liver scan images, consideration must be given to the space the liver occupies. With elevation of the right diaphragm, the liver moves superiorly with a clockwise rotation, since it is fixed medially by the falciform ligament, which is attached to the fixed central portion of the diaphragm and the anterior abdominal wall. This results in an apparent relative decrease in the size of the right lobe and an increase in the size of the left lobe, which rotates down and laterally to the right (Fig. 16-6). Conversely, when the right diaphragm is flattened, the liver descends with a "counterclockwise" rotation (Fig. 16-7), resulting in an apparent relative increase in the size of the right lobe and a decrease in the size of the left lobe.

Likewise, the effect of the approximation of other organs on the shape of the liver depends on the position of these structures in relation to the liver. For example, cardiac enlargement limits elevation of the left diaphragm and therefore alters the normal relative positions of the right and left lobes of the liver and spleen. Since the inferior-medial margin of the liver as seen on the posterior scan image is usually determined by the right kidney, any process that alters the

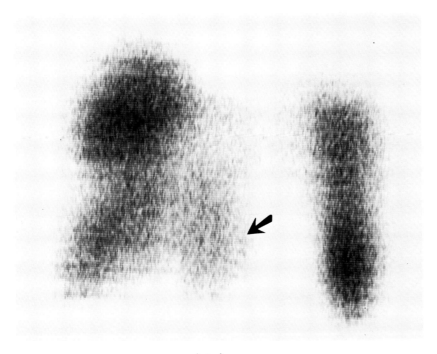

Anterior

Fig. 16-5. Extreme example of enlarged quadrate lobe (arrow) resulting in "cloverleaf" appearance of liver image on anterior view.

Right

Anterior

Fig. 16-6. Elevation of right hemidiaphragm causes liver to rotate clockwise (arrow) about its central fixation at the falciform ligament, resulting in an apparent relative decrease in size of right lobe and increase in size of left lobe.

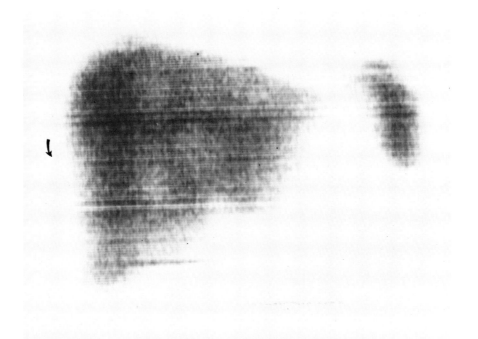

Fig. 16-7. Flattening of right hemidiaphragm causes liver to rotate counterclockwise (arrow) about its central fixation at the falciform ligament, resulting in an apparent relative increase in size of right lobe.

cephalocaudal relationship of kidney and liver will impose changes on the contour of the liver.

Patient position must also be considered. It should be remembered that the diaphragm is high in a supine patient breathing quietly, and therefore the relationships of liver and diaphragm cannot be compared with those on the routine posteroanterior chest radiograph made with the patient erect and in deep inspiration. During scanning also, patient positioning affects the relationship of these organs to one another. In a patient lying on his side the dependent hemidiaphragm rises while the contralateral hemidiaphragm encroaches on the space of the abdominal cavity. Therefore patient positioning is an important factor to be reckoned with in the interpretation of scan images and radiographic examinations.

Determination of hepatic size. The traditional clinical method of liver size evaluation by palpation of its inferior margin is so dependent on the shape and position of the liver and diaphragm that the method is unreliable at best. Estimation of liver size by the experienced observer viewing the scan image in the routine four views is probably sufficient clinically, except in borderline cases. Because of these cases, several investigators have been stimulated to devise mathematical models by which the actual weight of the liver in grams can be

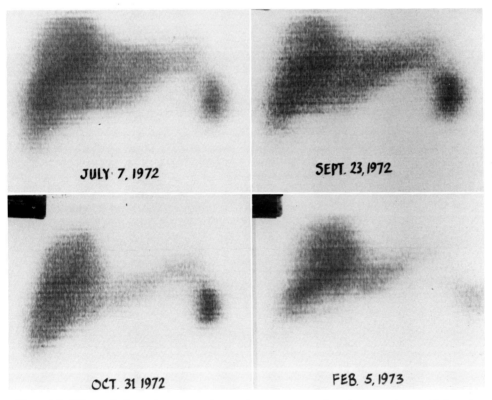

Fig. 16-8. Effect of chemotherapy on liver-spleen sizes in a lymphoma patient with hepatosplenic involvement. To evaluate changes in organ size, scanning parameters must be standardized.

estimated with a relatively high degree of accuracy.[53, 54] It should be emphasized, however, that although these techniques may prove accurate in the hands of one investigator using a certain set of scanning parameters, similar accuracy with another set of parameters cannot be assured.

Estimation of liver size must be correlated with body weight. In the adult the liver represents approximately 2.5% of the total body weight; in the infant, about 5% to 6%. Estimation of progressive enlargement, involution, or regeneration of the liver during the course of disease has been extremely useful clinically (Fig. 16-8).

Extrahepatic lesions. An extrahepatic lesion should be suspected whenever the liver shape and its relationship to adjacent structures varies from the expected norm. When this occurs, additional views with altered positioning of the patient or combination scans (e.g., transmission-emission, liver-lung, liver-blood pool, liver-kidney, and liver-stomach) often are helpful in delineating the character of extrahepatic masses. Obviously the selection of the technique to be used must be tailored to the problem at hand. As a specific example, transmission-emission scanning and combination liver-lung scanning (Fig. 16-9) have been found very useful in the diagnosis of subphrenic abscess. It must be emphasized that careful correlation with the radiographic findings in the chest and abdomen is necessary, since the technique merely shows separation between the lung parenchyma and the liver, which may result from other causes within the chest, abdomen, or diaphragm.

Focal disease. Focal areas of decreased uptake on the liver scan may have many causes, including metastatic and primary tumor, cysts, abscesses, trauma, and infarcts. Making the specific diagnosis from the liver scan alone is usually

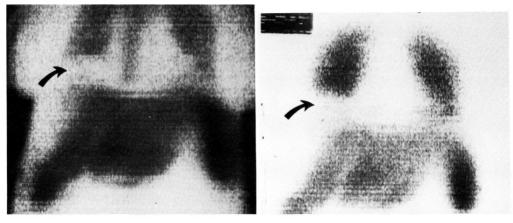

Fig. 16-9. Transmission-emission scan with 4 mCi of ^{99m}Tc-sulfur colloid (IV) and an external source of 4 mCi of ^{99m}Tc compound showing separation between right lung and liver (left, arrow). Combination liver-lung scans performed with 4 mCi of ^{99m}Tc-sulfur colloid and 4.0 mCi ^{99m}Tc-MAA shows separation of liver and lung (arrow) due to a sub-diaphragmatic abscess (right).

impossible; however, when the scan is viewed in the context of the patient's overall clinical presentation, the diagnosis is generally not difficult.

Liver scans are performed most commonly for the detection of metastatic tumor. Lesions may be discrete, single (Fig. 16-10), or multiple (Fig. 16-11). In many instances of numerous, multiple metastases, discrete lesions cannot be identified because the liver scan shows primarily a gross irregularity in colloid distribution. The proliferation of chemotherapeutic agents for the treatment of malignant disease has placed increased emphasis on the detection of metastatic tumor within the liver. It must be emphasized that a positive scan carries a high degree of reliability, but a negative scan in no way excludes metastatic disease. Superficial liver lesions smaller than 2 cm cannot be identified, and larger lesions lying only 1 or 2 cm below the surface of the liver are often obscured by the overlying normal liver tissue. The assessment of the progression or regression of a known metastatic tumor following systemic or intra-arterial infusion therapy can be determined by interval scanning (Fig. 16-12). A flow study using radio-

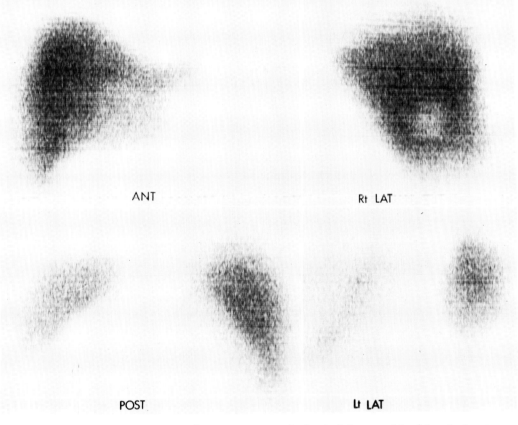

ANT   Rt LAT

POST   Lt LAT

Fig. 16-10. Liver scan images demonstrate a single focal defect in right lobe. Lesion is visualized only on right lateral view. Overlying normal liver obscures lesion on anterior and posterior views.

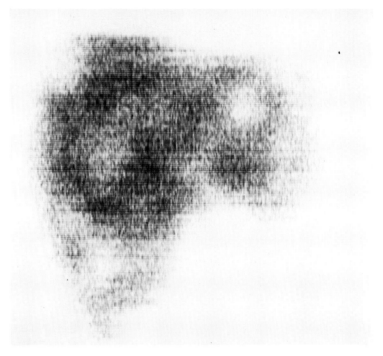

Fig. 16-11. Characteristic appearance of a liver with multiple metastatic lesions. Scan findings are nonspecific and must be correlated with other clinical findings.

pharmaceuticals injected through the intra-arterial catheter can be helpful in determining the proper placement of the catheter for infusion therapy.

The liver scan has proved especially useful in the early detection of amebic or pyogenic abscesses, thereby substantially reducing mortality. In amebic abscesses the progress of therapy can be monitored (Fig. 16-13), and identification of the pyogenic abscess assists the surgeon in the proper approach for drainage.

The inherent limitations of the scanning system and an understandable zeal to make correct diagnoses has in some centers led to an unacceptable number of false positive examinations. This has proved to be counterproductive by detracting from the true usefulness of the liver scan. There is no easy solution to this problem. The most common false positive focal defects are caused by the gallbladder fossa, the interlobar notches, the varying size of the porta hepatis, and the costal margin impression. These areas all have one common characteristic—they are peripheral. Often additional views with the patient turned 5° or 10° more obliquely are helpful. Adjunctive scan studies (e.g., using ^{131}I rose bengal to demonstrate the gallbladder) may offer an alternative solution to the problem.

Diffuse hepatocellular disease. Early radiocolloid scan manifestations of diffuse hepatocellular disease are characterized by a relative increase in spleen uptake as compared to the liver (Fig. 16-14), with or without associated liver enlargement. The spectrum of scan change due to diffuse hepatic disease is wide. There may be practically no uptake in the advanced stage of liver disease and marked

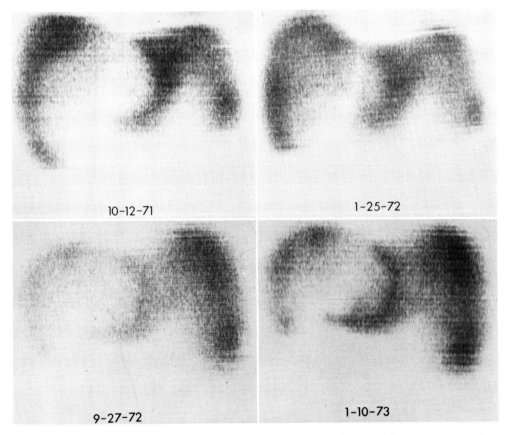

Fig. 16-12. Assessment of effect of intra-arterial infusion of 5-fluorouracil in a patient with primary hepatoma.

uptake in the spleen and bone marrow (Fig. 16-15). The many and varied causes of diffuse hepatocellular disease include cirrhosis, metabolic diseases, and infections. Scan findings are nonspecific, and clinical history, physical examination, laboratory findings, and often liver biopsy are required before a specific diagnosis can be established.

Alcoholic cirrhosis in its various stages is the most common cause of diffuse hepatocellular disease in the United States. The liver may be large, normal, or small. In early cirrhosis with typical fatty infiltration, the liver is enlarged and the spleen normal or enlarged, with a relative increase in colloid deposition. As the disease progresses, the right lobe may decrease in size because of fibrosis and scarring, and there may be a compensatory increase in size of the left lobe and occasionally the quadrate lobe. Radiocolloid uptake in the right lobe is decreased, which results in a relative increased deposition in the left lobe, often referred to as a "shift to the left."[13] The spleen is usually enlarged, and increased uptake is evident in both spleen and bone marrow.

These changes in radiocolloid uptake by the liver, spleen, and bone marrow

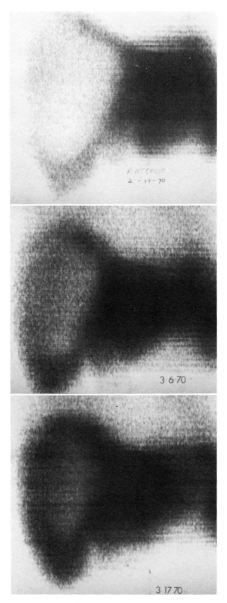

Fig. 16-13. Serial liver scans demonstrate resolution of an amebic abscess with therapy.

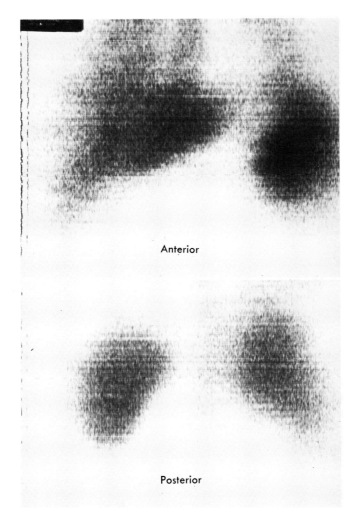

Anterior

Posterior

Fig. 16-14. Characteristic liver appearance of a patient with alcoholic cirrhosis and marked impairment of liver function. Radiocolloid uptake and size of right lobe are decreased; radiocolloid uptake and size of left lobe are increased (shift to left) with marked extrahepatic radiocolloid uptake in spleen and bone marrow.

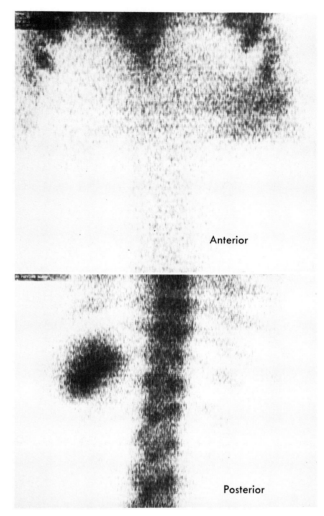

Fig. 16-15. Advanced stage of portal cirrhosis shows practically no uptake of radiocolloid in liver and marked uptake in spleen and bone marrow.

are secondary to alterations in blood flow and are not due to a relative decrease of hepatic and increase of extrahepatic reticuloendothelial cells. A positive correlation between the portohepatic pressure gradient and the extrahepatic uptake of radiocolloids has been shown.[20] Although the blood clearance rate of radiocolloids and the extrahepatic uptake of radiocolloid independently may not be a reflection of the degree of portal hypertension, in combination they can be helpful in identifying patients with a significant degree of portal hypertension.[47] The absence of significant extrahepatic uptake of radiocolloids has been reported in patients with presinusoidal portal hypertension,[50] and persistence of extrahepatic uptake has been observed in patients with normal portal pressures following surgical portosystemic shunts.[43] These findings suggest that portal hypertension per se is not the cause of the increased extrahepatic uptake of the radiocolloids, but that the latter is due to decreased sinusoidal blood flow. Uncorrected portal hypertension is merely a reflection of this decreased flow.

Budd-Chiari syndrome and portal vein thrombosis. The Budd-Chiari syndrome (hepatic vein thrombosis) and portal vein thrombosis result in scan findings very similar to those of advanced cirrhosis.[6, 9] The acute onset of the disease along with a rapidly deteriorating liver uptake of colloid on repeat scans (as soon as within a week) permits a differential diagnosis. In addition, the spleen is normal or only slightly enlarged, and uptake is more pronounced in the bone marrow. Demonstrable uptake by the reticuloendothelial cells within the lung is not uncommon.

Lymphoma. The scan findings in a liver involved by lymphoma may be entirely normal[44] or show only nonspecific enlargement. As with other metastatic tumors to the liver, it is rare to have impairment of the blood supply, and therefore the ratio of uptake within the liver and the spleen remains normal. Rarely, the liver will show a focal defect, or, with extensive involvement uptake, may become irregular; these changes are nonspecific. In contrast to one report,[40] it has been suggested that focal defects, and/or mottled, irregular colloid uptake within the liver are unreliable indicators of involvement by lymphoma.[46] Lymphoma patients are subject to other liver diseases, which can cause similar scan findings. Although this is true of scan diagnoses in general, the impact of liver involvement with lymphoma on therapy requires more than presumptive evidence of involvement.

At present, the open liver biopsy appears to be the technique of choice to exclude liver involvement, though this technique is not 100% reliable. It remains to be seen whether a negative liver biopsy at laparotomy is sufficiently reliable to eliminate the possibility of hepatic relapse. It is possible that a combination of indirect indexes obtained from liver imaging and laboratory tests may eventually prove to be of greater prognostic significance than biopsy alone.

Lung uptake of radiocolloids. Lung uptake of radiocolloids is not an uncommon finding. Often it can be traced to improper colloid particle size, which should be suspected if lung uptake occurs in more than one patient or if it occurs several hours after the preparation of the radiocolloid. However, true lung uptake of radiocolloids can occur in patients with portal or hepatic vein thrombosis and in patients with advanced cirrhosis, probably because of a relative rather than absolute increase in reticuloendothelial cell function within the lung. Care must be taken not to confuse rib uptake with lung uptake, a distinction difficult to make in many instances.

Clinical studies using carefully prepared ^{99m}Tc sulfur colloid have demonstrated increased lung uptake of colloids in patients with primary liver disease and neoplastic processes[34] and in those with spleen and bone marrow transplant (Fig. 16-16).[36] The intraperitoneal injection of *Escherichia coli* endotoxins in animals causes an increase in reticuloendothelial cell activity and colloid uptake the lungs.[52] An absolute increase in the reticuloendothelial system function of the

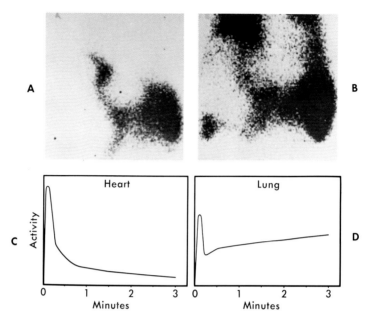

Fig. 16-16. Radiocolloid uptake in lungs following spleen and bone marrow transplantation. **A,** Pretransplantation anterior liver scan showing large hepatoma and clear lung fields (upper portion of scan). **B** to **D,** Anterior liver scan and corresponding time-activity curves 84 days after spleen and bone marrow transplant. Scan shows marked lung uptake. Heart time-activity curve is normal, but lung time-activity curve is unusual because it shows increasing activity with time, even before subtracting blood pool activity. (From Klingensmith, W. C., III, and Ryerson, T. W.: J. Nucl. Med. **14:**201, 1973.)

lungs has also been described in animals challenged with estrogen.[45] This same mechanism and rapid in vivo clumping and secondary microembolization are believed to play a role in these clinical situations.[34, 36]

Malignant melanomas. A relative increase in splenic as compared to hepatic uptake has been observed in patients with malignant melanoma.[24] This increased splenic radioactivity is attributed to stimulation of splenic reticuloendothelial cell function, rather than a depressed hepatic reticuloendothelial cell function,[23] presumably secondary to immunologic factors. In one such patient a repeat liver-spleen scan following surgical removal of a malignant melanoma showed a reduction of spleen size and a return to a normal ratio of spleen-to-liver uptake.[35]

Focal areas of increased uptake in liver. Focal areas of increased colloid uptake are usually attributable to poorly tuned photomultiplier tubes in the scintillation camera (Fig. 16-2). Generally, although not always, recent reports of true localized areas of increased uptake associate this phenomenon with cases of superior vena caval obstruction.[14, 27-29, 31] In at least 2 of these cases the liver showed practically no abnormality on a repeat study when the radiocolloid was injected through a leg vein.[29] It is also to be emphasized that not all patients with superior vena caval obstruction exhibit this phenomenon.[27] Focal areas of increased radiocolloid uptake have also been observed when an injection has been

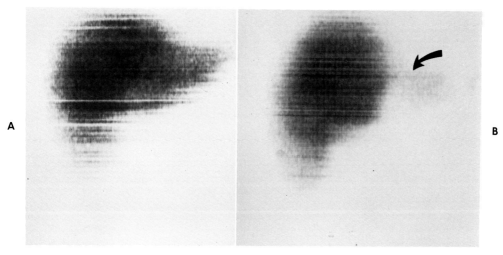

Fig. 16-17. Liver scans. **A,** Normal liver. **B,** Effect of radiation therapy in a patient treated for lymphoma.

made through a malpositioned central venous catheter with its tip in one of the hepatic vein tributaries.[28]

Liver scan changes secondary to radiation therapy. Changes in the function of the polygonal and reticuloendothelial cells secondary to radiation therapy can be documented earlier and more reliably by scanning than by the usual liver function tests.[4] Dual scanning with radiocolloids and ^{131}I BSP have shown that the reticuloendothelial cells are the most radiosensitive elements.[3] Decreased radiocolloid uptake has been demonstrated with fractionated radiation doses of 3000 rads in 28 days, and doses of 4000 rads will almost totally eliminate radiocolloid uptake (Fig. 16-17). With doses above 5000 rads, the changes are usually irreversible.[3]

HEPATOBILIARY IMAGING

Parenchymal cell function and biliary excretion. Although ^{131}I rose bengal has been replaced by the radioactive colloids for routine liver imaging, many workers consider it useful for evaluating hepatobiliary function and biliary excretion. [131]I rose bengal is cleared exponentially from the plasma by the parenchymal cells of the liver after injection, with a half-time clearance of about 7 to 8 minutes in normal individuals. Peak activity within the liver occurs at approximately 20 to 30 minutes. Secretion into the bile begins immediately, but is usually not appreciated within the gallbladder or gut until 1 to 2 hours after injection. Four hours after injection a large amount of the rose bengal has been excreted from the liver into the gut (Fig. 16-18).

Sequential scanning that includes the heart blood pool, liver, gut, and kidneys at intervals of 30 minutes, 2, 4, 24, and occasionally 48 and 72 hours after injection permits an evaluation of hepatobiliary function. In patients with recent ex-

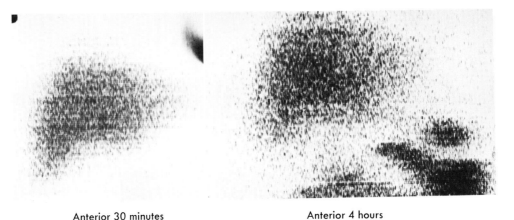

Anterior 30 minutes   Anterior 4 hours

Fig. 16-18. A normal ^{131}I rose bengal liver scan shows practically no activity in heart blood pool 30 minutes after injection. Gallbladder is not visualized. Free release of activity into gut is seen on 4-hour scan.

trahepatic biliary obstruction, plasma clearance is normal, and excretion into the gut is reduced or absent, depending on the degree of obstruction. As obstruction persists, there is subsequent impairment of hepatocellular function, resulting in delayed plasma clearance (Fig. 16-19). In patients with diffuse hepatocellular disease and patency of the biliary tree, plasma clearance is prolonged, as evidenced by increased heart blood pool activity and kidney extraction on early scans and delayed and decreased biliary excretion. It is reported that activity in the gut can always be observed within 24 hours in adults in spite of severe hepatocellular disease, provided the biliary tree is patent.[66] With increased renal extraction, care must be taken not to confuse uptake in the kidneys for gut radioactivity.[21] Posterior scans, which show kidney radioactivity to best advantage, are usually sufficient for this differentiation; occasionally sequential scans, which show unchanging position of renal activity, are necessary.

Theoretically, ^{131}I rose bengal imaging of the liver should be of especial value in the differential diagnosis of neonatal jaundice with high direct bilirubin, which can result from neonatal hepatitis (intrahepatic cholestasis) or biliary atresia. Bile excretion of less than 10% by stool measurements and lack of evidence of gut radioactivity within 48 to 72 hours after injection have been considered evidence of biliary atresia.[55] Unfortunately, bile excretion in neonatal hepatitis is so diminished that a differential diagnosis by this technique is not possible in a significant percentage of patients. Recently, investigators have shown that cholestyramine given orally for 2 weeks significantly increases biliary excretion in infants with neonatal hepatitis but has no effect on excretion in infants with biliary atresia.[5] Thus preoperative differential diagnosis is possible by comparing ^{131}I rose bengal scans and fecal excretion percentages before and after administration of cholestyramine.

Other applications of [131]***I rose bengal.*** In patients with cirrhosis and severe

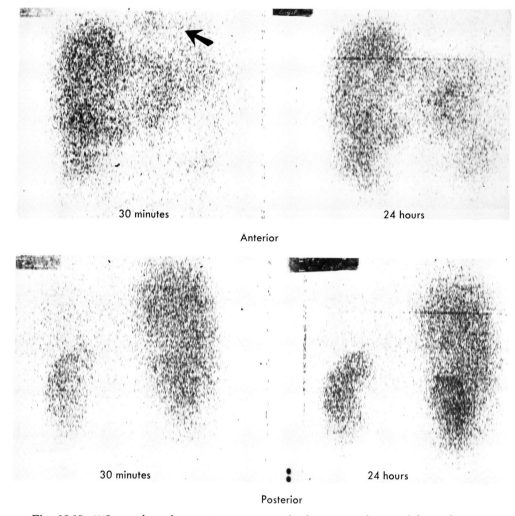

30 minutes   24 hours

Anterior

30 minutes   24 hours

Posterior

Fig. 16-19. [131]I rose bengal scan in a patient with chronic extrahepatic biliary obstruction shows delayed plasma clearance evidenced by persistence of heart blood pool activity (arrow) on 30-minute scan and absence of gut activity 24 hours later. Note kidney activity, which must not be mistaken for gut activity.

portal hypertension, ^{131}I rose bengal commonly permits better visualization of the liver than the radiocolloids. The total uptake of both ^{131}I rose bengal and the radiocolloids is dependent on organ blood supply and on the blood concentration of these agents. In contrast to the radiocolloids, ^{131}I rose bengal is almost entirely removed by the parenchymal cells of the liver only; therefore blood levels remain high and afford continued opportunity for removal by the liver.

Uptake in a primary hepatoma in a cirrhotic patient has been reported,[57] but this apparently is so rare as to negate the usefulness of ^{131}I rose bengal in the differential diagnosis of voids within a cirrhotic liver.

About 50% of choledochal cysts communicate with the biliary tract; progressive accumulation of ^{131}I rose bengal within the cyst on 4- to 24-hour delayed scans may fill an initially present void and thus facilitate correct diagnosis.[64]

ADJUNCTIVE STUDIES

To increase the specificity of the diagnosis of hepatic mass lesions, early flow studies[18, 63, 67] with ^{99m}Tc sulfur colloid and static blood pool scans with radiopharmaceuticals such as ^{99m}Tc human serum albumin[61] or [113m]In transferrin[41] have been shown to be useful in demonstrating the differential blood supply and the relative vascularity of the lesions. In general, cysts and abscesses are avascular. Metastatic tumors are usually less vascular than the surrounding liver, and most primary hepatomas show a vascularity similar to that of normal liver. Highly vascular tumors such as hemangiomas often show relatively greater blood pool than the normal liver. In addition to dynamic blood pool scanning (Fig. 16-20), tumor-seeking agents such as ^{75}Se selenomethionine, ^{67}Ga gallium citrate, ^{99m}Tc bleomycin, [87]Sr strontium citrate, and ^{99m}Tc phosphate compounds[9, 11, 32, 38, 65] have been shown useful in the diagnosis of mass lesions.

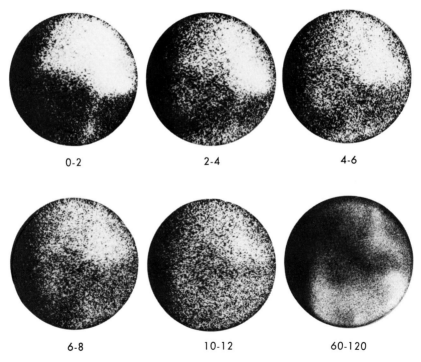

| 0-2 | 2-4 | 4-6 |
| 6-8 | 10-12 | 60-120 |

Fig. 16-20. Positioning film (60 to 120 seconds) outlines liver, lesion, heart, and right lower lung from anterior perspective. A tumor stain is first seen at 0 to 2 seconds and persists through 8 seconds. At 10 to 12 seconds (venous phase) decreased radioactivity is seen. (From DeNardo, G. L., et al.: Radiology **111**:135, 1974.)

THE PRESENT AND FUTURE

The clinical usefulness of liver scanning has been well documented through the vast experience accumulated over the past two decades. Even though morphologic alterations produced by diseases in the liver are generally nonspecific, correlation with other clinical findings usually permits a specific etiologic diagnosis. The developing independent confidence in the specificity of liver scan findings poses the potential hazard of diminishing, rather than enhancing, the clinical usefulness of the procedure. Therefore expectations must be kept within the inherent limitations of the technique if the credibility of its results is to be maintained.

At this time it appears unlikely that further technical refinement of present instrumentation will profoundly enhance the diagnostic capabilities of the procedure in the near future. The development of new tumor-seeking radiopharmaceuticals is accelerating, but major advances that might improve the specificity of liver scanning do not appear to be just beyond the horizon. Progress in ultrasound and the recent development of whole-body computerized tomography will certainly have an effect on the usefulness of radionuclide liver scanning, but in the foreseeable future these different approaches to the same diagnostic problem will probably remain complementary.

References

1. Aronow, S., Thors, R., and Brownell, G. L.: Positron scanning of the liver and pancreas. In Medical radioisotope scanning, International Atomic Energy Agency, 1959, Vienna.
2. Asard, P. E., and Bois-Svensson, I.: Preparation methods of liver and lung radiopharmaceuticals with Sr-87m, Tc-99m and In-113m, Acta Radiol. [Ther.] (Stockh.) 11:240, 1972.
3. Brase, A., Bockslaff, H., and Kauman, M.: Scintigraphic findings in the liver following partial irradiation with Cobalt-60, Strahlentherapie 143:41, 1972.
4. Brase, A., Bockslaff, H., and Kauman, M.: Scintigraphic follow-up studies following Cobalt-60 irradiation of liver tumors, Strahlentherapie 143:179, 1972.
5. Campbell, D. P., et al.: The differential diagnosis of neonatal hepatitis and biliary atresia, J. Pediatr. Surg. 9:699, 1974.
6. Carulli, N., et al.: Liver scans in the Budd-Chiari syndrome, J.A.M.A. 223: 1161, 1973.
7. Charkes, N. D., and Shansky, F.: Liver scanning with radioactive isotopes, J. Einstein Med. Cent. 12:126, 1964.
8. Chaudhuri, T. K., Chaudhuri, T. K., and Christie, J. H.: Two-stage liver and bone scanning with single dose of one isotope, Int. J. Appl. Radiat. Isot. 24:204, 1972.
9. Chaudhuri, T. K., et al.: Liver scan in Budd-Chiari syndrome, J.A.M.A. 221: 506, 1972.
10. Chaudhuri, T. K., et al.: Uptake of Sr-87m by liver metastasis from carcinoma of colon, J. Nucl. Med. 14:293, 1973.
11. Chaudhuri, T. K., et al.: Extraosseous noncalcified soft-tissue uptake of 99mTc-polyphosphate, J. Nucl. Med. 15:1054, 1974.
12. Chaudhuri, T. K., Evans, T. C., and Chaudhuri, T. K.: Autoradiographic studies of distribution in the liver of Au-198 and Tc-99m-sulfur colloid, Radiology 109:633, 1973.
13. Christie, J. H., et al.: Radioisotope scanning in hepatic cirrhosis, Radiology 81: 455, 1963.
14. Cole, M., et al.: Intrahepatic lesion presenting as an area of increased radiocolloid uptake on a liver scan, J. Nucl. Med. 13:221, 1972.
15. Cunningham, R. E.: Albumin flocculations in Tc-99m–labeled sulfur colloid preparation, communication from AEC to licensees, July 7, 1970.
16. Delaloye, B., Magnenat, P., and Cruehaurt, S.: L'hépatoscintillogramme après

injection d'albumine humaine denaturée marquée à I'I-131, Schweiz. Med. Wschr. **89**:1305, 1959.

17. DeLand, F. H., and Mauderli, W.: Gating mechanism for motion-free liver and lung scintigraphy, J. Nucl. Med. **13**: 939, 1972.

18. DeNardo, G. L., et al.: Hepatic scintiangiographic patterns, Radiology **111**: 135, 1974.

19. Endlich, H., et al.: The use of I-125 to increase isotope scanning resolution, Am. J. Roentgenol. Radium Ther. Nucl. Med. **87**:148, 1962.

20. Fernandez, J. P., et al.: The extrahepatic uptake of Au-198 as an index of portal hypertension, Am. J. Dig. Dis. **15**:883, 1970.

21. Freeman, L. M., Kay, C., and Derman, A.: Renal concentration of I-131 rose bengal confusing the interpretation of abdominal scans in liver disease, Br. J. Radiol. **41**:826, 1968.

22. Friedell, H. L., MacIntyre, W. J., and Rajali, A. M.: A method for the visualization of the configuration and structure of the liver, Am. J. Roentgenol. Radium Ther. Nucl. Med. **77**:455, 1957.

23. Gillette, R. W., and Lance, E. M.: Kinetic studies of macrophages. Distributional characteristics of radiolabeled peritoneal cells, J. Reticuloendothel. Soc. **10**:223, 1971.

24. Goldman, A. B., Braunstein, P., and Song, C.: Augmented splenic uptake of radiocolloid in patients with malignant melanoma, Lancet **1**:460, 1974.

25. Goodwin, D. A., et al.: Indium-113m: a new radiopharmaceutical for liver scanning, Nucleonics **24**:65, 1966.

26. Harper, P. V., et al.: Technetium-99m as a scanning agent, Radiology **85**:101, 1965.

27. Hattner, R. S., and Shames, D. M.: Nonspecificity of radiocolloid hepatic "hotspot" for superior vena caval obstruction, J. Nucl. Med. **15**:1041, 1974.

28. Helbig, H. D.: Focal iatrogenic increased radiocolloid uptake on liver scan, J. Nucl. Med. **14**:354, 1973.

29. Holmquest, D. L., and Burdine, J. A.: Caval-portal shunting as a cause of a focal increase in radiocolloid uptake in normal livers, J. Nucl. Med. **14**:348, 1973.

30. Jones, D. P., Terz, J., Laurence, W.,

Jr., and Pappel, J. W.: Extrahepatic clearance of I-131 rose bengal, Am. J. Physiol. **201**:1025, 1961.

31. Joyner, J. T.: Abnormal liver scan (radiocolloid "hot spot") associated with superior vena caval obstruction, J. Nucl. Med. **13**:849, 1972.

32. Kaplan, E., and Domingo, M.: Se-75-Selenomethionine in hepatic lesions, Semin. Nucl. Med. **2**:139, 1972.

33. Kelly, W. N., and Ice, R. D.: Pharmaceutical quality of Technetium-99m sulfur colloid, Am. J. Hosp. Pharm. **30**: 817, 1973.

34. Keyes, J. W., Wilson, G. A., and Quinones, J. D.: An evaluation of lung uptake of colloid during liver imaging, J. Nucl. Med. **14**:687, 1973.

35. Klingensmith, W. C., III: Resolution of increased splenic size and uptake of Tc-99m-sulfur colloid following removal of a malignant melanoma, J. Nucl. Med. **15**:1203, 1974.

36. Klingensmith, W. C., III, and Ryerson, T. W.: Lung uptake of Tc-99m-sulfur colloid, J. Nucl. Med. **14**:201, 1973.

37. Krishnamurthy, G. T., et al.: Cholescintigraphy with ^{99m}Tc-penicillamine, Radiology **115**:201, 1975.

38. Lin, M. S., Goodwin, D. A., and Kruse, S. L.: Bleomycin as a Tc-99m carrier in tumor visualization, J. Nucl. Med. **15**: 338, 1974.

39. Lin, T. H., Khentigan, A., and Winchell, H. S.: A 99MTc–labeled replacement for I-131-rose bengal in liver and biliary tract studies, J. Nucl. Med. **15**:613, 1974.

40. Lipton, M. J., et al.: Evaluation of the liver and spleen in Hodgkin's disease. I. The value of hepatic scintigraphy, Am. J. Med. **52**:256, 1972.

41. Lubin, E., et al.: Radioisotopic study of the blood pool of space-occupying lesions of the liver, J. Nucl. Med. **11**: 334, 1970.

42. MacIntyre, W. J., and Houser, T. S.: A method for the visualization of the configuration and structure of the liver, Am. J. Roentgenol. Radium Ther. Nucl. Med. **77**:471, 1957.

43. Magnenat, P., and Delaloye, B.: La scintigraphie du foie et de la rate dans la cirrhose, Bull. Schweiz. Acad. Med. Suisse **19**:20, 1963.

44. McCready, V. R., Swyther, M. M., and

Stringer, A. M.: Organ visualization and function in the lymphomata, Br. J. Radiol. **40**:316, 1967.

45. Mikhael, M. A., and Evans, R. G.: Migration and embolization of macrophages to the lung—a possible mechanism for colloid uptake in the lung during liver scanning, J. Nucl. Med. **16**:22, 1975.

46. Milder, M. S., et al.: Liver-spleen scan in Hodgkin's disease, Cancer **31**:826, 1973.

47. Millette, B., et al.: The extrahepatic uptake of radioactive colloidal gold in cirrhotic patients as an index of liver function and portal hypertensions, Am. J. Dig. Dis. **18**:719, 1973.

48. Mould, R. F.: An investigation of the variation in normal liver shape, Br. J. Radiol. **45**:586, 1972.

49. Nordyke, R. A., and Blahd, W. H.: The differential diagnosis of biliary tract obstruction with radioactive rose bengal, J. Lab. Clin. Med. **51**:565, 1958.

50. Papanicolaou, N., et al.: Étude de la fixation extrahépatique au cours de la scintigraphie à l'or colloidal radioactif. Valeur clinique. Essai de'étude physiopathologique, Rev. Medicochir. Mal. Foie **41**:219, 1966.

51. Potchen, E. J., and Adatepe, M.: Liver and spleen scintiscanning with indium-113m. A clinical and pathologic correlation, Am. J. Roentgenol. Radium Ther. Nucl. Med. **106**:739, 1969.

52. Quinones, J. D.: Localization of Technetium-sulfur colloid after RES stimulation, J. Nucl. Med. **14**:443, 1973.

53. Rollo, F. D., and DeLand, F. H.: The determination of liver mass from radionuclide images, Radiology **91**:1191, 1968.

54. Rosenfield, A. T., and Schneider, P. B.: Rapid evaluation of hepatic size on radioisotope scan, J. Nucl. Med. **15**:237, 1974.

55. Rosenthall, L.: The application of radioiodinated rose bengal and colloidal radiogold in the detection of hepatobiliary disease, St. Louis, 1969, Warren H. Green, Inc.

56. Sapirstein, L. A., and Simpson, A. M.: Plasma clearance of rose bengal (tetraiodotetrabromfluorescein), Am. J. Physiol. **182**:337, 1955.

57. Shoop, J. D.: Functional hepatoma demonstrated with rose bengal scanning, Am. J. Roentgenol. Radium Ther. Nucl. Med. **107**:51, 1969.

58. Sorensen, L. B., and Archambault, M.: Visualization of the liver by scanning with Mo-99 molybdate as tracer, J. Lab. Clin. Med. **62**:330, 1963.

59. Stirrett, L. A., Yuhl, E. T., and Cassen, B.: Clinical applications of hepatic radioactive surveys, Am. J. Gastroenterol. **21**:310, 1954.

60. Suwanik, R., et al.: I-BSP scanning of the liver, Am. J. Proctol. **17**:462, 1966.

61. Taplin, G. V.: Dynamic studies of liver function with radioisotopes. In Proceedings of Symposium on Dynamic Studies with Radioisotopes in Medicine, International Atomic Energy Agency, 1971, Vienna.

62. Taplin, G. V., Meredith, O. M., and Kade, H.: The radioactive (I-131–tagged) rose bengal uptake-excretion test for liver function using external gamma-ray scintillation counting techniques, J. Lab. Clin. Med. **45**:665, 1955.

63. Waxman, A. D., Apau, R., and Siemsen, J. K.: Rapid sequential liver imaging, J. Nucl. Med. **13**:522, 1972.

64. Williams, L., Fischer, J., Courtney, R., and Darling, D.: Preoperative diagnosis of choledochal cyst by hepatoscintigraphy, New Engl. J. Med. **283**:85, 1970.

65. Winchell, H. S., et al.: Visualization of tumors using Ga-67-citrate and the Anger whole-body scanner, scintillation camera and tomographic scanner, J. Nucl. Med. **11**:459, 1970.

66. Winston, M. A., and Blahd, W. H.: I-131 rose bengal imaging techniques in differential diagnosis of jaundiced patients, Semin. Nucl. Med. **2**:167, 1972.

67. Witek, J. T., and Spencer, R. P.: Clinical correlation of hepatic flow studies, J. Nucl. Med. **16**:71, 1975.

17 Evaluation of diagnostic screening tests: a case study in hypertension

Barbara J. McNeil and S. James Adelstein

In a thought-provoking article written several years ago entitled "Radiology—a Case Study in Technology and Manpower," John Knowles made the following statement: "One could and should ask how many renal arteriograms in patients with hypertension have resulted directly in the surgical or medical cure of the patient's hypertension. . . . Increasingly we shall be asked to answer such questions, for our resources are not infinite nor is our share of the Gross National Product."[11]

This statement focuses on one of the central problems in medicine today: Can we measure the impact of our current diagnostic modalities in medical management? This "impact" could be measured in three ways. First, we need to determine the fraction of patients with a given disease; second, we need to identify those patients who do not have the disease; and third, we need to estimate the gain to the individual and society of classifying patients with and without disease.

All these measures are associated with costs—a financial cost and a life cost. The financial cost is obviously the dollar cost of diagnostic workups of all patients afflicted with, or thought to be afflicted with, the disease in question. In practice, this financial cost should be a realistic one in terms of the total financial allotment for medical care. The second cost is the life cost. The meaning of this cost is not so simple. In its most fundamental aspects, however, it involves the lives lost in and the morbidity associated with the diagnostic workup—lives not only of those patients who have disease but also of those who are thought to have disease but do not. This life cost should not be greater than the potential number of lives saved by the identification and treatment of those with the disease.

We selected the problem of hypertension as a case study to exemplify some of the techniques that can be employed in measuring the utility of various diagnostic modalities. We wished to answer four questions:

1. How good are the intravenous pyelogram (IVP) and the iodohippurate renogram (RG) in searching for patients with renovascular disease (RVD)?
2. How much does it cost to find a patient with renovascular disease?
3. How much does it cost to surgically cure a patient with renovascular disease?

4. Is it worth searching for patients with renovascular disease, or can they be treated just as well medically without identifying them?

All calculations were made using a representative hypertensive population as follows:

No identifiable cause (RVD−)	90%	
Renovascular disease (RVD+)	10%	
Atherosclerotic	6.7%	
Operative mortality		9%
Surgical cures		44%
Fibromuscular	3.3%	
Operative mortality		3%
Surgical cures		60%

As shown here, in most hypertensive patients there is no identifiable cause of hypertension; that is, they have essential hypertension. A smaller percentage have an identifiable cause; for this case study we have assumed that all these individuals have renovascular disease.

HOW GOOD ARE RADIOGRAPHIC SCREENING MODALITIES?

For these calculations we assumed that hypertensive patients were screened with the intravenous pyelogram, the renogram, or both and that all patients with an abnormal screening examination would have arteriography to delineate the cause of their abnormal screening examination.[3, 13]

Intravenous pyelogram. The Cooperative Study of Renovascular Disease provided information on the characteristics of the IVP in patients with and without renovascular disease.[1-3] IVPs were considered abnormal when one or more of the following signs occurred: significant disparity in the length of the two kidneys, delayed calyceal appearance time, and ipsilateral hyperconcentration of contrast media on delayed films. By these criteria, 78.2% of patients with renovascular disease and 11.4% of patients without renovascular disease have abnormal studies. Thus in a representative hypertensive population, 7.8 out of 10 patients with renovascular disease are found by the IVP, but 9.9 out of 90 patients without disease are falsely included.[15]

Renogram. The iodohippurate renograms from the Cooperative Study were analyzed according to the method of Burrows and Farmelant[4, 5] in order to quantitate differences in the degree of asymmetry of renal function. The percentages of patients with these diseases were related to a discriminant ratio (R)*, which measures this asymmetry. For two kidneys functioning symmetrically, R is close to 1, whereas in renovascular disease, R decreases and approaches 0 in the most severe cases. Low R values are found in a large percentage of patients with renovascular disease and a small percentage of patients without renovascular disease; with larger R values the percentage of patients in each group increases.

---

*R is defined as the ratio of two quantities A to B (or B to A) that is less than or equal to 1. A is the ratio of counts (kidney 1 to kidney 2) at the time of the first peak. B is the ratio of counts (kidney 1 to kidney 2) at the time that this value has dropped to 50% of its maximum.

Different cutoff values for R are thus associated with varying proportions of patients from each disease category. Graphically these results can be portrayed by a receiver operating characteristic (ROC) curve, that is, a plot of the true positive (TP) ratio versus the false positive (FP) ratio.[15] Each point corresponds to a different R value or, in other words, to different degrees of asymmetry of renal function (Fig. 17-1).

A number of discrete values on the renogram can be used as the cutoff points in differentiating patients with renovascular disease from those without. We carried out calculations at two points. One point was sensitive but not specific and had a TP ratio of 0.85 and an FP ratio of 0.10. The other was specific but not sensitive and had TP and FP ratios of 0.62 and 0.03, respectively. Thus in a representative hypertensive population, use of the sensitive operating position results in the discovery of 8.5 out of 10 patients with renovascular disease and 9.0 out of 90 without renovascular disease.[15] When the renogram is made more specific, the number of patients found drops to 6.2, but the number of patients falsely identified also drops to 2.7 out of 90.

Obviously, both the intravenous pyelogram and the renogram can be used in the same patient to search for renovascular disease. The number of patients found by this technique depends on two factors: (1) the operative position selected for the renogram and (2) the criteria required for arteriography (i.e., whether one or both examinations must be abnormal for arteriography to be performed). The greatest number of patients are found with these combined techniques if the renogram is evaluated at a sensitive operating position (TP ratio = 0.85) and if arteriography is performed when either examination is abnormal. Under these conditions one or both tests are abnormal in 9.1 out of 10

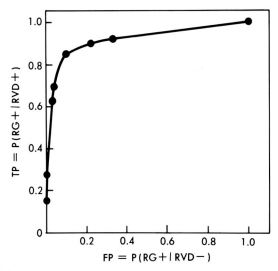

Fig. 17-1. ROC curve for the renogram (RG). True positive (TP) ratio is plotted against false positive (FP) ratio.

patients with renovascular disease and in 16.2 out of 90 without renovascular disease. On the other hand, when the renogram is evaluated at a more strict operating position (TP ratio = 0.62) and arteriography is performed only when both are abnormal, only 4.6 out of 10 patients with renovascular disease are found, but *no* patients are falsely identified.[15]

HOW MUCH DOES IT COST TO FIND A PATIENT WITH RENOVASCULAR DISEASE?

The financial costs of various scintigraphic and radiographic procedures were obtained from the Massachusetts Relative Value Scale.[12] The hypertensive IVP served as baseline at $83 per examination. The relative cost of the renogram, including data analysis and radiopharmaceuticals, was $100, and the cost of selective arteriography of both renal arteries was $375. The total cost of diagnosis included the costs of the primary screening modality (IVP, renogram, or both) and arteriography. Thus the total cost of diagnosis was the number of patients screened times the cost of screening plus the number of patients undergoing arteriography times the cost of arteriography. The cost of identifying a patient with renovascular disease by means of a primary diagnostic modality (IVP, renogram, or both) and continuing through arteriography then becomes:

$$\frac{\text{Total cost of diagnosis}}{\text{Number of patients with RVD+ found}}$$

The relative cost of finding patients with renovascular disease varied with the screening modality used (Table 17-1). When a *single* radiographic or scintigraphic examination was used for screening, the IVP had the lowest cost per patient diagnosed ($1915); 7.8 of 10 patients were found. The renogram alone at a relatively sensitive position (TP ratio = 0.85) found the most patients (8.5) for a single examination, and the cost per patient found was $1948. When two examinations were used in combination, the costs varied considerably, depending on whether one or both examinations were required to be abnormal for arterio-

Table 17-1. Relative costs of case finding of patients with RVD (100 patients screened; 10 assumed to have RVD)

Test	Number of RVD+ patients found	Total cost (in dollars)	Cost per positive diagnosis (in dollars)
IVP (TP = 0.78)	7.8	14,938	1915
RG (TP = 0.85)	8.5	16,562	1948
RG (TP = 0.62)	6.2	13,338	2151
IVP and RG (TP = 0.62)			
Both +	4.6	20,025	4353
Either or both +	8.5	22,012	2590
IVP and RG (TP = 0.85)			
Both +	6.9	23,662	3429
Either or both +	9.1	27,787	3053

graphy to be performed; in all instances the costs were higher than with only one diagnostic examination.

HOW MUCH DOES IT COST TO SURGICALLY CURE A PATIENT WITH RENOVASCULAR DISEASE?

The cost of surgery was set at $5000 for these calculations. The cost of each identification and surgical cure was calculated as follows:

$$\frac{\text{Total cost of diagnosis and surgery}}{\text{Number of patients with RVD+ cured surgically}}$$

We assumed that the operative mortality in patients with atherosclerotic disease was 9% and that 44% of these were cured surgically and that the operative mortality in patients with fibromuscular disease was 3% and 60% of these were cured surgically.[7, 8] Under these conditions the cost of a surgical cure was between $14,000 and $20,000 per patient, depending on whether one or two radiographic examinations were used for screening.[15]

These calculations on the cost of finding and curing a patient with renovascular disease were extended to include the total American hypertensive population (23 million individuals). The total cost of screening then became billions of dollars (Table 17-2). The total number of deaths associated with diagnosis and surgery varied from 75,000 to about 141,000 in the American hypertensive population. The smallest number (75,000) of deaths resulted when the IVP and renogram (TP ratio = 0.62) were used for detection and arteriography was reserved for patients in whom both examinations were abnormal. Simultaneously the number of potential cures dropped from over 900,000 when either screening procedure was used alone to 494,000 when both studies were employed. Approximately 150 deaths occurred for every 1000 surgical cures regardless of the initial screening test(s) employed.

IS IT WORTH IT?

Determination of the value of case finding depends on how well patients do when they are treated surgically in comparison to how well they would have

Table 17-2. Cost-effectiveness analysis for the total American hypertensive population for diagnostic workup and surgery for renovascular disease*

	Screening modality		
	IVP (TP = 0.78)	RG (TP = 0.85)	IVP and RG (TP = 0.62)
Total dollar cost	12.5×10^9	13.6×10^9	9.90×10^9
Number of deaths	130,000	140,600	75,000
Surgical cures—60% of those operated on	827,000	912,000	494,000
Cost/surgical cure	$15,100	$14,100	$20,000
Deaths/1000 surgical cures	157	154	152

*Reprinted by permission from McNeil, B. J., Varady, P. D., Burrows, B. A., and Adelstein, S. J.: N. Engl. J. Med. **293:**216, 1975.

done had their hypertension been treated medically without regard to its cause. Our approach to this problem is expressed in the decision flow diagrams (Figs. 17-2 and 17-3).[14] The first decision is a choice of screening all hypertensive patients with the intravenous pyelogram (strategy 1) or of not screening and thus instituting drug treatment without regard for cause (strategy 2). Since the intravenous pyelogram detects 78% of patients with renovascular disease, one third of whom have fibromuscular disease, this diagnostic strategy identifies 2.6% of hypertensive patients as having fibromuscular renovascular disease and 5.2% as having atherosclerotic renovascular disease.[15] These patients are then treated surgically (node S, Fig. 17-2) and either live or die (node A, Fig. 17-3). At the next chance node (B) those patients surviving the operation are either cured or not cured. Those not cured by surgery may be either improved or unchanged; in either case they receive medical therapy, which results in medical cure, improvement, or failure (node C_1). If the initial treatment is medical, either because screening was not performed or because the patients screened were not suitable surgical candidates, then the results are also cure, improvement, or failure (node C_2).

A patient was considered a *surgical cure* when the average diastolic blood pressure became 90 mm Hg or less and was at least 10 mm Hg less than the

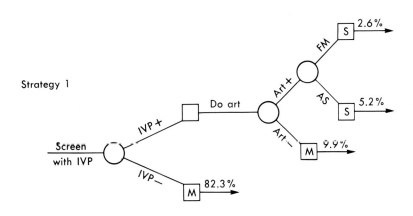

Fig. 17-2. Decision flow diagrams for treatment of patients with hypertensive disease. *Strategy 1:* Screening is performed on all patients with hypertension. If intravenous pyelogram *(IVP)* is abnormal *(IVP+),* arteriography *(Art)* is always performed. When IVP and arteriogram are negative, medical therapy *(M)* is followed. When arteriogram is positive *(Art+),* surgery is chosen *(S).* The outcomes of surgery and medicine are shown in Fig. 17-3. *Strategy 2:* No screening intravenous pyelograms are done, and all patients are treated medically *(M).*

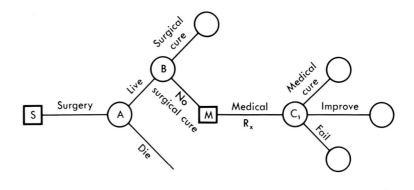

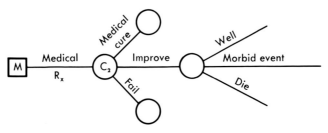

Fig. 17-3. Outcomes associated with surgical and medical regimens. Results of surgery on patients with renovascular disease are detailed at chance nodes *A* and *B*. Results of primary or supplemental medical therapy are expressed at nodes C_1 and C_2. All terminal chance nodes are associated with three possible outcomes: well, morbid event, or die. (From McNeil, B. J., Varady, P. D., Burrows, B. A., and Adelstein, S. J.: N. Engl. J. Med. **293**:216, 1975.)

preoperative level.[7] A patient was considered a *medical cure* when the posttreatment diastolic blood pressure became 90 mm Hg or less; a drop in diastolic blood pressure of at least 10% was considered an *improvement;* maintenance of the pretreatment pressure was considered a treatment *failure.*

The results of medical antihypertensive therapy (nodes C_1 and C_2) were assumed to be affected by only two factors: (1) patient compliance (i.e., the number of patients following the recommended medical regimen) and (2) the degree to which vigorous therapy was used for the control of hypertension. Two extremes were investigated. The first and probably the most common is a typical population in which 50% of known hypertensive patients are lost to follow-up, 25% are cured, and 25% are improved. The second population is an unusual one found in specially designed hypertensive programs in which 84% are cured and 16% are lost to follow-up.[6]

At the end of all of the branches in the decision diagram (Fig. 17-3), except that associated with death, is a terminal chance node with three components: those patients who suffer no complications secondary to hypertension, those who suffer a nonfatal morbid event, and those who die from their morbid event. Calculations of the probabilities determining the proportion of patients in the three branches of the terminal node were made from the epidemiologic data on cardiovascular disease collected by the Framingham Study.[9, 10] Although several morbid events associated with hypertension were investigated by the Framingham Study Group, we studied two common complications—coronary heart disease (CHD) and cerebrovascular accidents (CVA). The probability of each of these events, P (CHD) and P (CVA), was calculated as a function of initial diastolic blood pressure for men and women 45 to 54 years of age. The probability of each was calculated independently of the other. The probabilities of death from these events—P (Death|CHD) and P (Death|CVA)—were obtained from the Framingham Life Table Analysis.

These two strategies (Fig. 17-2) were compared in patients with renovascular disease by evaluating the number of patients without any complication, the number of patients suffering a nonfatal morbid event, and the number of patients dying from a morbid event. We calculated these numbers, assuming that the patients were followed for 16 years after they were seen initially by the Framingham Study Group.

The outcomes of these two strategies depended on the compliance of the patient and his initial diastolic blood pressure (Tables 17-3 and 17-4). For low compliance rates (50%), nonfatal morbid events affected 19% to 37% of the treated men and 12% to 27% of the treated women. Deaths occurred in 14% to 22% of the men and 8% to 15% of the women. At a higher compliance rate (84%) the number of nonfatal morbid events dropped to 16% to 21% for men and 9% to 14% for women for both medical and surgical therapy (Tables 17-3 and 17-4). Deaths occurred in 12% to 17% of men and 6% to 11% of women.

The difference in number of deaths for the two therapeutic regimens varied strikingly with initial blood pressure and compliance. At compliance rates of both 84% and 50% for patients with diastolic blood pressures of 110 to 135 mm Hg,

Table 17-3. Comparison of surgical and medical regimens in 45- to 54-year-old male hypertensive patients with renovascular disease*†

	Surgical regimen Initial diastolic blood pressure			Medical regimen‡ Initial diastolic blood pressure		
	110	120	135	110	120	135
50% compliance						
No complications	63%	59%	50%	63%	55%	41%
Nonfatal morbid events	19%	22%	28%	23%	28%	37%
Death from morbid events	18%	19%	22%	14%	17%	21%
84% compliance						
No complications	68%	67%	65%	70%	68%	65%
Nonfatal morbid events	16%	17%	18%	18%	19%	21%
Death from morbid events	16%	16%	17%	12%	13%	14%

*Reprinted by permission from McNeil, B. J., Varady, P. D., Burrows, B. A., and Adelstein, S. J.: N. Engl. J. Med. **293**:216, 1975.
†The exact numbers of patients in each category for this table are available from the authors.
‡These same values apply to *all* hypertensives treated with drugs alone.

Table 17-4. Comparison of surgical and medical regimens in 45- to 54-year-old female hypertensive patients with renovascular disease*†

	Surgical regimen Initial diastolic blood pressure			Medical regimen‡ Initial diastolic blood pressure		
	110	120	135	110	120	135
50% compliance						
No complications	77%	73%	66%	76%	70%	59%
Nonfatal morbid events	12%	14%	19%	16%	20%	27%
Death from morbid events	11%	13%	15%	8%	10%	14%
84% compliance						
No complications	81%	80%	78%	83%	83%	79%
Nonfatal morbid events	9%	10%	11%	11%	11%	14%
Death from morbid events	10%	10%	11%	6%	6%	7%

*Reprinted by permission from McNeil, B. J., Varady, P. D., Burrows, B. A., and Adelstein, S. J.: N. Engl. J. Med. 293:216, 1975.
†The exact numbers of patients in each category for this table are available from the authors.
‡These same values apply to *all* hypertensives treated with drugs alone.

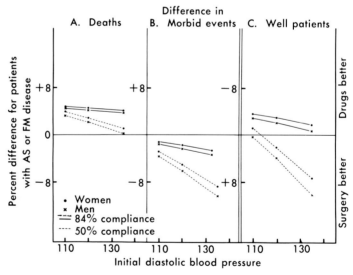

Fig. 17-4. Difference in number of deaths (panel *A*), nonfatal morbid events (panel *B*), and well patients (panel *C*) as a function of sex, compliance, and initial diastolic blood pressure. The ordinate represents the percent difference in results of surgical and medical therapy in patients with renovascular disease. Note that negative differences in deaths or nonfatal morbid events favor surgical treatment. Therefore the signs of the ordinate in the right panel *(C)* have been reversed to simplify presentation of results. (From McNeil, B. J., Varady, P. D., Burrows, B. A., and Adelstein, S. J.: N. Engl. J. Med. **293:**216, 1975.)

there were more deaths in the surgery group than in the medical group (Fig. 17-4, panel *A*), that is, drug therapy was better than surgery. When the difference between the number of nonfatal morbid events was examined, surgery appeared better than drug treatment regardless of diastolic pressure and the compliance rate (Fig. 17-4, panel *B*). The difference in the number of well patients in the two therapeutic regimens was fixed by the number of patients suffering or dying from a morbid event and reflected the effects of both blood pressure and compliance (Fig. 17-4, panel *C*). For patients with a high compliance rate, more patients on drug therapy were well, whereas for patients with a low compliance rate, the surgical regimen generally kept more patients well, especially those with diastolic blood pressures over 115 mm Hg (Fig. 17-4, panel *C*).

SUMMARY

This study demonstrates that there is some potential benefit to the identification and surgical treatment of patients with renovascular disease but that the mode of treatment contributes much less to the ultimate prognosis than does compliance, initial diastolic blood pressure, and sex. The results further suggest that in patients with renovascular disease and a low diastolic blood pressure, surgery may not be recommended if its only purpose is blood pressure control. In light of the minor gain to be derived from screening all hypertensive patients for renovascular disease, some means of selecting patients for testing is desirable.

References

1. Bookstein, J. J., et al.: Radiologic aspects of renovascular hypertension. I. Aims and methods of the radiology study group, J.A.M.A. **220**:1218, 1972.
2. Bookstein, J. J., et al.: Radiologic aspects of renovascular hypertension. II. The role of urography in unilateral renovascular disease, J.A.M.A. **220**:1225, 1972.
3. Bookstein, J. J., et al.: Radiologic aspects of renovascular hypertension. III. Appraisal of arteriography, J.A.M.A. **221**:368, 1972.
4. Farmelant, M. H., et al.: Radioisotopic renal function studies and surgical findings in 102 hypertensive patients, Am. J. Surg. **107**:50, 1964.
5. Farmelant, M. H., Sachs, C., and Burrows, B. A.: Prognostic value of radioisotopic renal function studies for selecting patients with renal arterial stenosis after surgery, J. Nucl. Med. **11**:743, 1970.
6. Finnerty, F. A., Jr., Shaw, L. W., and Himmelsbach, C. K.: Hypertension in the inner city. I. Detection and follow-up, Circulation **47**:76, 1973.
7. Foster, J. H., et al.: Cooperative study of renovascular hypertension. Results of operative treatment of renovascular occlusive disease, J.A.M.A. **231**:1043, 1975.
8. Franklin, S. S., et al.: Operative morbidity and mortality in renovascular disease, J.A.M.A. **231**:1148, 1975.
9. Kannel, W. B., and Gordon, T., editors: The Framingham study. An epidemiological investigation of cardiovascular disease. Section 25. Survival following certain cardiovascular events, Washington, D.C., 1970, U.S. Government Printing Office.
10. Kannel, W. B., and Gordon, T., editors: The Framingham study. An epidemiological investigation of cardiovascular disease. Section 26. Some characteristics related to the incidence of cardiovascular disease and death, Washington, D.C., 1970, U.S. Government Printing Office.
11. Knowles, J. H.: Radiology—a case study in technology and manpower, N. Engl. J. Med. **280**:1323, 1969.
12. Massachusetts relative value study, Boston, 1971, Massachusetts Medical Society.
13. McAfee, J. H.: Complications of abdom-

inal aortography and arteriography. In Abrams, H. L., editor: Angiography, Boston, 1971, Little, Brown & Co.

14. McNeil, B. J., and Adelstein, S. J.: Measures of clinical efficacy. II. The value of cost-finding in hypertensive renovascular disease, N. Engl. J. Med. **293:**221, 1975.

15. McNeil, B. J., Varady, P. D., Burrows, B. A., and Adelstein, S. J.: Measures of clinical efficacy. I. Cost-effectiveness calculations in the diagnosis and treatment of hypertensive renovascular disease, N. Engl. J. Med. **293:**216, 1975.

INDEX